Methods in Neurosciences

Volume 16

Neurobiology of Cytokines
Part A

Methods in Neurosciences

Editor-in-Chief

P. Michael Conn

Methods in Neurosciences

Volume 16
Neurobiology of Cytokines
Part A

Edited by
Errol B. De Souza
Neurocrine Biosciences, Inc.
La Jolla, California

ACADEMIC PRESS, INC.
A Division of Harcourt Brace & Company

San Diego   New York   Boston   London   Sydney   Tokyo   Toronto

Front cover photograph: A dark-field photomicrograph of an emulsion autoradiogram demonstrating type I interleukin 1 receptor messenger RNA in mouse testis. Dense autoradiographic signal is seen over interstitial cells, most of which are known to be of the Leydig, or testosterone-producing, type. In contrast, signal intensity over the epithelium of seminiferous tubules is comparable to background. The section has been counterstained with hematoxylin–eosin. Courtesy of Dr. Emmett T. Cunningham, Jr., Department of Ophthalmology, School of Medicine, University of California, San Francisco.

This book is printed on acid-free paper. ∞

Academic Press, Inc.
1250 Sixth Avenue, San Diego, California 92101

United Kingdom Edition published by
Academic Press Limited
24–28 Oval Road, London NW1 7DX

International Standard Serial Number: 1043-9471

International Standard Book Number: 0-12-185281-4

PRINTED IN THE UNITED STATES OF AMERICA
93 94 95 96 97 98   E B   9 8 7 6 5 4 3 2 1

Table of Contents

Contributors to Volume 16   ix
Preface   xiii
Volumes in Series   xv

Section I General Aspects

1. Pharmacological, Biochemical, and Molecular Biological
   Studies on Cytokine Receptors
   Steven K. Dower   3

2. Genetic Regulation and Activities of an Interleukin 1
   Receptor Antagonist Protein
   Donald B. Carter, Ann E. Berger, and Daniel E. Tracey   33

3. Identification of Intracellular Mediators of the Actions of
   Cytokines: Identifying Proteins Involved in Kinase
   Signaling Pathways
   Gerald A. Evans, Hallgeir Rui, and William L. Farrar   49

4. Measurement of Transport of Cytokines across the
   Blood–Brain Barrier
   William A. Banks and Abba J. Kastin   67

Section II Anatomical Localization Studies

5. *In Situ* Hybridization Techniques for Localization of
   Interleukin 1 and Interleukin 1 Receptor Antagonist mRNA
   in Brain
   Ma-Li Wong, Philip W. Gold, and Júlio Licinio   81

6. Immunocytochemical Methods for Localization of
   Cytokines in Brain
   John A. Olschowka   100

7. Localization of Type I Interleukin 1 Receptor mRNA in
   Brain and Endocrine Tissues by *in Situ* Hybridization
   Histochemistry
   Emmett T. Cunningham, Jr., and Errol B. De Souza   112

8. Identification, Autoradiographic Localization, and Modulation of Interleukin 1 Receptors in Brain–Endocrine–Immune Axis: Methodology and Overview
Toshihiro Takao, Dimitri E. Grigoriadis, and Errol B. De Souza   128

9. c-*fos*-Based Functional Mapping of Central Pathways Subserving Effects of Interleukin 1 on the Hypothalamo–Pituitary–Adrenal Axis
Anders Ericsson and Paul E. Sawchenko   155

10. Anatomical and Functional Approaches to Study of Interleukin 2 and Its Receptors in Brain
David Seto, Uwe Hanisch, Françoise Villemain, Alain Beaudet, and Rémi Quirion   173

Section III Neuroendocrine Actions

11. Endocrine Aspects of Neuroimmunomodulation: Methods and Overview
Samuel M. McCann, Ljiljana Milenkovic, M. Carmen Gonzalez, Krzysztof Lyson, Sharada Karanth, and Valeria Rettori   187

12. Determining Role and Sources of Endogenous Interleukin 1 in Pituitary–Adrenal Activation in Response to Stressful and Inflammatory Stimuli
Frank Berkenbosch, Nico Van Rooijen, and Fred J. H. Tilders   211

13. *In Vivo* and *in Vitro* Methods for Studying Effects of Cytokines on Adrenocorticotropic Hormone, Arginine Vasopressin, and Oxytocin Secretion
Junichi Fukata, Hajime Segawa, Yoshiyuki Naito, Norihiko Murakami, Hiromasa Kobayashi, Osamu Ebisui, Takeshi Usui, and Hiroo Imura   232

14. *In Vivo* and *in Vitro* Models for Evaluating Effects of Interleukin 1 on Hypothalamic–Pituitary–Gonadal Axis
Pushpa S. Kalra and Satya P. Kalra   248

15. Methodological Evaluation of Sites and Mechanisms of Action Involved in Neuroendocrine Effects of Cytokines
Akira Arimura and Paul E. Gottschall   269

16. *In Vivo* and *in Vitro* Methods for Studying Effects of
    Tumor Necrosis Factor on Pituitary Cells
    Alberto E. Panerai, Vittorio Locatelli, and Paola Sacerdote   294

17. Determination of Direct Effects of Cytokines on Release of
    Neuropeptides from Rat Hypothalamus by an *in Vitro*
    Method
    *Ashley Grossman, Stylianos Tsagarakis, Marta Korbonits, and
    Alfredo Costa*   302

18. Effects of Interleukin 1 on β-Endorphin Secretion in
    AtT-20 Pituitary Cells: Methods and Overview
    Mirela O. Făgărăşan   327

Index   343

Contributors to Volume 16

Article numbers are in parentheses following the names of contributors. Affiliations listed are current.

AKIRA ARIMURA (15), U.S.–Japan Biomedical Research Laboratories, Tulane University Hebert Center, Belle Chasse, Louisiana 70037

WILLIAM A. BANKS (4), Veterans Affairs Medical Center, New Orleans, Louisiana 70146, and Tulane University School of Medicine, New Orleans, Louisiana 70118

ALAIN BEAUDET (10), Montreal Neurological Institute, Montréal, Québec, Canada H3A 2B4

ANN E. BERGER (2), Cell Biology Research Upjohn, Kalamazoo, Michigan 49007

FRANK BERKENBOSCH* (12), Departments of Pharmacology and Histology, Medical Faculty, Free University, 1081 BT Amsterdam, The Netherlands

DONALD B. CARTER (2), CNS Research Upjohn, Kalamazoo, Michigan 49007

ALFREDO COSTA (17), Divisione di Neurologio C, Fondazione "Istituto Neurologico Casimiro Mondino," 27100 Pavia, Italy

EMMETT T. CUNNINGHAM, JR. (7), Department of Ophthalmology, School of Medicine, University of California, San Francisco, San Francisco, California 94143

ERROL B. DE SOUZA (7, 8), Neurocrine Biosciences, Inc., La Jolla, California 92037

STEVEN K. DOWER (1), Department of Biochemistry, Immunex Research and Development Corporation, Seattle, Washington 98101

OSAMU EBISUI (13), Second Division, Department of Internal Medicine, Kyoto University Faculty of Medicine, Kyoto 606, Japan

ANDERS ERICSSON (9), Laboratory of Neuronal Structure and Function, The Salk Institute for Biological Studies, and The Foundation for Medical Research, La Jolla, California 92037

* Deceased.

GERALD A. EVANS (3), Biological Carcinogenesis and Development Program, PRI/DynCorp, Frederick Cancer Research and Development Center, National Cancer Institute, Frederick, Maryland 21702

MIRELA O. FĂGĂRĂȘAN (18), Department of Biochemistry and Molecular Biology, George Washington University Medical Center, Washington, D.C. 20037

WILLIAM L. FARRAR (3), Laboratory of Molecular Immunoregulation, Biological Response Modifiers Program, Frederick Cancer Research and Development Center, National Cancer Institute, Frederick, Maryland 21702

JUNICHI FUKATA (13), Second Division, Department of Internal Medicine, Kyoto University Faculty of Medicine, Kyoto 606, Japan

PHILIP W. GOLD (5), Clinical Neuroendocrinology Branch, National Institute of Mental Health, National Institutes of Health, Bethesda, Maryland 20892

M. CARMEN GONZALEZ (11), Universidad de La Laguna, Departamento de Fisiologia, E-38320 Tenerife, Spain

PAUL E. GOTTSCHALL (15), Department of Pharmacology and Therapeutics, University of South Florida College of Medicine, Tampa, Florida 33612

DIMITRI E. GRIGORIADIS (8), Central Nervous System Diseases Research, The DuPont Merck Pharmaceutical Company, Wilmington, Delaware 19880

ASHLEY GROSSMAN (17), Department of Endocrinology, St. Bartholomew's Hospital, London EC1A 7BE, England

UWE HANISCH (10), Douglas Hospital Research Centre, and Departments of Psychiatry, Pharmacology and Therapeutics and of Neurology and Neurosurgery, Faculty of Medicine, McGill University, Montréal, Québec, Canada H4H 1R3

HIROO IMURA (13), Second Division, Department of Internal Medicine, Kyoto University Faculty of Medicine, Kyoto 606, Japan

PUSHPA S. KALRA (14), Department of Obstetrics and Gynecology, University of Florida College of Medicine, Gainesville, Florida 32610

SATYA P. KALRA (14), Department of Obstetrics and Gynecology, University of Florida College of Medicine, Gainesville, Florida 32610

SHARADA KARANTH (11), Department of Physiology, University of Texas Southwestern Medical Center, Dallas, Texas 75235

ABBA J. KASTIN (4), Veterans Affairs Medical Center, New Orleans, Louisiana 70146, and Tulane University School of Medicine, New Orleans, Louisiana 70118

HIROMASA KOBAYASHI (13), Second Division, Department of Internal Medicine, Kyoto University Faculty of Medicine, Kyoto 606, Japan

MARTA KORBONITS (17), Department of Endocrinology, St. Bartholomew's Hospital, London EC1A 7BE, England

JÚLIO LICINIO (5), Department of Psychiatry, Yale University School of Medicine, and Affective Disorders Program, West Haven Veterans Affairs Medical Center, West Haven, Connecticut 06516

VITTORIO LOCATELLI (16), Department of Pharmacology, School of Medicine, University of Milan, 20129 Milan, Italy

KRZYSZTOF LYSON (11), Department of Physiology, University of Texas Southwestern Medical Center, Dallas, Texas 75235

SAMUEL M. MCCANN (11), Neuropeptide Division, Department of Physiology, University of Texas Southwestern Medical Center, Dallas, Texas 75235

LJILJANA MILENKOVIC (11), Department of Obstetrics/Gynecology and Reproductive Sciences, University of California, San Francisco, San Francisco, California 94143

NORIHIKO MURAKAMI (13), Second Division, Department of Internal Medicine, Kyoto University Faculty of Medicine, Kyoto 606, Japan

YOSHIYUKI NAITO (13), Department of Anesthesia, Kyoto University Faculty of Medicine, Kyoto 606, Japan

JOHN A. OLSCHOWKA (6), Department of Neurobiology and Anatomy, University of Rochester School of Medicine and Dentistry, Rochester, New York 14642

ALBERTO E. PANERAI (16), Department of Pharmacology, School of Medicine, University of Milan, 20129 Milan, Italy

RÉMI QUIRION (10), Department of Psychiatry, McGill University, Douglas Hospital Research Centre, Verdun (Québec), Canada H4H 1R3

VALERIA RETTORI (11), Neuropeptide Division, Department of Physiology, University of Texas Southwestern Medical Center, Dallas, Texas 75235

HALLGEIR RUI (3), Laboratory of Molecular Immunoregulation, Biological Response Modifiers Program, Frederick Cancer Research and Development Center, National Cancer Institute, Frederick, Maryland 21702

PAOLA SACERDOTE (16), Department of Pharmacology, School of Medicine, University of Milan, 20129 Milan, Italy

PAUL E. SAWCHENKO (9), Laboratory of Neuronal Structure and Function, The Salk Institute for Biological Studies, and The Foundation for Medical Research, La Jolla, California 92037

HAJIME SEGAWA (13), Department of Anesthesia, Kyoto University Faculty of Medicine, Kyoto 606, Japan

DAVID SETO (10), Douglas Hospital Research Centre, and Departments of Psychiatry, Pharmacology and Therapeutics and of Neurology and Neurosurgery, Faculty of Medicine, McGill University, Montréal, Québec, Canada H4H 1R3

TOSHIHIRO TAKAO (8), Kochi Medical School, Okohcho, Nankoku, Kochi 783, Japan

FRED J. H. TILDERS (12), Departments of Pharmacology and Histology, Medical Faculty, Free University, 1081 BT Amsterdam, The Netherlands

DANIEL E. TRACEY (2), BASF Bioresearch Corporation, Cambridge, Massachusetts 02139

STYLIANOS TSAGARAKIS (17), Department of Endocrinology, Evangelismos Hospital, Athens, Greece

TAKESHI USUI (13), Second Division, Department of Internal Medicine, Kyoto University Faculty of Medicine, Kyoto 606, Japan

NICO VAN ROOIJEN (12), Departments of Pharmacology and Histology, Medical Faculty, Free University, 1081 BT Amsterdam, The Netherlands

FRANÇOISE VILLEMAIN (10), Montreal Neurological Institute, Montréal, Québec, Canada H3A 2B4

MA-LI WONG (5), Department of Psychiatry, Yale University School of Medicine, and Affective Disorders Program, West Haven Veterans Affairs Medical Center, West Haven, Connecticut 06516

Preface

One of the most exciting recent developments in biology has been a growing awareness that nerves, endocrine cells, and immune cells share common communication molecules and receptors and are functionally linked to form a brain–endocrine–immune axis that integrates the physiological responses of the organism. This neuroendocrine–immune interaction is bidirectional. That is, immune and endocrine responses are modulated by the brain, and, in turn, by-products of the immune responses alter brain and endocrine activities. The cytokines provide a classic example of products of the immune system which alter brain and endocrine activities. A variety of cytokines, including interleukin 1, interleukin 2, interleukin 6, and tumor necrosis factor α, have been traditionally associated with peripheral control of the immune system, inflammation, and the acute phase response. More recent data suggest a critical role for the cytokines in regulating brain and endocrine function under normal physiological conditions. The cytokines are synthesized in brain by neurons, glia, endothelial cells, and invading macrophages, and receptors have been identified in discrete areas of the central nervous system. Cytokines act directly within the central nervous system to alter growth and differentiation, to modulate neuronal and neuroendocrine activities, and to produce pyrogenic, somnogenic, thermogenic, anorexigenic, and behavioral effects. Aberrant regulation of cytokines in brain has been implicated in the development of pathological conditions seen in Alzheimer's disease, Down's syndrome, multiple sclerosis, AIDS, tissue injury, and neurodegeneration.

The goal of "Neurobiology of Cytokines," Volumes 16 and 17 of *Methods in Neurosciences*, is to provide an overview of the effects of cytokines in brain and in the endocrine system. The focus is on methodological aspects that will enable the reader to get an appreciation for the field and the methods utilized. Each volume is divided into three major sections. This volume focuses on general aspects of cytokines, including the endogenous agonists and antagonists, their receptors, their second messengers, and transport mechanisms for cytokines across the blood–brain barrier. In addition, the anatomical localization of cytokines, cytokine receptors, and their respective mRNA in brain and in endocrine tissues is described. Next, the methods for evaluating the *in vivo* as well as *in vitro* actions of cytokines on hormone secretion are covered. Volume 17 focuses on the synthesis and release of cytokines and their central nervous system actions. Methodology for studying the role of cytokines in human neuropathological conditions is also described.

I wish to express my appreciation to Dr. P. Michael Conn and the staff of Academic Press for their continued support and efficient coordination of production. I would also like to thank the many contributors for their excellent chapters and, in particular, for meeting the deadlines allowing for the timely publication of these volumes.

ERROL B. DE SOUZA

Methods in Neurosciences

Volume 1 Gene Probes
Edited by P. Michael Conn

Volume 2 Cell Culture
Edited by P. Michael Conn

Volume 3 Quantitative and Qualitative Microscopy
Edited by P. Michael Conn

Volume 4 Electrophysiology and Microinjection
Edited by P. Michael Conn

Volume 5 Neuropeptide Technology: Gene Expression and Neuropeptide Receptors
Edited by P. Michael Conn

Volume 6 Neuropeptide Technology: Synthesis, Assay, Purification, and Processing
Edited by P. Michael Conn

Volume 7 Lesions and Transplantation
Edited by P. Michael Conn

Volume 8 Neurotoxins
Edited by P. Michael Conn

Volume 9 Gene Expression in Neural Tissues
Edited by P. Michael Conn

Volume 10 Computers and Computations in the Neurosciences
Edited by P. Michael Conn

Volume 11 Receptors: Model Systems and Specific Receptors
Edited by P. Michael Conn

Volume 12 Receptors: Molecular Biology, Receptor Subclasses, Localization, and Ligand Design
Edited by P. Michael Conn

Volume 13 Neuropeptide Analogs, Conjugates, and Fragments
Edited by P. Michael Conn

Volume 14 Paradigms for the Study of Behavior
Edited by P. Michael Conn

Volume 15 Photoreceptor Cells
Edited by Paul A. Hargrave

Volume 16 Neurobiology of Cytokines (Part A)
Edited by Errol B. De Souza

Volume 17 Neurobiology of Cytokines (Part B) (in preparation)
Edited by Errol B. De Souza

Volume 18 Lipid Metabolism in Signaling Systems (in preparation)
Edited by John N. Fain

Volume 19 Ion Channels of Excitable Membranes (in preparation)
Edited by Toshio Narahashi

Section I

General Aspects

[1] Pharmacological, Biochemical, and Molecular Biological Studies on Cytokine Receptors

Steven K. Dower

Introduction

The molecular characterization of cytokine receptors has proceeded rapidly over the last 5 years, in large part due to the advent of expression cloning methods of sufficient sensitivity to allow the isolation of cDNAs corresponding to rare mRNAs encoding receptors expressed at low levels in tissues or cultured cell lines (1–4). The expression cloning methods in turn have been dependent on the characterization of the binding properties of the receptors and some estimation of the molecular size of receptor subunits. These data are obtained by more classic receptor biochemical techniques, which will be covered in detail in the next section of this chapter.

The primary sequence data that have been obtained from the cloning studies have identified five separate families of cytokine receptors (4). The largest family has been termed the hematopoietin or type I cytokine receptor family (5), and includes the receptors for interleukin 2 (IL-2) (6, 7), IL-3 (8), IL-4 (9), IL-5 (10), IL-6 (11), IL-7 (12), IL-9, granulocyte–macrophage colony-stimulating factor (GMCSF) (13), granulocyte colony-stimulating factor (GCSF) (14), leukemia inhibitory factor (LIF) (15), oncostatin M (16), ciliary neurotrophic factor (CNTF), erythropoietin (EPO) (17), growth hormone (18), and the product of a receptor-like protooncogene (c-mpl) (19) found after isolation of its viral counterpart (v-mpl); no ligand has yet been identified for this molecule. Within this family, a subgroup of "large cytokine receptors" can be discerned, composed of the receptors for GCSF, LIF, and oncostatin M. The oncostatin M receptor polypeptide, called gp130, is also the β chain of the LIF and IL-6 receptors (16, 20). In addition, one subunit of the IL-12 heterodimer is clearly related to the type I cytokine receptors (21). All of the type I receptors share in common a domain structure consisting of approximately 130 residues in the extracellular ligand-binding region, which is repeated two or more times. The membrane-proximal domain of type I receptors has a characteristic sequence WSXWS close to its C terminus and an imperfect version of this motif can also be found in the more membrane-distal regions. In addition, several of these receptors, most

Methods in Neurosciences, Volume 16

notably the "large" subset, contain fibronectin type III motifs. The solution of the X-ray structure of the complex of a soluble fragment of the growth hormone receptor with growth hormone confirms that the hematopoietin domain sequence repeats do indeed correspond to relatively independently folded structures (18).

The receptors for the interferons (IFN-α, IFN-β, and IFN-γ) form a distinct second set of two receptors (IFN-α and IFN-β share a common receptor) that are distantly related to one another, and even more distantly related to the type I receptors (4). There is indirect evidence that the functional receptors include additional subunits. For example, the human IFN-γ gene, which maps to chromosome 6, will not reconstitute signaling when transfected into murine cells unless those cells also contain a copy of human chromosome 21.

The tumor necrosis factor (TNF) receptors [type I or p60 (22, 23) and type II or p80 (24)], the low-affinity nerve growth factor (NGF) receptor (25), and the cell surface proteins CD40 (26), CD27 (27), FAS, CD30 (28), and OX40 (29) form another family characterized by an approximately 40-residue cysteine-rich repeat in the extracellular ligand-binding region. The TNF and NGF receptors were originally identified as receptors for soluble ligands, but cloning of TNF-α revealed that it is synthesized as a membrane-bound precursor of the type II receptor (30), and the soluble form is generated by proteolytic cleavage. A type II integral membrane protein ligand has been identified for the CD40 antigen (31); whether this or a soluble cleavage product is the biologically relevant form remains to be established. No ligands have been identified for the other members of this family of putative receptors.

There is also a group of cytokine receptors that have extracellular regions composed of approximately 110-residue immunoglobulin-like domains. This family includes the two IL-1 receptors (type I and type II) (2, 32), the macrophage colony-stimulating factor receptor (MCSF or CSF-1) or c-*fms* protooncogene product (33), and the steel factor/mast cell growth factor/ stem cell factor receptor or c-*kit* protooncogene product (34). These last two receptors are structurally related to one another and to the two platelet-derived growth factor (PDGF) receptors (α and β). In addition, fibroblast growth factor (FGF) receptors also belong to this group of immunoglobulin-like regulatory factor receptors (35). The subgroup composed of c-Fms, c-Kit, the PDGF receptors, and some forms of FGF receptor all have large cytoplasmic domains with intrinsic protein tyrosine kinase activity. This subgroup is further distinguished from other receptor protein tyrosine kinases such as the epidermal growth factor receptor by having an insert in the kinase domain. The evolutionary relationship between them is underscored by the finding that the genes for c-Fms and PDGF receptor β subunit (PDGFRβ) map next to one another on human chromosome 5 (36).

Finally, cDNA clones have been isolated for IL-8 receptors (37). Interleukin 8 is a member of a large family of mediators termed small inflammatory cytokines. The IL-8 receptor is a member of the β-adrenergic receptor family, being composed of seven membrane-spanning regions connected by a series of short loops. Like other members of this receptor family, IL-8 receptors activate intracellular signals by coupling through heterotrimeric G proteins. Presumably, the other members of the small inflammatory cytokine family bind to receptors of similar structure.

In the preceding summary the receptors for cytokines were described as if each polypeptide were a discrete entity. This is not the case. In most instances it has become clear that these receptor polypeptides are subunits of multi-chain complexes. Indeed, in many instances individual chains are shared between receptors, so that binding of a cytokine to a cell leads to recruitment of subunits from a common pool in a combinatorial fashion to form a final structure that transduces the signal for that cytokine. Thus, for example, the receptors for IL-3, IL-5, and GMCSF are formed by association of cytokine-specific α chains with a common β subunit (38, 39), and the receptors for IL-6, LIF, oncostatin M, and CNTF are formed by combinatorial assembly from the subunits IL-6Rα, gp130, LIFR, and CNTFR [the IL-6R being IL6Rα/gp130 (20), the LIFR and oncostatin M receptors being gp130/LIFR (16), and the CNTFR being gp130/LIFR/CNTFR]. There is also evidence that as these complexes assemble, in a ligand-driven fashion, that other subunits associate with the complex. Thus when NGF binds to its receptor, a tyrosine kinase subunit, the c-*trk* protooncogene product, binds to the complex and is involved in transducing signals (40). There is also a growing body of evidence that following ligand binding, there are subunits with protein tyrosine kinase activity that associate with many of the hematopoietin family of receptors (41, 42). In addition to heterologous cross-linking of subunits, it is clear for many cytokine receptor systems that ligand binding leads to homologous cross-linking. For example, TNF is a trimer and has been shown to cause dimerization and trimerization of its receptors when it binds. Similarly, PGDF in all three forms (AA, AB, and BB) is a dimer and causes receptors to dimerize when it binds (43). Furthermore, in what may well be a paradigm for the hematopoietin receptor family, the binding of growth hormone to its receptor leads to receptor dimerization (18). The notion that lateral aggregation is a general mechanism for transmembrane signaling has been well established for many years. It now appears that cytokine receptors also employ this mechanism to deliver signals.

Finally, an intriguing finding in the cytokine receptor field is the existence of soluble receptors in many systems. It is clear that alternatively spliced mRNAs exist that encode soluble forms of a number of cytokine receptors. For example, soluble forms of IL-5R (44), IL-7R (12), IL-1R type II (45), IL-2Rα, IL-6R, IFN-γR, TNFRI, and TNFRII have all been found (46, 47).

In this last group of systems, no evidence for alternatively spliced mRNAs encoding these soluble receptor forms has been detected and the presumption is that they are derived from the integral membrane-bound forms by proteolysis. The physiological functions of soluble forms of cytokine receptors remain to be established. It has been suggested, on the basis of experiments in which pharmacological doses of soluble receptors administered to animals can be shown to inhibit cytokine action (48), that endogenously produced soluble receptors act as antagonists, but this remains to be proved. In at least one case this is not so; the soluble IL-6 receptor α chain when complexed with IL-6 will act as an agonist by signaling through the IL-6 receptor β chain (gp130) (49). Neither soluble IL-6 receptor α chain nor IL-6 alone are capable of this; thus the heterodimeric complex might be regarded as a ligand for gp130, allowing cells that express this protein but not the IL-6 receptor α chain to respond to IL-6. The IL-12 receptor system is a different variation on this theme. Interleukin 12 is a stable heterodimer of a chain that is homologous to IL-6 and a chain that is homologous to IL-6 receptor α chain (21). The IL-12 receptor, for which no cDNA clones have yet been isolated, has a size, as estimated by cross-linking, that suggests that it will be related to the gp130/LIFR/GCSFR subgroup of the hematopoietin receptor family.

The remainder of the chapter focuses on the methods that have been used to generate the data reviewed above.

Analysis of Binding Properties of Cytokine Receptors

Production and Radiolabeling of Recombinant Cytokines

Most of the studies of the binding properties of cytokine receptors have been carried out with recombinant cytokines. Cytokines purified from natural sources were used in early studies. Thus, for example, the original experiments with IL-1 and IL-2 receptors were done with natural forms of the molecules purified from activated human peripheral blood monocytes (IL-1β) (50) and human Jurkat T cell (IL-2) (51) supernatants, respectively. In general, this is not a practical approach as most cytokines have high specific biological activities and are hence produced in small amounts by natural sources. Thus, to generate the quantities (10- to 100-μg range) needed for chemical labeling requires large amounts of natural starting materials. Recombinant cytokines have been generated from cloned cDNAs in a variety of expression systems, yeast and *Escherichia coli* being the most common hosts. A description of the expression vectors, host systems, fermentation procedures, and purification schemes is beyond the scope of this review.

Purified recombinant cytokines in quantities sufficient for labeling can be obtained from a variety of commercial sources.

The most commonly employed radiolabeling methods utilize ^{125}I as a tracer and introduce the label into the protein with either Bolton–Hunter reagent, which labels lysine ε-amino groups, or the Enzymobead (glucose oxidase-lactoperoxidase; Bio-Rad, Richmond, CA) method, which labels tyrosine residues in the ortho position relative to the hydroxyl on the phenol ring. Typical procedures would be as follow.

Bolton–Hunter Reagent

One to 10 μg of cytokine (e.g., IL-1β) in 10–20 μl of borate (0.05 M, pH 8.5)-buffered saline (0.15 M) is labeled with 1 mCi (0.23 nM) of ^{125}I-labeled diiodo-Bolton–Hunter reagent (New England Nuclear, Boston, MA). The reagent is supplied as a dry benzene solution and is prepared for use by evaporation of the solvent with a stream of dry nitrogen. The reagent is hydrolyzed and hence inactivated by moisture in the air; thus, the reagent must be used immediately after the vial is opened, with minimal handling. The protein solution is introduced into the vial containing the dried reagent and the reaction is allowed to proceed at 4–8°C for 30 min or overnight. Subsequently, 30 μl of 2% gelatin is added as a carrier [the reagent will bind noncovalently to bovine serum albumin (BSA)], and the labeled protein is separated from the hydrolyzed label by gel filtration on a 1-ml bed volume column with either Sephadex G-25 or BioGel P10. The column is preblocked with protein by running 2 ml of a 10% BSA or gelatin solution through, and then washing with 10–20 ml of PBS. The labeled protein is eluted with PBS and collected in 0.1-ml fractions. The ^{125}I-labeled protein will elute in fractions 3 and 4. The specific activity estimated for the protein (cpm/unit of protein) will clearly be dependent on the recovery. The most convenient way to estimate this is to carry the same amount of unlabeled cytokine through the procedure after spiking it with a small amount of ^{125}I-labeled cytokine, and either omit the Bolton–Hunter reagent or use noniodinated Bolton–Hunter reagent [3-(p-hydroxyphenyl)propionic acid N-hydroxysuccinimide ester] in the first step. Protein recovery can be estimated as input counts/output counts. Because this is an external, not internal, correction, the procedure should be recalibrated with each new cytokine or at any time when the protocol is modified significantly (e.g., scaled up, scaled down, column material changed, or source of cytokine changed). An alternative is to measure the total recovery of protein (i.e., carrier). This is also, of course, subject to sources of error. The presumption is that the labeled cytokine will behave like the carrier in sticking to glass, the column bed, and so on. In addition, if any blocking protein leaches off the column it can lead to an overestimate of recovery. Furthermore, for gelatin carrier, absorbance at 280 nm is a poor method for estimating concentration, because the tryptophan content of this protein is low. Chemical methods, which are more sensitive and accurate, consume labeled protein, and also involve handling of relatively high quantities of label. For all these reasons, we prefer the simpler external estimation method. Finally, it is important to check that all the label in the preparation is covalently attached to protein by performing a trichloroacetic acid precipitation (10%) on an aliquot. For IL-1β, this method routinely gives 1–3 $\times$ 10^{15} dpm/mmol or approximately 0.5–1.5 atoms ^{125}I per molecule protein.

Enzymobead (Glucose Oxidase-Lactoperoxidase) Method

Protein [1–10 μg in 50 μl of sodium phosphate (0.2 M, pH 7.2)] is combined with 50 μl of Enzymobead reagent reconstituted according to manufacturer (Bio-Rad) instructions. Then 20 μl of the same buffer containing 2 mCi (0.8 nmol) of Na^{125}I is added and the reaction is started by adding 10 μl of β-D-glucose, and allowed to proceed for 10 min at room temperature. The reaction is terminated by adding sodium azide (20 μl, 25 mM) and then sodium metabisulfite (10 μl, 5 mg/ml). Incubation is continued for a further 5 min at room temperature to allow enzyme inactivation and reduction of residual peroxide and I$_3^+$ to occur. The entire reaction mixture is applied to a small column and separated as described above for the Bolton–Hunter reaction, except that BSA (1%, w/v) may be used as a carrier. The initial characterization of the preparation is done essentially as described for the Bolton–Hunter method.

There are several other radiolabeling techniques that we have used less frequently in the laboratory: these include two other tyrosine-directed methods, a modified chloramine-T method, and the Iodogen (Pierce) method. In principle, these two methods and the Enzymobead method described above, by oxidizing I$^-$ and generating I$_3^+$, the species that gives rise to electrophilic substitution at the ortho position relative to the hydroxyl on tyrosine, should be equally effective at labeling any protein. Many cytokines that can be labeled with full retention of activity by the Enzymobead method suffer significant losses of activity with chloramine-T, which is a strong oxidizing agent that can damage proteins through side reactions; Iodogen is intermediate in harshness, as is the immobilized form of this reagent (Iodobeads). Finally, we have on occasion used Woods reagent to label the N-terminal free α-amino group.

The concern over labeling damage necessitates determination of the activity of the labeled relative to the unlabeled cytokine. Ideally, the labeled material should be 100% active relative to the unlabeled material both in a standard bioassay and in a radioreceptor assay. In practice, this may not always be possible and in that case the use for which the material is intended should be considered. The requirement for 100% bioactivity of the cytokine can be applied less than rigorously for at least two reasons. First, many bioassays are simply not quantitative enough to be able to determine with any confidence that two preparations of cytokine have relative activities that are closer than a factor of 2. Furthermore, because most bioassays are carried out for 12 hr or more at 37°C, factors such as stability to proteases and intracellular trafficking pattern might affect the activity of a molecule in the assay. It is therefore reasonable to argue that even if there is some loss of bioactivity, the reagent should be satisfactory for characterizing receptor binding if the affinity constant of the labeled protein [K_A (M^{-1})] is the same as the inhibition constant of the unlabeled protein [K_I (M^{-1})] under the conditions of the receptor-binding assays.

Another measure that is often used to determine the quality of a labeled preparation of cytokine is the maximum percentage of radioligand that can be bound to receptor-bearing cells. The format of the experiment is simply to choose a concentration of labeled protein that is 10–30% of the K_D (i.e., $1/K_A$) and to titer cells bearing receptors against the labeled ligand. By plotting % cpm$_{bound}$ [bound cpm/(bound cpm + free cpm)] vs cell concentration or, more quantitatively, by plotting % cpm$_{bound}$/cell concentration (y) vs % cpm$_{bound}$ (x), essentially a Scatchard plot, one can extrapolate to percentage label bound at infinite cell concentration. This is a useful parameter to measure, and clearly if percentage label bound at infinite cell concentration is significantly less than 100%, then quantitative data obtained with that material should be regarded as suspect. However, if this value is low, it is difficult to make a simple correction to data obtained with the preparation in the absence of several other pieces of information:

1. Is the failure of the labeled preparation to bind 100% a consequence of damage during the labeling or due to a preexisting inactive fraction of protein?

2. Is there a correlation between the extent of labeling and activity? In general, one might assume that more heavily labeled molecules might be less active. However, in the absence of data this remains an assumption.

3. What is the average level of labeling? If, for example, labeling does indeed decrease the binding activity of a cytokine to 10% of that of the unlabeled material, and in the simplest case there is one site on the protein that can be modified, the preparation will have an apparent K_A that is the same as that of the unlabeled protein but will give an apparent maximal level of binding that is only 10% of the true value. By contrast, if the same labeling procedure yields a preparation that is 90% modified, the apparent K_A will be 10% that of the unlabeled protein but the estimated maximal binding will be approximately correct.

4. At an average level of labeling, what is the distribution of label? It is possible that two different cytokines labeled by the same method might have

different fractions of a labeled preparation, with zero, one, two, or more atoms of iodine per molecule of protein, with an average of one atom per molecule.

5. Are the receptors being studied themselves a homogeneous population, or are there subpopulations of receptors that can differentially bind subpopulations of the ligand preparation?

It is of course possible to write down systems of equilibria that model each of these situations, and determine how one might correct the binding data. It is frankly best to attempt to find a source of cytokine/labeling method that yields a relatively high fractional substitution, at least as estimated by atoms iodine per molecule protein, while retaining a K_A that is close to the K_I of the unlabeled material.

Binding and Kinetic Assays: Phthalate Oil Method

In this section, the approach used for characterizing the binding properties of receptors is summarized. The method that we routinely use is based on a phthalate oil technique developed by Segal and Hurwitz (52). A typical experiment is carried out as follows.

Materials

Polyethylene centrifuge tubes (400 μl) (Brinkmann, Westbury, NY)
Eppendorf microfuge
Razor blades (single edge)
Household slip joint pliers
Bis(2-ethylhexyl)phthalate and dibutyl phthalate (Eastman-Kodak, Rochester, NY): The oils are mixed at a ratio of 1.5 parts dibutyl phthalate to 1.5 parts bis(2-ethylhexyl)phthalate to yield a density that is less than that of the cells but more than that of the binding medium, in the range 4–20°C
Round-bottomed microtiter plates (96 well; available from several manufacturers)
Orbital shaker (Bellco)
Binding medium: RPMI-1640 containing 1% BSA, 0.1% sodium azide, and 20 mM N-2-hydroxyethylpiperazine-N'-2-ethanesulfonic acid (HEPES) (pH 7.2)
Glass or polypropylene disposable test tubes (12 × 75 mm)

Procedure

Cells at a concentration range of 1–10 × 10^7 cells/ml (50 μl) are mixed with 125I-labeled ligand (50 μl) and either binding medium (50 μl) or unlabeled ligand (50 μl) in the control wells of 96-well plates. The plates are placed on an orbital shaker and incubated at the desired temperature for the desired time (see below). At the end of the incubation, duplicate 60-μl aliquots are removed from each well and each aliquot is transferred to an Eppendorf tube containing 200 μl of phthalate oil mixture. Irrespective of the incubation temperature, the prefilled oil tubes are stored in the refrigerator and either moved to the bench top just before use or placed in an ice water bath. Once the cell suspension is placed in the tubes, they are quickly transferred to the microfuge, which is kept in a cold box, and spun for approximately 1 min. The cells sediment to the tip, and the medium remains on top of the oil. To separate the bound from free radioligand, the tube is pinched firmly with the pliers, and the tip sliced off with a razor blade so that it falls into a 12 × 75 mm tube placed in a test tube rack. Sufficient pressure is maintained on the cut tube so that the bulk of the oil and the supernatant do not leak out; the cut tube is held over a second 12 × 75 mm tube and the grasp rapidly released so that it drops in. The tubes are then counted on a γ counter, typically for 1–5 min/tube or with a 1–2% counting error terminator.

Some Practical Tips

1. The cell concentration range is somewhat arbitrary and may need to be determined empirically. Several factors should be borne in mind. First, in contrast to an aqueous separation method, the cells do not pass through the oil layer singly but first accumulate at the oil–water interface as a layer that breaks up into spherical aqueous droplets lined with cells that sediment to the bottom of the tube and break up, releasing smaller droplets of medium without cells that return to the top. Consequently, a minimum cell mass and thus cell concentration must be placed in each tube. Second, the calculation of the data presumes that the cells occupy a negligible fraction of the volume of the suspension. This assumption can be avoided by removing a known volume of the supernatant (e.g., 25 μl) from the tube prior to cutting, although this makes the procedure somewhat more labor intensive. In this case, however, much higher cell concentrations may be used, which may be useful when receptor numbers and/or affinities are low. The method can be made more accurate by labeling the cells first with ^{51}Cr sodium chromate and counting each sample for both ^{51}Cr and ^{125}I, and using the ^{51}Cr counts as an internal control for cell number. However, test experiments have shown that in general this only marginally improves the quality of the data.

2. The oil mixture is of relatively high viscosity and it is important that no bubbles are left in the 400-μl tubes as they are filled. The most convenient method of rapidly filling a large number of the tubes is to fill a disposable 20-ml syringe with the mixture, and fit it with a wide-gauge needle cut and blunted so it just reaches the bottom of the 400-μl tubes.

3. The oil mixture has a higher coefficient of thermal expansion than water. Thus, the mixture will need to be adjusted if one wishes to use tubes warmed to 37°C for any reason. If no adjustments are made, the entire aqueous phase will sediment to the bottom of the tube if the oil is warm.

4. In general, it will be easier if 12 × 75 mm polypropylene tubes are used, as there is a tendency to strike the razor blade against the lip of the tubes and the blades become blunted less rapidly if plastic tubes are used, rather than glass ones.

5. The single largest source of error in the assay is retention of trapped medium containing unbound ligand in the cell pellet. The major causes of this are the presence of dead cells, cell aggregates, or debris in the stock cell suspension. It is critical therefore to prepare at the outset of the experiment a single cell suspension of high viability. If some lysis has occurred, the cells should be treated with DNase.

First-Stage Data Reduction

The bound and free counts can be converted into whatever concentration units the user desires. Our laboratory chooses to express free concentrations in molar and bound concentrations in molecules per cell. The merit of the latter is that saturation values give a direct measure of receptor numbers per cell independent of the cell concentration in the assay. These are calculated as shown in Eqs. (1) and (2):

$$\text{Free } (M) = \text{cpm} \times 1000/(\text{spA} \times 60) \tag{1}$$

where specific activity (spA) is expressed as counts per minute per millimole.

$$\text{Bound (molecules/cell)} = \text{cpm} \times N/(C \times 60 \times \text{spA}) \tag{2}$$

where N is Avogadro's number (6.03×10^{23}) and C is cell concentration in the assay (cells/ml); in both instances 60 is the aliquot size in microliters. To calculate the specific binding, the amount bound at any given concentration of ^{125}I-labeled cytokine must be corrected for the amount ''bound'' in the presence of an approximately 100-fold excess of unlabeled cytokine. Most of this so-called nonspecific binding represents trapped free ligand present in a small volume of liquid that cosediments with the cells. This is one drawback of the oil method because no washing is possible as the cells sediment. This contamination of bound ligand by free is cell-type dependent, but for any given cell type it is characterized by a cell concentration-independent value of x μl/cell. For this reason, if receptor numbers and/or affinity of a given cell type are low the signal-to-noise ratio is unlikely to improve by increasing the cell density in the assay.

For adherent cells, it may be preferable to assay binding *in situ*, because removal from monolayer cultures by limited protease treatment may damage receptors, and simply using ethylenediaminetetraacetic acid (EDTA) often gives preparations that are aggregated and have extracellular matrix associated with the cells. We describe an *in situ* binding assay for IL-1 in Qwarnstrom *et al.* (53). It is similar to many others described for other growth factors and cytokines. Briefly, cells are grown in 6-well trays, which we use rather than 24- or 48-well trays because IL-1 receptor levels are low. After incubation with ^{125}I-labeled IL-1α or ^{125}I-labeled IL-1β (0.5–1 ml/well in binding medium), 100 μl of medium is removed to determine free IL-1, the remainder of the medium is discarded, and the wells are washed several times with binding medium and PBS. The cells plus bound ligand are released by trypsin treatment and the contents of the wells are removed for counting. Each six-well plate gives two duplicate data points plus two wells for cell counts. This procedure is more labor intensive than the oil assay and therefore used only when unavoidable.

Strategy for Binding Analysis of a Novel Cytokine Receptor

The previous section has outlined the mechanics of binding assays in two standard formats, the most broadly useful format being described in the most detail. In this section, the overall approach to obtaining the most accurate overall estimates of binding properties will be summarized.

The initial approach to identifying the presence of receptors on cells for a recombinant cytokine will depend on how cDNA clones for it were isolated. For example, as was the case for IL-7, if the cytokine was isolated on the basis of a bioassay with a cell line, then that cell line represents a logical starting place for receptor characterization. If, by contrast, a cytokine is identified as a cDNA in an activation library, as were several members of the small inflammatory cytokine family, then some kind of crude screen must be done to find cells with receptors. In this latter case, the cytokine might be labeled by several methods, and then some arbitrary concentration incubated with a cell line or a population of primary cells such as spleen cells or peripheral blood mononuclear cells ± a 100-fold excess of unlabeled ligand to find some evidence for specific binding. It is probably advisable in the latter case to use cells from the same species as the cytokine to avoid failing to detect receptors due to species differences in receptors. Once some evidence of specific binding of a radiolabeled cytokine to cells has been obtained, it is worthwhile to pursue the semiquantitative screen to the point at which a cell line easily propagated in culture and expressing a reasonable number of receptors can be identified. The definition of "reasonable" is somewhat arbitrary: the original characterization of IL-1 receptors was done on a cell line expressing 200–500 receptors/cells. Once a cell line has been chosen, it should be decided whether further assays should be done at 4–8 or 37°C. In principle, it is better to do the binding assays at 37°C; however, there may be several artifacts that prevent assays done at this temperature from being easily interpretable. The following issue should be addressed.

1. At 37°C does the ligand become partially or completely degraded in the assay?
2. At 37°C do the receptors internalize, desensitize, or shed from the cells in response to ligand binding, even in the presence of sodium azide or other inhibitors such as bacitracin?
3. Does the ligand cause lysis or death of the cells at 37°C?
4. Does the system ever reach equilibrium at 4–8°C? If so, are the equilibrium binding properties of the system at 4–8°C essentially the same as those at 37°C?

Depending on the answers to these questions, a temperature can be selected to perform most of the characterization experiments. Ideally, 37°C is preferable as it is more physiological. However, because there are more potential complexities at 37°C than at 4–8°C the latter may be simpler in practice.

To establish conditions for equilibrium binding, association kinetics experiments are first done. These are done at a minimum of three different concentrations of ^{125}I-labeled cytokine, because in even the simplest case of a bimolecular reaction, the reaction rate is concentration dependent. The most convenient way to carry out the experiments is to prepare each of the ^{125}I-labeled cytokine solutions in a separate 15-ml centrifuge tube with a paired tube containing a large excess of unlabeled cytokine. At $t = 0$ cells are added to all six tubes, and duplicate 60-μl samples withdrawn at various times, and placed in 400-μl tubes with 200 μl of oil prepared prior to starting the experiment. The time when the centrifuge is started should be taken as the time at which the measurement was actually made. Typical time points would be 2, 5, 10, 20, 30, 45, 60, 90, 120, 180, and 240 min. Typical radioligand concentrations would be 3×10^{-10}, 1×10^{-9}, and $3 \times 10^{-9} M$. The forward and reverse rates can be estimated from the slope and intercept of the rate vs concentration plot. The reverse rate can also be determined directly by a dissociation kinetics experiment; cells are first incubated with ^{125}I-labeled cytokine for a time estimated to reach equilibrium based on the association kinetics data. The cells are then sedimented by centrifugation, the supernatant withdrawn, and the cells suspended without washing in the same volume of either medium or medium containing a large concentration of unlabeled cytokine. A sample of the cells should be taken before the centrifugation/resuspension to serve as the zero time point. The amount bound as a function of time can again be measured by transferring samples to the 400-μl tubes containing oil. If the system follows a simple bimolecular reaction mechanism, the value for k_r (min^{-1}) measured in this experiment will be the same in the medium and medium plus unlabeled cytokine experiments and also the same as the value estimated from the association experiment. Differences in the values are indicative of complexity in the ligand–receptor interaction.

With a cell line that gives a reasonable signal-to-noise ratio in hand and the kinetics experiments done so that the conditions of temperature and time for attainment of equilibrium are defined, the next step is to run inhibition experiments to determine precisely the concentrations of unlabeled cytokine needed to inhibit specific binding completely. The expected K_D can be estimated as the ratio of the forward to the reverse rate constants. Two concentrations of ^{125}I-labeled cytokine should be used (one concentration of about 20% of the K_D and one of about 500% of the K_D) and a complete dose–response curve of unlabeled competitor, with 10–15 data points covering a 1000- to 10,000-fold concentration range being carried out. Finally, a dose of unlabeled competitor can be selected and a titration of ^{125}I-labeled cytokine is run to generate a data set for determining the binding parameters of the labeled material.

Analysis of Binding Data

A comprehensive description of mechanisms of receptor binding, how to derive models based on them, and how to fit these to binding data is beyond the scope of this review. However, the basic analyses for the simplest model will be summarized, giving some hints as to what points are critical and/or useful. Furthermore, a description of how the data may deviate from the model and their implications about the underlying mechanisms of ligand–receptor interactions will be provided.

1. A simple bimolecular reaction is

$$\begin{array}{cccc} L & + & R & = & LR \\ (z) & & (r) & & (B) \end{array} \qquad (3)$$

where L is the ligand, R is the receptor, and LR is the ligand–receptor complex; z, r, and B are the concentrations of free ligand, free receptor, and receptor–ligand complex, respectively. The affinity constant can be defined by Eq. (4):

$$K_A = k_f/k_r = B/z(r) \tag{4}$$

where k_f is the association rate constant in units of concentration$^{-1} \times$ time^{-1} and k_r is the reverse rate constant in units of time^{-1}. We conventionally express r and B in units of molecules per cell, z in units of molarity, and time in units of minutes. K_A therefore has units of M^{-1}.

2. The association reaction can be described by Eq. (5):

$$B_t = B_\infty(1 - e^{-kt}) \tag{5}$$

when B_t (molecules per cell) is the amount bound at time t, B_∞ (molecules per cell) is the amount bound at infinite time, and k (minute^{-1}) is the reaction rate constant. This constant can in turn be defined as

$$k = k_f z + k_r \tag{6}$$

3. The dissociation reaction can be described by Eq. (7):

$$B_t = B_0 e^{-kt} \tag{7}$$

when B_t is the amount bound at time t, B_0 is the amount bound at time zero, and $k = k_r$ (minute^{-1}).

4. Inhibition of labeled cytokine by unlabeled cytokine can be described by Eq. (8):

$$I\ (\%) = I_{max}K_I i/(1 + K_I i + K_A z) \tag{8}$$

In the instance in which labeled and unlabeled cytokines are identical, with the exception of the labeling, I_{max} is by definition set equal to 100%, and the remainder of the binding is assumed to be nonspecific (see below). i is the unlabeled cytokine concentration (in units of molarity), and z is the labeled cytokine concentration (M). K_I and K_A are the inhibition constant and binding constant, respectively, in M^{-1}. Note that the equation predicts that if $z > 1/K_A$ (i.e., if $K_A z > 1$) then the midpoint of the inhibition dose–response curve will be dependent on z.

5. Binding of labeled cytokine to cells can be described by Eq. (9):

$$B_{tot} = r_0 K_A z/(1 + K_A z) + A_{ns} z \tag{9}$$

where B_{tot} is the total observed binding, r_0 is the total receptor concentration (in sites per cell), K_A and z are as defined earlier, and A_{ns} is the nonspecific binding coefficient. Binding in the presence of a large excess of unlabeled ligand as defined by Eq. (8) is given by

$$B_{ns} = A_{ns}z \qquad (10)$$

and therefore if binding is truly nonspecific, all the data points will lie on a straight line of slope A_{ns} (molecules cell^{-1} M^{-1}) that passes through the origin. Then

$$B = B_{tot} - B_{ns} = r_0K_Az/(1 + K_Az) \qquad (11)$$

Note that as K_A tends to zero $K_Az \ll 1$ and hence Eq. (11) becomes

$$B = r_0K_Az \qquad (12)$$

Equation (12) has the same form as Eq. (10). This is logical because nonspecific binding represents weak binding to a large number of sites. Equation (12) is also the limit that Eq. (11) approaches as z tends to 0, that is, it represents the slope of the binding curve at low ligand concentrations. It is thus a measure of the binding activity of the cells. Also, the ratio (r_0K_A/A_{ns}), which is a dimensionless number, is a good measure of the signal-to-noise ratio for a system. One final standard piece of algebra to be noted is the Scatchard equation, which is a transformation of Eq. (11):

$$B/z = B(r_0 - K_A) \qquad (13)$$

This shows that if binding data from a system that follows Eq. (3) are plotted in the form of bound/free against bound, the points fall on a straight line, the slope of which is the affinity constant and the x axis intercept the number of sites per cell. This method of analysis was used extensively prior to the general availability of personal computers and nonlinear least-squares curve-fitting programs because it converts the data into a format than can be analyzed by linear regression or more simply with graph paper and a ruler. The graphic analyses of these equilibrium binding data in both the bound vs free and Scatchard coordinate systems are illustrated in Fig. 1.

As indicated in the previous paragraph, there are now a variety of programs available for desktop and mainframe computers for nonlinear least-squares curve-fitting models of binding data. The programs allow the user to take a mathematical model with unknown parameters, defined on the basis of a compartmental model of the type given in Eq. (3), and to determine the

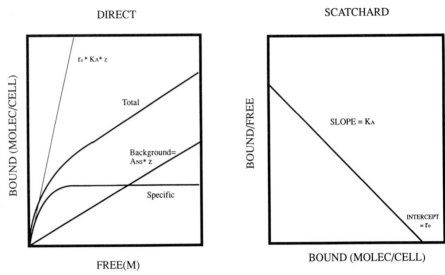

Fig. 1   Graphic analyses of binding data from a simple bimolecular ligand–receptor interaction.

numerical values of the parameters at which the model best fits a set of data. We use RS/1 (Bolt, Beranek, and Newman) run on a VAX cluster, or Mathematica (Wolfram Associates) running on a Macintosh IIx with 8 Mbytes of RAM. There are several other such programs available, among them the LIGAND (54) and DESIGN (55, 56) programs written by P. Munson, D. Rodbard, and collaborators and the MS-DOS version of MLAB (Civilised Software). The availability of these tools makes use of the Scatchard plot superfluous except for illustrative purposes. Thus we fit Eqs. (5–11) to data in the format of bound vs free or bound vs time to obtain estimates for rate constants or binding constants.

The model described above is consistent with the receptors behaving as a set of identical sites. The simplest type of deviation from the behavior described in this set of equations is that the receptors behave as a set of n subpopulations with distinct affinities and rate constants (57). Thus, for example, the equilibrium binding equation becomes

$$B_s = r_0 \, \Sigma_i \, F_i K_i z/(1 \, + \, K_i z) \tag{14}$$

where F_i is the fraction of the total receptor population with affinity K_i and i runs from 1 to n. Similar versions can be written for the association and dissociation rate equations and the inhibition equation. In practice, these equations become of little use beyond $n = 3$, since as the number of parameters becomes sufficiently large, any one of them will be determined with a low degree of accuracy. This type of model is also unsatisfactory in that it make no real reference to any particular type of mechanism. More complex models can be built that account for cooperativity between receptors, in which the affinity of unoccupied receptor sites is affected by the binding of ligand to receptors. These types of models allow for effects of ligand binding on ligand already bound. Thus, for example, in the dissociation experiments, resuspending cells preloaded to a low fractional receptor occupancy with ^{125}I-labeled ligand in medium with sufficient unlabeled cytokine to occupy the remaining receptors rapidly can cause the prebound ligand to dissociate more quickly (negative cooperativity) or more slowly (positive cooperativity). These kinetic effects also correlate with complex binding behavior, as illustrated in Fig. 2. The mechanistic origins of such binding properties are varied. They may arise from multisubunit receptors and multivalent ligands as seems to be the case for growth hormones for example TNF and PDGF or by intramolecular conformational effects as has been postulated for insulin. In some parameter value domains, complex binding properties can arise from

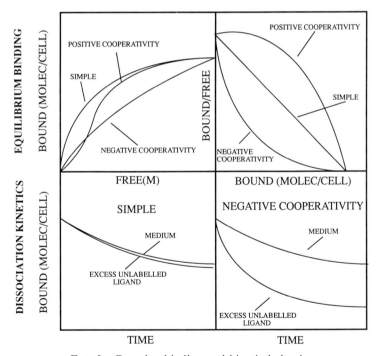

FIG. 2   Complex binding and kinetic behavior.

a system in which, were the ligand and receptor-isolated molecules reacting in solution, the system would behave as the ideal case described in Eqs. (3–12). However, by virtue of the reaction occurring at a surface, they would behave as a complex system with occupancy dependent rate constants. The interested reader is referred to the many review articles and textbooks that deal with the modeling of such complex systems.

Other Types of Binding Assay: Flow Cytometry and Autoradiography

In many instances, rather than having a precise description of the site numbers and/or affinities of receptors for a particular cytokine, it may be more important to know what fraction of the cell types in a mixed population of cells or a solid tissue express receptors. These data can be obtained for some cell populations (e.g., bone marrow cells and other hematopoietic tissues) by flow cytometry with labeled cytokines. Interleukin 1α, for example, can be labeled directly with fluorescein isothiocyanate and used to detect receptors on some cell types by flow cytometry. Several dye-labeled cytokines are available from R&D Biosystems. In most instances, these reagents are of limited use in staining for fluorescence microscopy as the levels of cytokine receptor expression on most cell types are too low to detect by this method.

Autoradiography has been used to look at cytokine receptor distribution in a variety of cell preparations, such as bone marrow, thymus, whole brain, and adherent cultured cells. The protocols have been based on those developed for the adherent cell and suspension ^{125}I-labeled cytokine binding. Usually, cells are incubated at 4–8°C with a concentration of radiolabel three times that of the K_D for the system, for a time determined from previous experiments to allow equilibrium to be reached. Subsequently, the cells if incubated in suspension are washed several times and then spun onto slides with a cytocentrifuge. Adherent cells can be grown in slide chambers and then incubations carried out in the chambers, and the slides subsequently washed several times. In either case, the slides are then dipped in photographic emulsion in the dark, dried and exposed at 8°C for 1 to 30 days, and subsequently developed. A picture of such a monolayer autoradiograph is shown in Fig. 3. This method has also been adapted to detect receptors in expression screening (see below).

Characterization of Cytokine Receptors by Affinity Cross-Linking

Approaches to the characterization of the structure of cytokine receptors are limited by the low levels of expression in most cells. The method that has proved most generally useful is affinity cross-linking of radiolabeled cytokine to cells. In this technique, the signal-to-noise ratio is high because the only label in the system is covalently bound to the high specific activity radioligand. The structure of the receptor is inferred from the generation of high molecular weight covalent complexes of the ligand and cellular proteins when cells with ligand bound to them are treated with bivalent, usually lysine-directed, chemical modification reagents. These complexes are detected by gel electrophoresis of detergent-extracted proteins. In general, such methods, which rely on the fortuitous apposition of appropriate side chains, can be subject to several artifacts. First, the ligand may not be efficiently cross-linked to the protein with which it forms the most intimate noncovalent interactions. Second, the receptor chains themselves may be cross-linked to one another or to other cellular proteins with varying degrees of efficiency.

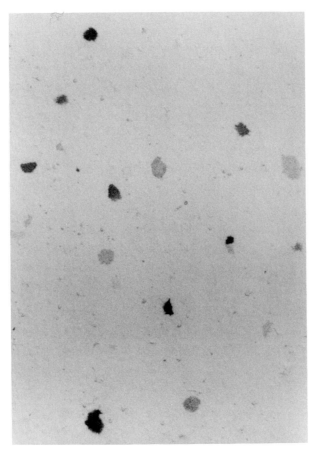

FIG. 3 Detection of receptors by autoradiography.

Finally, once the covalent bonds are formed, structural and functional integrity of ligand and receptor are not required for continued association. Hence, when cells are extracted with detergent, release of intracellular proteases and partial degradation of the complex may occur. Nevertheless, the method has proved remarkably robust, in that the sizes of individual subunits of receptors and even the composition of multichain receptor complexes, as determined early on in the characterization of most cytokine receptors, have been confirmed by later cDNA cloning studies and once antibodies to receptors have been developed by surface and/or biosynthetic labeling and immunoprecipitation studies.

A typical cross-linking experiment is carried out in the following fashion. Cells (10^7/ml) are incubated in binding medium (100–200 μl) (see Analysis of Binding Properties of Cytokine Receptors, above) with ^{125}I-labeled cytokine at a concentration of $3–10 \times K_D$ at 8°C, for a time known to allow the system to reach equilibrium. Use of low temperature is important, as even limited proteolysis or internalization could produce uninterpretable or misleading results. As a specificity control, a parallel incubation can be done with a 100-fold excess of unlabeled ligand. Subsequently the cells are washed several times with phosphate-buffered saline (PBS), pH 7.4, resuspended in 100 μl of PBS, and treated with cross-linking reagent for 1 hr at 8°C. The cross-linker is added as 2 μl of a $50\times$ stock, typically 5–50 mg/ml in dimethyl sulfoxide (DMSO). Samples are then washed twice with PBS and solubilized in the same buffer (50 μl) containing 1% Triton X-100 and protease inhibitors (e.g., phenylmethylsulfonyl fluoride; 2 mM final concentration), incubated on ice for 5 min, and clarified by centrifugation for 15 min in a microfuge at 8°C. Ten microliters of the sample is taken for counting to determine how much ^{125}I-labeled cytokine is present and 10–40 μl is used for sodium dodecyl sulfate-polyacrylamide gel electrophoresis (SDS-PAGE), depending on the number of counts present.

A variety of cross-linking reagents are available from Pierce Chemical Company (Rockford, IL). We have used disuccinimidyl suberate (DSS), disuccinimidyl tartrate (DST), bis(succinimidyl) suberate (BS^3), and dithiobis(succinimidyl)propionate (DSP). The first three reagents are ranked in order of increasing hydrophilicity, and hence one might choose BS^3 when it is important to minimize penetration into the membrane. DSP can be used to give an additional control because it contains a disulfide in the bridge, so cross-linked species present on nonreducing gels will be cleaved and appear different when the same sample is analyzed on reducing gels. The best reagent to use for any particular system must be established empirically, as must the optimal concentrations. The details of how the electrophoresis is done is again dependent on the system. We typically use 8% Hoefer (San Francisco, CA) slab gels and apply approximately 10–30 μl of sample per lane.

The Triton X-100 extracts are mixed with an equal volume of $2\times$ sample buffer and heated to 100°C for 3–5 min to denature proteins prior to electrophoresis. The gels are then run with stackers, soaked, dried and exposed to film, or placed in a phosphorimager cassette. We have begun to analyze most of our data quantitatively with a phosphorimaging system (Molecular Dynamics), which also yields data approximately 10 times faster than film.

Molecular Cloning of Cytokine Receptors

With a radioreceptor assay developed and some notion of the probable structure of the receptor based on cross-linking experiments, the next logical step is to obtain cDNA clones encoding it. There are currently a variety of potential routes from radioreceptor assay to cDNA clones, although broadly these may be broken down into two generic approaches, protein purification and expression cloning. The first uses some form of ligand-binding assay in conjunction with biochemical purification techniques to obtain a homogeneous protein preparation with ligand-binding activity. The second identifies DNA sequences directly on the basis of their ability to encode expressible ligand-binding activity, or potentially to confer hormone responsiveness on cells.

Three components are needed to implement a purification strategy, a cell line/tissue source of receptor, an assay for receptor once the cells are disrupted, and a method of purification. The source can be identified by radioreceptor assays and by selecting that cell or tissue showing the highest level of ligand binding in picomoles per gram cellular protein; at present >10–100 pmol/g wet weight is a practical source concentration. Tracking receptor requires that it bind ligand after cells are solubilized in detergent. This solubilization step is the first in purifying receptor away from other integral membrane proteins, as it potentially stabilizes the receptor and dilutes the membrane lipids and other proteins with detergent molecules. It is the step at which this approach succeeds or fails. Specifically, this approach will fail if the receptor contains two or more chains, neither of which alone binds ligand and which separate when solubilized, or if the structure is highly sensitive to the lipid environment. If, however, binding activity is retained, then affinity chromatography on a ligand column is a logical choice as a first step in purification. It should also be straightforward to determine the size of any protein binding specifically to the hormone or antibody column, and to compare these data with those from cross-linking experiments to confirm that the membrane proteins being purified are of the expected size(s). At this stage, a combination of standard chromatographic and/or gel electrophoresis steps should, in principle, permit purification of quantities of protein sufficient for sequencing. The final step in cloning is to use a suitable stretch of protein sequence to construct oligonucleotide probes and screen a cDNA library made from poly(A)$^+$ mRNA prepared from the same source as the receptor protein. By way of examples, this method was used to clone the α subunit of IL-2 receptor (58–60). The purification of TNF receptors has also been successful because human serum and urine, particularly from patients with systemic inflammatory diseases such as sepsis, contain soluble TNF receptors at relatively high concentrations (10–100 ng/ml).

In practice, purification and sequencing of receptor proteins on the picomolar scale is laborious, technically demanding, and requires complex and expensive equipment. It is being superceded by expression cloning methods. There are three basic protocols: (1) prokaryotic expression with cDNA libraries constructed in λ phage-based vectors such as λgt11, (2) eukaryotic expression, the system of choice being COS cells, and using libraries made in vectors based on that originally designed by Okayama and Berg (3), and (3) expression from genomic DNA transfected, for example, into L cells. In addition, one cytokine receptor, the IL-4 receptor, was cloned by a strategy that employed subtractive hybridization (61). In this instance, attempts to enrich the best cell source of receptor (the murine cell line CTLL-2) by staining with fluorescein-labeled IL-4 and sorting, generated the line CTLL-19.4 with approximately 10^6 receptors/cell compared to approximately 10^3 on the parental line. This level of enrichment was sufficient to allow the generation of a subtractive probe that identified receptor cDNAs. Unfortunately, it has not been our experience that this level of enrichment can be generally attained by cell sorting.

Each of these approaches has its own drawbacks and merits. Because λ-based expression systems use *E. coli* as a host organism and express the product of a cDNA as a fusion protein with β-galactosidase, it is unlikely that the protein will be present in the native conformation. It is, therefore, unlikely to be successful unless an antibody that will recognize denatured protein is available. Monoclonal or polyclonal antibodies raised against the natural protein can be screened by Western blots to determine if they are suitable. If such a reagent is available, then this is the method of choice as the vectors are well tested, easy to use, and a large number of cDNAs can be screened rapidly. Unfortunately, it has proved difficult to generate antibodies against most cytokine receptors, using natural sources as immunogens, primarily because expression levels are low. This method was used to clone the human IFN-γ receptor (62).

Genomic cloning offers one potential advantage over cDNA expression methods, and several drawbacks. The advantage is that if the mRNA for the protein of interest is present at low levels in the best source, the gene may be a better source of the sequences coding for the protein. The major drawbacks are that many genes are too large to be transfected in their entirety, in sheared DNA because of the presence of intervening sequences, the efficiency of expression is low compared to that of cDNAs in specifically tailored expression vectors (25). Furthermore, the screens are laborious.

Eukaryotic expression cloning has proved to be the most successful method for receptor cloning. Indeed, a number of studies by Seed and collaborators have shown that if antibodies are available, it is possible to clone virtually any cell surface protein by a preparative panning method that is simple and rapid (1, 26–28, 63–69). Without antibodies, it is also possible to isolate receptor cDNA clones by transient expression of pools of cDNAs in COS cells and assaying for ligand binding directly (2, 13). Because most cytokine receptors have been cloned this way, the method will be described in more detail.

Both the direct ligand-binding method and the panning method rely on the use of a variety of vectors that are based on the original design by Okayama and Berg (3). A schematic is shown in Fig. 4. The vectors contain four basic elements, a high-expression cassette containing a cloning site, a viral origin of replication, an *E. coli* origin of replication, and bacterial drug resistance

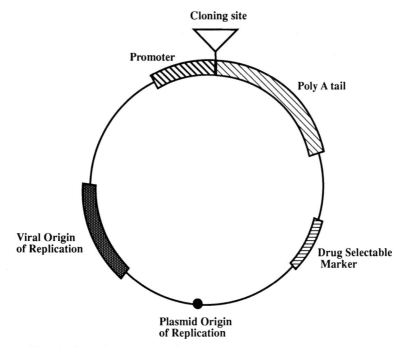

FIG. 4 Generic structure of a mammalian high-expression vector.

genes. The basic strategy for using such vectors is as follows: vector DNA is linearized by restriction enzyme digestion, and a cDNA library ligated into the cloning site. The library is then used to transform *E. coli,* and the library titrated to determine the number of drug (usually ampicillin)-resistant colonies. The library is then plated in pools of 100–10,000 colonies on selection plates containing ampicillin and grown overnight. Colonies are scraped and "miniprep" DNAs are prepared.

COS cells are cultured either on plates or slides for 12–24 hr after plating, and subsequently transfected with 1–10 μg of vector DNA by one of several methods. For example, the DEAE-dextran method involves incubating the cells with the vector DNA in the presence of 67 μM chloroquine and dextran. The DNA is premixed with the DEAE-dextran (100 μg) in approximately 100 μl of medium containing chloroquine, and then added to the cells. The culture is then incubated for 5 hr, washed, and shocked with medium containing 10% DMSO for 5 min. The medium is then changed, and the cultures are incubated at 37°C for 72 hr. During this time, the plasmid replicates to a high copy number and the transcription unit drives production of a high level of mRNA from the inserts. At the end of this time, the expression of receptor is assayed. We have used two methods for assaying receptor expression (2, 13). In both methods, the cell monolayers are washed and then overlaid with binding medium containing ^{125}I-labeled cytokine at a concentration approximately equal to the K_D for receptors and the cultures are then incubated at 4–8°C for a time previously determined to allow equilibrium to be reached. The cells are then washed. In the first method, the cells cultured in tissue culture dishes are fixed, dried, the sides of the dishes cut away, and the plates placed cell side down on X-ray film (2). Individual cells expressing receptors appear as dark spots. In the second method, cells are cultured in chamber slides, and after the ^{125}I-labeled cytokine incubation the chambers are removed and the slides dipped in emulsion (GTNB-2; Kodak) (13). Cells expressing receptors show clusters of grains over them after development (see Fig. 3). In either case, a cDNA pool that gives positive cells must contain a receptor cDNA. In this case, the *E. coli* glycerol pool from this stock is further fractionated into subpools and the procedure repeated. After several cycles, the individual colonies are grown, "miniprep" DNA made, and a single clone identified that encodes the receptor. The insert can then be excised and sequenced by standard methods. At this stage a large quantity of the pure vector DNA can be grown and transfections performed to analyze the binding properties and size, by cross-linking, of the recombinant receptor.

We have used two vector systems in our laboratory. The first, like the original Okayama and Berg (3) vector, is based on simian virus 40 (SV40); the vector contains the SV40 origin and the host cells are COS cells that are a derivative of the CV-1 monkey kidney cell line that stably expresses the

SV40 large T antigen, allowing vector replication. More recently, we have switched to an analogous system based on Epstein–Barr virus (EBV). The vectors contain the EBV origin, and the host cell CV-1/EBNA stably expresses the Epstein–Barr virus nuclear antigen-1 (EBNA-1) antigen, which serves the same function as large T in the SV40 system. The difference in practice is that the EBV-based system gives a larger percentage of cells transfected at any DNA dose, but a lower level of expression on each expressing cell. Because the emulsion autoradiography method is more sensitive than the plate method, the combination of this detection method and the EBV-based vector system generates a screen that uses fewer cells and reagents and can detect cDNAs in larger pools. The COS/film method can handle pool sizes in the 100–1000 range, and the CV-1/EBNA/emulsion method can handle pool sizes in the 1000–10,000 range. The simple consequence of this is that libraries can be screened 10 times faster with the newer method. A typical library might contain 2×10^6 individual clones or approximately 10,000 pools by the old method vs 1000 pools by the new one. At a maximal throughput of 2–300 pools a week, the old method would take approximately 6 months to run through the library vs 3 weeks by the new method. The new method is hence clearly superior.

We have had little direct experience with the Seed method (26) in our laboratory because, for the most part, we have been attempting to clone receptors for which we did not have antibodies. But in outline the vector construction, library preparation, and screening are similar to those described above. However, after culture of transfected COS cells, the cells are harvested by EDTA treatment and scraping, pooled, and incubated with a monoclonal antibody to the molecule of interest. The cells are then washed and transferred to panning plates coated with anti-immunoglobulin. After allowing the cells to adhere, the plates are washed gently to remove the nonadherent cells and the adherent cells are subsequently removed by scraping, and plasmid DNA prepared. The plasmid DNA is then grown in *E. coli* and the transfection/panning procedure repeated. Usually after two or more rounds an aliquot of the transfected cells is stained with antibody and analyzed by flow cytometry to determine if the procedure has enriched for cDNA(s) that drive a high level of expression of the antigen. The anticipated result is the presence of a small subpopulation of brightly staining cells. Eventually individual colonies are isolated and the cDNA characterized as above.

In conclusion, it is our experience that with the current technologies, if a novel cytokine is cloned and a radioreceptor assay developed, that the direct expression method by labeled ligand binding provides the most rapid means to isolate cDNAs encoding the receptor. With a precise understanding of the binding properties of multisubunit receptors and cDNA clones for one of those subunits in hand, it is also proving useful as a cloning method for additional subunits. Thus subunits for both the LIF and GMCSF/IL-3 systems that are required for high-affinity binding have been isolated by using concentrations of ligands in the screen that are too low to give significant binding to low-affinity sites, and "doping" all pools in the library with cDNA encoding the low-affinity receptor (16, 70). Thus the screen allows detection of pools of cDNA that contain an affinity converter protein. For the LIF system, for example, this method allowed the cloning of the β chain, which transpired to be gp130, the β chain of the IL-6 receptor.

Production of Monoclonal Antibodies to Cytokine Receptors

Because cytokine receptors are expressed at low levels in natural sources, and with the ease of cloning offered by the direct ligand-binding expression methods, we usually wait until we have receptor cDNAs or recombinant protein in hand to generate antibodies. We routinely use four sources of antigen for immunizations: (1) CV-1/EBNA or COS cells transfected with the cDNA (these cells express on average 100,000 to 10 million receptors, many times the natural receptor levels); (2) we also use purified soluble receptor ectodomains made by expressing truncated receptor cDNAs in mammalian cells; (3) in addition, for making high-titer rabbit polyclonal antibodies, we use synthetic peptides based on predicted immunogenic epitopes in the predicted protein sequence. These are coupled to ovalbumin for immunization; (4) finally, we have had considerable success with vaccinia virus immunization vectors into which we introduce cloned receptor cDNAs. An example of the last method follows.

To generate antibodies to the human type II IL-1 receptor a Lewis rat was immunized intradermally with 10^8 plaque-forming units (pfu) of recombinant human IL-1RII (71) vaccinia virus. Three weeks later, the animal was boosted with 10^6 primary rat dermal fibroblasts infected with the recombinant human IL-1RII vaccinia virus at approximately 5 pfu/cell. One week after boosting, peroxidase dot-blot assays with recombinant soluble human type II IL-1 receptor, and inhibition assays with ^{125}I-labeled IL-1β binding to CV-1/EBNA cells transfected with human type II IL-1 receptor cDNA, showed a significant (>1/100) titer of anti-receptor antibody in the serum. Three days prior to sacrifice and fusion, the animal was boosted with 5 mg of recombinant soluble human type II IL-1 receptor protein. The spleen cells were fused to the X63-Ag8.653 mouse myeloma cell line by standard methods. After hybridoma cultures were established, supernatants were tested by an antigen capture assay with ^{125}I-labeled soluble type I or type II IL-1 receptor protein. Wells that scored positive were subcloned and retested until stable clones were isolated. The supernatants were then tested in several assays, including direct labeled antigen capture, antigen capture followed by labeled IL-1, flow cytometry with natural type I and type II receptor-bearing cells and CV-1 EBNA cells, and inhibition of IL-1 binding to various target cells. For generation of large quantities, antibody was purified from spent bulk culture supernatants from cells grown in roller bottles. Antibody was purified on a protein G affinity matrix with an automated purification system (Bio-Rad MAPS system). Protein concentration was determined by absorbance at 280 nm and purity assessed by SDS–polyacrylamide gel electrophoresis and silver staining. Concentrations were adjusted to approximately 1 mg/ml and the purified antibodies were stored frozen at $-20°C$ in 0.05 M citrate buffer (pH 7.0) until use. Thawed vials were not refrozen.

Concluding Remarks

The methods and general approaches reviewed in this article provide a complete overview of how to begin with a radiolabeled cytokine and proceed to the isolation of cDNA clones for its receptor and hence determine the primary sequence and generate antibodies to it. This general approach has led successfully in the last 4 years to the isolation of cDNAs for more than 20 cytokine receptors, and is now allowing the cloning of additional receptor subunits that may not even bind ligand themselves. In the last year, these approaches have been taken a further step by using essentially the same methods to isolate ligands for receptor-like molecules. This method led to the isolation of the ligand for the B cell surface molecule CD40. In principle the expression cloning methodology can be combined with any assay capable of identifying expression of product in single cells to allow isolation of cDNAs, and hence this technology is likely to continue to play a major role in the elucidation of the molecular mechanisms underlying the functioning of cytokine receptors.

References

1. A. Aruffo and B. Seed, *Proc. Natl. Acad. Sci. U.S.A.* **84,** 8573 (1987).
2. J. E. Sims, C. J. March, D. Cosman, M. B. Widmer, H. R. MacDonald, C. J. McMahan, C. E. Grubin, J. M. Wignall, S. M. Call, D. Friend, A. R. Alpert, S. Gillis, D. L. Urdal, and S. K. Dower, *Science* **241,** 585 (1988).
3. H. Okayama and P. Berg, *Mol. Cell. Biol.* **3,** 280 (1983).
4. A. Miyajima, T. Kitamura, N. Harada, T. Yokata, and K.-I. Arai, *Annu. Rev. Immunol.* **10,** 295 (1992).
5. D. Cosman, S. Lyman, R. Izerda, M. P. Beckmann, L. S. Park, R. Goodwin, and C. March, *Trends Biochem. Sci.* **15,** 265 (1990).

6. T. Takeshita, H. Asao, K. Ohtani, N. Ishii, S. Kumaki, N. Tanaka, H. Munakata, M. Nakamura, and K. Sugamura, *Science* **257**, 379 (1992).

7. M. Hatakeyama, M. Tsudo, S. Minamoto, T. Kono, T. Doi, T. Miyata, M. Miyasaka, and T. Taniguchi, *Science* **244**, 551 (1989).

8. N. Itoh, S. Yonehara, J. Schreurs, D. M. Gorman, K. Maruyama, A. Ishii, I. Yahara, K. Arai, and A. Miyajima, *Science* **247**, 324 (1990).

9. B. Mosley, A. Alpert, D. M. Anderson, J. Jackson, J. M. Wignall, C. Smith, B. Gallis, J. E. Sims, D. L. Urdal, M. B. Widmer, D. Cosman, and L. S. Park, *Cell (Cambridge, Mass.)* **59**, 335 (1989).

10. S. Takaki, A. Tominaga, Y. Hitoshi, S. Mita, E. Sonoda, N. Yamaguchi, and K. Takatsu, *EMBO J.* **9**, 4367 (1990).

11. K. Yamasaki, T. Taga, Y. Hirata, H. Yawata, Y. Kawanishi, B. Seed, T. Taniguchi, T. Hirano, and T. Kishimoto, *Science* **241**, 825 (1988).

12. R. G. Goodwin, D. Friend, S. F. Zeigler, R. Jerzy, B. A. Falk, S. Gimpel, D. Cosman, S. K. Dower, C. J. March, A. E. Namen, and L. S. Park, *Cell (Cambridge, Mass.)* **60**, 941 (1990).

13. D. P. Gearing, J. A. King, N. M. Gough, and N. A. Nicola, *EMBO J.* **8**, 3667 (1989).

14. R. Fukunaga, I. E. Ishizaka, Y. Seto, and S. Nagata, *Cell (Cambridge, Mass.)* **61**, 341 (1990).

15. D. P. Gearing, C. J. Thut, T. VandeBos, S. D. Gimpel, P. B. Delaney, J. King, V. Price, D. Cosman, and M. P. Beckmann, *EMBO J.* **10**, 2839 (1991).

16. D. P. Gearing, M. R. Comeau, D. J. Friend, S. D. Gimpel, C. J. Thut, J. McGourty, K. K. Brasher, J. A. King, S. Gillis, B. Mosley, S. F. Ziegler, and D. Cosman, *Science* **255**, 1434 (1992).

17. A. D. D'Andrea, H. F. Lodish, and G. G. Wong, *Cell (Cambridge, Mass.)* **57**, 277 (1989).

18. A. M. DeVos, M. Ultsch, and A. A. Kossiakoff, *Science* **255**, 306 (1992).

19. I. Vigon, J.-P. Mornon, L. Cocault, M.-T. Mitajavila, P. Tambourin, S. Gisselbrecht, and M. Souyri, *Proc. Natl. Acad. Sci. U.S.A.* **89**, 5640 (1992).

20. M. Hibi, M. Murakami, M. Saito, T. Hirano, T. Taga, and T. Kishimoto, *Cell (Cambridge, Mass.)* **63**, 1149 (1990).

21. D. P. Gearing and D. Cosman, *Cell (Cambridge, Mass.)* **66**, 9 (1991).

22. H. Loetscher, Y. C. Pan, H. W. Lahm, R. Gentz, M. Brockhaus, H. Tabuchi, and W. Lesslauer, *Cell (Cambridge, Mass.)* **61**, 351 (1990).

23. T. J. Schall, M. Lewis, K. J. Koller, A. Lee, G. C. Rice, G. H. Wong, T. Gatanaga, G. A. Granger, R. Lentz, H. Raab, W. J. Kohr, and D. V. Goeddel, *Cell (Cambridge, Mass.)* **61**, 361 (1990).

24. C. A. Smith, T. Davis, D. Anderson, L. Solam, M. P. Beckmann, R. Jerzy, S. K. Dower, D. Cosman, and R. G. Goodwin, *Science* **248**, 1019 (1990).

25. M. J. Radeke, T. P. Misko, C. Hsu, L. A. Herzenberg, and E. M. Shooter, *Nature (London)* **325**, 593 (1987).

26. I. Stamenković, E. A. Clark, and B. Seed, *EMBO J.* **8**, 1403 (1989).

27. D. Camerini, G. Walz, W. A. Loenen, J. Borst, and B. Seed, *J. Immunol.* **147**, 3165 (1991).

28. H. Durkop, U. Latza, M. Hummel, F. Eitelbach, B. Seed, and H. Stein, *Cell* (*Cambridge, Mass.*) **68,** 421 (1992).
29. S. Mallett, S. Fossum, and A. N. Barclay, *EMBO J.* **9,** 1063 (1990).
30. A. M. Wang, A. A. Creasey, M. B. Ladner, L. S. Lin, J. Strickler, A. J. Van, R. Yamamoto, and D. F. Mark, *Science* **228,** 149 (1985).
31. R. J. Armitage, W. C. Fanslow, L. Strockbine, T. Sato, K. N. Clifford, B. M. MacDuff, D. M. Anderson, S. D. Gimpel, T. Davis-Smith, C. R. Maliszewski, E. A. Clark, C. A. Smith, K. H. Grabstein, D. Cosman, and M. K. Spriggs, *Nature* (*London*) **357,** 80 (1992).
32. C. J. McMahan, J. L. Slack, B. Mosley, D. Cosman, S. D. Lupton, L. L. Brunton, C. E. Grubin, J. M. Wignall, N. A. Jenkins, C. I. Brannan, N. Copeland, K. Huebner, C. M. Croce, L. Cannizzaro, D. Benjamin, S. K. Dower, M. K. Spriggs, and J. E. Sims, *EMBO J.* **10,** 2821 (1991).
33. C. J. Sherr, C. W. Rettenmier, R. Sacca, M. F. Roussel, A. T. Look, and E. R. Stanley, *Cell* (*Cambridge, Mass.*) **41,** 665 (1985).
34. D. E. Williams, J. Eisenman, A. Baird, C. Rauch, N. K. Van, C. J. March, L. S. Park, U. Martin, D. Y. Mochizuki, H. S. Boswell, G. S. Burgess, D. Cosman, and S. D. Lyman, *Cell* (*Cambridge, Mass.*) **63,** 167 (1990).
35. K. Keegan, D. E. Johnson, L. T. Williams, and M. J. Hayman, *Proc. Natl. Acad. Sci. U.S.A.* **88,** 1095 (1991).
36. W. M. Roberts, A. T. Look, M. F. Roussel, and C. J. Sherr, *Cell* (*Cambridge, Mass.*) **55,** 655 (1988).
37. P. M. Murphy and H. L. Tiffany, *Science* **253,** 1280 (1991).
38. T. Kitamura, K. Hayashida, K. Sakamaki, T. Yokota, K. Arai, and A. Miyajima, *Proc. Natl. Acad. Sci. U.S.A.* **88,** 5082 (1991).
39. S. Takaki, S. Mita, T. Kitamura, S. Yonehara, N. Yamaguchi, A. Tominaga, A. Miyajima, and K. Takatsu, *EMBO J.* **10,** 2833 (1991).
40. F. Lamballe, R. Klein, and M. Barbacid, *Cell* (*Cambridge, Mass.*) **66,** 967 (1991).
41. A. O. Morla, J. Schreurs, A. Miyajima, and J. T. Wang, *Mol. Cell. Biol.* **8,** 2214 (1988).
42. M. Hatakeyama, T. Kono, N. Kobayashi, A. Kawahara, S. D. Levin, R. M. Perlmutter, and T. Taniguchi, *Science* **252,** 1523 (1991).
43. C.-H. Heldin, A. Ernlund, C. Rorsman, and L. Ronnstrand, *J. Biol. Chem.* **264,** 8905 (1989).
44. J. Tavernier, R. Devos, S. Cornelis, T. Tuypens, J. Van der Heyden, W. Fiers, and G. Plaetinck, *Cell* (*Cambridge, Mass.*) **66,** 1175 (1991).
45. J. G. Giri, R. C. Newton, and R. Horuk, *J. Biol. Chem.* **265,** 17416 (1990).
46. D. Novick, H. Engelman, D. Wallach, and M. Rubinstein, *J. Exp. Med.* **170,** 1409 (1989).
47. H. Engelmann, D. Novick, and D. Wallach, *J. Biol. Chem.* **265,** 15311536 (1990).
48. W. C. Fanslow, J. E. Sims, H. Sassenfeld, P. J. Morrissey, S. Gillis, S. Dower, and M. B. Widmer, *Science* **248,** 739 (1990).
49. M. Hibi, M. Murakami, M. Saito, T. Hirano, T. Taga, and T. Kishimoto, *Cell* (*Cambridge, Mass.*) **63,** 1149 (1990).

50. S. K. Dower, S. Kronheim, C. J. March, T. Hopp, P. J. Conlon, S. Gillis, and D. L. Urdal, *J. Exp. Med.* **162,** 501 (1985).
51. R. J. Robb, A. Munck, and K. A. Smith, *J. Exp. Med.* **154,** 1455 (1981).
52. D. M. Segal and E. Hurwitz, *J. Immunol.* **118,** 1338 (1977).
53. E. E. Qwarnstrom, R. C. Page, S. Gillis, and S. K. Dower, *J. Biol. Chem.* **263,** 8261 (1988).
54. P. J. Munson and D. Rodbard, *Anal. Biochem.* **107,** 220 (1980).
55. G. E. Rovati, D. Rodbard, and P. J. Munson, *Anal. Biochem.* **174,** 636 (1988).
56. G. E. Rovati, D. Rodbard, and P. J. Munson, *Anal. Biochem.* **184,** 172 (1990).
57. A. K. Thakur, P. J. Munson, D. L. Hunston, and D. Rodbard, *Anal. Biochem.* **103,** 240 (1980).
58. T. Nikaido, A. Shimizu, N. Ishida, H. Sabe, K. Teshigawara, M. Maeda, T. Uchiyama, J. Yodoi, and T. Honjo, *Nature (London)* **311,** 631 (1984).
59. W. J. Leonard, J. M. Depper, G. R. Crabtree, S. Rudikoff, J. Pumphrey, R. J. Robb, M. Kronke, P. B. Svetlik, N. J. Peffer, T. A. Waldmann, *et al., Nature (London)* **311,** 626 (1984).
60. D. Cosman, D. P. Cerretti, A. Larsen, L. Park, C. March, S. Dower, S. Gillis, and D. Urdal, *Nature (London)* **312,** 768 (1984).
61. B. Mosley, M. P. Beckmann, C. J. March, R. L. Idzerda, S. D. Gimpel, T. VandenBos, D. Friend, A. Alpert, D. Anderson, J. Jackson, J. M. Wignall, C. Smith, B. Gallis, J. E. Sims, D. L. Urdal, M. B. Widmer, D. Cosman, and L. S. Park, *Cell (Cambridge, Mass.)* **59,** 335 (1989).
62. M. Aguet, Z. Dembič, and G. Merlin, *Cell (Cambridge, Mass.)* **55,** 273 (1988).
63. B. Seed and A. Aruffo, *Proc. Natl. Acad. Sci. U.S.A.* **84,** 3365 (1987).
64. A. Aruffo and B. Seed, *EMBO J.* **6,** 3313 (1987).
65. S. Stengelin, I. Stamenkovič, and B. Seed, *EMBO J.* **7,** 1053 (1988).
66. A. Aruffo, I. Stamenkovič, M. Melnick, C. B. Underhill, and B. Seed, *Cell (Cambridge, Mass.)* **61,** 1303 (1990).
67. B. J. Classon, A. F. Williams, A. C. Willis, B. Seed, and I. Stamenkovič, *J. Exp. Med.* **172,** 1007 (1990).
68. I. Stamenkovič and B. Seed, *Nature (London)* **345,** 74 (1990).
69. D. L. Simmons, A. B. Satterthwaite, D. G. Tenen, and B. Seed, *J. Immunol.* **148,** 267 (1992).
70. T. Kitamura, N. Sato, K. Arai, and A. Miyajima, *Cell (Cambridge, Mass.)* **66,** 1165 (1991).
71. C. J. McMahan, J. L. Slack, B. Mosley, D. Cosman, S. D. Lupton, L. L. Brunton, C. E. Grubin, K. Huebner, C. M. Croce, L. A. Cannizzano, D. Benjamin, S. K. Dower, M. K. Spriggs, and J. E. Sims, *EMBO J.* **10,** 2821 (1991).

[2] Genetic Regulation and Activities of an Interleukin 1 Receptor Antagonist Protein

Donald B. Carter, Ann E. Berger, and Daniel E. Tracey

Introduction

The cytokine interleukin 1 (IL-1) plays an important role in the response to infection and injury. Gram-negative bacterial endotoxin is a potent inducer of IL-1 production (1). Interleukin 1, in turn, can affect the central nervous system [resulting in fever and adrenocorticotropic hormone (ACTH) production (2)], the liver [resulting in the acute-phase response (3)], the hematopoietic system [resulting in neutrophilia (4)], and the vasculature [resulting in leukocyte adherence (5) and release of prostaglandins (6)]. In addition, IL-1 can have positive effects on events in the immune response, including T, B, and natural killer (NK) cell activation (7). Many cell types, therefore, are targets for the action of IL-1 and, indeed, IL-1 receptors are found on almost all cell types examined (8).

What is known about the actions of IL-1 imply that the regulatory mechanisms controlling the pleiomorphic effects of IL-1 must be complex. Although physiological IL-1 regulation is not well understood, the studies to date describing IL-1 regulatory mechanisms bear out the prediction of complexity. For example, *in vivo* studies have demonstrated that ACTH, acting through the adrenal–pituitary axis, induces the production of glucocorticoids. Glucocorticoids inhibit both the synthesis of IL-1 and its action on glucocorticoid-sensitive IL-1-responsive cells (9, 10).

The production of IL-1 is also regulated at several levels. Transcription of IL-1α and IL-1β mRNA are not coordinately regulated (11, 12), posttranscriptional modifications occur (13), transcription of IL-1 mRNA and its translation to protein can be uncoupled (14, 15), and posttranslational proteolytic cleavage of pro-IL-1β appears to determine the release of IL-1β from cells (16). Cleavage lacking the necessary protease(s), such as keratinocytes, can retain IL-1β intracellularly (17). The activation of kinases, which rapidly follows IL-1 binding to its receptor (18, 19), implies that IL-1 effects are initiated extracellularly, but the finding that IL-1 is retained intracellularly, that extracellular IL-1 can be internalized and retained in the nucleus (20, 21), and that anti-sense to IL-1 mRNA affects fibroblast survival (22) suggests that IL-1 may also be an intracellular ligand.

Another mechanism of IL-1 regulation has been described in the form of

Methods in Neurosciences, Volume 16
Copyright © 1993 by Academic Press, Inc. All rights of reproduction in any form reserved.

a third member of the IL-1 family, IRAP or IL-1ra (23–26). This protein has no agonist activity, but acts as a receptor-level antagonist of IL-1. IRAP was originally isolated from monocytes and monocytic cell lines (22, 23, 27), and an intracellular variant IRAP molecule has also been cloned from keratinocytes (28). Thus it appears that at least some of the cell types that produce IL-1 are also capable of producing a receptor-level antagonist.

This apparently paradoxical situation could result from differential regulation of IL-1 and IRAP, depending on the state of differentiation of the cell, on time, or on stimulus. Differences in Il-1α and IRAP production from monocytes cultured for various periods of time have been reported (29, 30), as have differences between cells stimulated with adherent IgG or lipopolysaccharide (LPS) (31). Positive effects of granulocyte–macrophage colony-stimulating factor (GM-CSF) and TGFα on IRAP production have also been noted (29, 30, 32), making it clear that cytokines or other stimuli, as well as the differentiative state, contribute to the net production of IL-1 and IRAP.

Both U937 and THP-1 monocytic cell lines require differentiation with phorbol ester before IRAP can be detected in their supernatants, but U937 cells require subsequent stimulation with GM-CSF (24, 26). These results suggest that monocytic cell lines share IRAP regulatory mechanisms with their untransformed counterparts. The possible interaction of IRAP in central nervous system (CNS) tissues is dependent on the presence of IL-1 receptors. A number of radioligand-binding studies have used ^{125}I-labeled forms of IL-1 to localize receptors that might mediate the above-mentioned effects of the cytokine IL-1 and its antagonist in the rodent CNS (33–36). In addition, *in situ* histochemical localization of type I IL-1 receptor mRNA in the murine CNS and pituitary has been described (37). It has also been shown that radiolabeled IRAP in CNS tissues could be important for suppressing the effects of IL-1 in the brain and spinal cord. Methods for detection of IRAP mRNA synthesis in primary or transformed cultured cells and the protein from tissue fluids as well as culture media are described.

Cell Culture for Production of Native IRAP

Culture of U937 Cells

U937 cells were obtained from the American Type Culture Collection (ATCC; Rockville, MD) and were maintained in RPMI 1640 (Irvine Scientific, Santa Ana, CA) containing 10% fetal bovine serum (FBS; Irvine Scientific), 2 mM L-glutamine (Irvine Scientific), and 1% Fungi-Bact (Irvine Scientific) (hereafter, medium). U937 cells were differentiated by culture at a starting cell concentration of 1×10^6 cells/ml in medium containing 100 nM phorbol

12-myristate 13-acetate (PMA) for 48 hr. The cells were then adherent and somewhat flattened. For stimulation with cytokines, the adherent U937 cells were washed twice with phoshate-buffered saline (PBS) and recultured in medium containing 1% low-endotoxin FBS (HyClone, Logan, UT) with cytokines. All media contained <5 pg/ml endotoxin a measured by the *Limulus* amebocyte lysate assay (Whittaker Bioproducts, Walkersville, MD). Undifferentiated U937 cells produced no detectable IRAP protein.

Optimal induction of IRAP synthesis from U937 cells was obtained with either GM-CSF (80 U/ml) (Amgen, Thousand Oaks, CA) or IL-4 (100 U/ml) (Genzyme, Boston, MA), with peak mRNA levels produced at 12 hr after addition to cells. Addition of the two cytokines together resulted in increases that were approximately the sum of the individual responses.

Determination of IRAP mRNA

Determination of IRAP mRNA per unit of total RNA in tissue or cultured cells can be carried out after RNA extraction by using the RNAzol (Cinna/Biotecx Labs International, Inc., Friendswood, TX) method, which is a modification of the Chomczynski and Sacchi single-step procedure (38). One 10-cm dish of tissue culture cells at confluence (2–4 $\times$ 10^6 cells) yields between 50 and 100 μg of total RNA, and the extraction and preparation of RNA by the Cinna/Biotecx method can be carried out in a single 1.5-ml Eppendorf tube. The RNA is quantitated by absorbance at 260 nm and denatured with glyoxal and dimethyl sulfoxide, and applied to 1.2% agarose gels (39). Usually 10- to 15-μg aliquots of RNA are denatured and applied in each well of agarose gel poured into the tray of an 11.14 Horizon (Bethesda Research Laboratories, Gaithersburg, MD) horizontal gel electrophoresis tray. The gel-fractionated RNA was electrophoretically transferred to nylon membranes (Nytran; Schleicher & Schuell, Keene, NH). Membranes were hybridized and washed by the conditions and wash buffers of Church and Gilbert (40).

The IRAP probe can be generated from a 1.8-kb *Eco*RI insert fragment from a plasmid containing the human IRAP cDNA (24), and the probe for the metabolic enzyme triosephosphate isomerase (TPI) is a 1.6-kb *Pst*I insert fragment from a plasmid containing the TPI cDNA (41).

The insert fragments were labeled with [α-^{32}P]dATP (300 Ci/mmol; Amersham, Arlington Heights, IL), using the Prime-It random priming kit (Stratagene, La Jolla, CA), to a specific activity of 5 $\times$ 10^8–10^9 dpm/μg. Because the level of TPI mRNA remains unchanged during cell proliferation, the TPI signal detected can be used as an internal reference standard for each sample of RNA analyzed. Quantitation of IRAP and TPI hybridization signals is done with a Betascope 603 blot analyzer (Betagen Corp., Waltham, MA). For normalization, all blots are first hybridized with probe to TPI and scanned and then, without further treatment, the blots are hybridized with the IRAP probe and scanned for signal at the IRAP mRNA position. The ratio of the counts per minute detected in the IRAP band to the TPI band is calculated and used to compare with other samples on the same or other blots. An example of a blot hybridized with TPI and IRAP as described below is shown in Fig. 1.

Detection of IRAP Protein

Necessary for the detection of IRAP protein is a specific high-affinity antibody. The methodology of preparation of a panel of monoclonal antibodies that have been effective in enzyme-linked immunosorbent assays (ELISAs), Western blots, and immunoprecipitation of IRAP protein will be discussed below.

Generation of Hybridomas

Female CAF_1 mice (Jackson Laboratories, Bar Harbor, ME) were immunized subcutaneously five times over a 6-month period with 5–10 μg of IRAP. The first injection was in Freund's complete adjuvant (CFA; GIBCO, Grand Island, NY); all others were in Freund's incomplete adjuvant (GIBCO). IRAP purified from U937 cells was used for the first two immunizations, and recombinant IRAP was used for subsequent immunizations (24). The last immunization was 3 days before fusion. Splenic lymphocytes from one mouse were fused with SP2/0 myeloma cells and the cells cultured in Dulbecco's

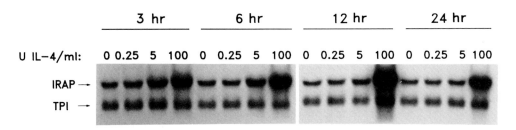

FIG. 1   Interleukin 4 increased IRAP mRNA levels in a time- and dose-dependent manner. PMA-differentiated U937 cells were cultured in the presence or absence of the indicated concentrations of IL-4 for the times indicated. RNA was prepared and Northern blots run as described.

modified Eagle's medium with glucose (4500 mg/liter) ((Irvine Scientific) containing 20% controlled process serum replacement (CPSR3; Sigma Chemical Co., St. Louis, MO), 4 mM L-glutamine, penicillin (100 U/ml), streptomycin (100 μg/ml), and Fungizone (0.25 μg/ml) (Irvine Scientific) and HAT (hypoxanthine–aminopterin–thymidine) medium supplement (Sigma). Cells were fed twice weekly until tested (see below). Positive hybridomas were cloned twice by limiting dilution. Ascites fluids were generated by growth of the hybridoma cells (5 × 10^6) as ascitic tumors in CAF$_1$ mice that had been injected intraperitoneally with 0.5 ml of 2,6,10,14-tetramethyl pentadecane (Pristane; Sigma) 7 days earlier.

ELISA for Identifying Anti-IRAP Antibodies

Wells of half-area 96-well plates (Costar 3690; Cambridge, MA) were coated with 100 ng of IRAP in 50 μl of 0.015 M sodium carbonate, pH 9.6, overnight at 4°C. The plates were then washed three times with 100 μl of Dulbecco's PBS (GIBCO) containing 0.05% Tween-20 (Sigma) (PBS-T) and blocked for 1 hr at room temperature with PBS-T (100 μl/well) containing 1% gelatin (Sigma). The blocked plates were washed three times with PBS-T and 50 μl of antibody/well (either as serum or tissue culture supernatant) was added for 1 hr at room temperature. The plates were then washed three times with PBS-T, and 50 μl/well of a 1/1000 dilution of goat anti-mouse IgG conjugated to horseradish peroxidase (Kirkegaard & Perry, Gaithersburg, MD) was added for 1 hr at room temperature. The plates were washed three times with PBS-T and 50 μl of 2,2'-azino-d-[3-ethylbenzthiazoline sulfonate 6] per well (ABTS; Kirkegaard & Perry) was added, and the OD$_{405}$ read.

Western Blots

Nitrocellulose strips (Schleicher & Schuell) onto which approximately 30 ng of rIRAP had been transferred were blocked with PBS-T for 15 min at room temperature, and then incubated for 1 hr at room temperature with 10 ml of tissue culture supernatants containing antibodies. After three washes with 15 ml of PBS-T, a 1/1000 dilution of biotinylated goat anti-mouse IgG (Bethesda Research Laboratories) was added for 1 hr at room temperature. After washing with PBS-T, the strips were incubated with 10 ml of a 1/750 dilution of avidin conjugated to alkaline phosphatase in PBS-T (Vector Laboratories, Burlingame, CA). The substrate BCIP/NBT (Bethesda Research Laboratories) was prepared by the addition of 44 μl of nitroblue tetrazolium (NBT) solution to 10 ml of 0.2 M Tris-HCl–0.1 M NaCl–50 mM MgCl$_2$ followed, after mixing, by the addition of 33 μl of 5-bromo-4-chloro-3-indolylphosphate toluidinium (BCIP). Visualization of the antigen–antibody complexes was completed in approximately 10 min at room temperature.

Immunoprecipitation

[^{35}S]IRAP (50,000 cpm) in 10 mM Tris, 150 mM NaCl, 5% gammaglobulin-free FBS, pH 7.4, was added to 100 μl of tissue culture supernatant and incubated overnight at 4°C. Protein A–Sepharose (Pharmacia, Piscataway, NJ) was washed three times with Tris–NaCl–FBS. A one-tenth volume of rabbit anti-mouse IgG (Cappel Laboratories) was added to a 10% slurry (v/v) in Tris–NaCl–FBS for 30 min at 4°C. The rabbit anti-mouse-coated Protein A–Sepharose was pelleted by centrifugation, resuspended to 50% (v/v) in Tris–NaCl–FBS, and 100 μl was added to the IRAP–antibody mixture. After 1 hr at 4°C, the Sepharose beads were washed three times with 1 ml of 100 mM Tris-HCl, 1% deoxycholine, 1% Nonidet P-40 (NP-40), pH 8.0, and once with distilled water. Sodium dodecyl sulfate-polyacrylamide gel electrophoresis (SDS-PAGE) sample buffer (50 μl) was added to the pellet, and the mixture boiled for 5 min. Supernatants were applied to a 12% SDS-PAGE gel. After electrophoresis and drying, the gel was exposed to film (SAR-Omat; Kodak, Rochester, NY) for 40 hr at −70°C.

Figure 2 shows a Western blot of immunoprecipitated IRAP protein from media of PMA-induced U937 cells treated with various cytokines. The medium was immunoprecipitated at 24 and 48 hr postcytokine treatment in each case. Detection of protein was done with monoclonal I5 anti-IRAP antibody.

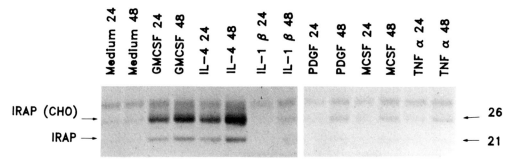

FIG. 2   Western blot of IRAP from U937 cells. Supernatants from PMA-stimulated U937 cells cultured with cytokines for 24 or 58 hr were concentrated, immunoprecipitated, electrophoresed, and transferred as described. The Western blot was probed with anti-IRAP antibody I5.

The *n*-glycanase-treated IRAP protein migrates aberrantly at 21 kDa and the non-glycanase-treated IRAP migrates at 26 kDa, implying that both forms of IRAP are secreted by GM-CSF- or IL-4-stimulated adherent U937 cells.

Induction of IRAP in Human Monocytes

To evaluate whether the above observations with U937 cells also pertained to the regulation of IRAP in normal human monocytes, we performed similar studies with mononuclear cells and monocytes isolated from normal human peripheral blood. However, instead of measuring the induction of IRAP mRNA and protein by Northern blotting, Western blotting, and immunoprecipitation, we measured the biological activity of IRAP released into the supernatants of cultured human mononuclear cells. The activity measured was the inhibition of IL-1 activity in murine T cells. We tested a variety of stimuli for their ability to induce IL-1 antagonist activity. A precedent for the induction of IRAP in human mononuclear cell cultures is the work of Arend *et al.* (42), using immobilized IgG or immobilized immune complexes as inducing agents.

Human Mononuclear Cell Cultures

Depending on the number of cells desired, two alternative procedures were used to prepare human peripheral blood mononuclear cells (HPBMCs). The low-yield method utilized 400- to 500-ml "units" of whole blood from healthy donors and yielded an average of 3.9×10^8 HPBMCs ($n = 16$). The high-yield method utilized leukocytes collected from healthy donors by leukapheresis and yielded an average of 4.1×10^9 HPBMCs ($n = 30$) from 5 to 7 liters of processed blood. In both cases, the HPBMCs must be prepared within 12 hr of blood or leukocyte collection in order to generate good yields of IRAP.

   The whole-blood method of HPBMC preparation was carried out as follows. A 400- to 500-ml unit of blood was drawn from healthy donors and 3.8% sodium citrate was added as an anticoagulant. The red blood cells were separated from the leukocytes by first centrifuging 50-ml aliquots of whole blood for 20 min at 300f *g* at room temperature in 50-ml polyethylene tubes. The platelet-rich plasma was removed from each tube and saved for later use. Five milliliters of a 6% solution of dextran in saline was added to the remaining cell pellets. Saline was added to fill the tubes, their contents were gently mixed, and the tubes were allowed to stand at room temperature for 1 hr to allow the red blood cells to settle. The supernatants were removed and the tubes were centrifuged at 275 g for 15 min at room temperature. The cell pellets in each tube were resuspended in 10 ml of a fourfold dilution in saline of platelet-free plasma, prepared from the saved plasma by centrifugation at 2500 g for 15 min at 10°C. The 10-ml leukocyte suspensions were layered onto 5 ml of LSM (lymphocyte separation medium; Organon Teknika, Durham, NC) in clear 10 × 75 mm tubes and centrifuged at 400 g for 20 min at room temperature. The mononuclear cells were aspirated from the density gradient interfaces and pooled. The pooled HPBMCs were washed three times by centrifugation and resuspension with 45 ml of Hanks' balanced salt solution (HBSS; GIBCO-Bethesda Research Laboratories, Grand Island, NY) and then resuspended in 20 ml of serum-free RPMI 1640 medium (GIBCO) at 4°C. The cells were counted in a hemacytometer by trypan blue dye exclusion and adjusted to 8 × 10^6 cells/ml in serum-free RPMI 1640 medium.

The leukapheresis method of HPBMC preparation was carried out as follows. Mononuclear leukapheresis was performed on healthy donors, using a Fenwal CS3000 blood cell separator according to the standard operating procedures provided by the manufacturer (Fenwal, Inc., Ashland, MA). For most procedures, between 5 and 7 liters of whole blood was processed for each donor. Anticoagulation used during the pheresis procedure was achieved with sodium citrate. Platelets were partially removed by a special spin cycle in the pheresis machine as a final step at the end of the pheresis procedure. Mononuclear cells from each donor, in an approximately 125-ml final volume, were divided into four equal portions in 50-ml polypropylene centrifuge tubes. The cells in each tube were diluted to 50 ml with cold Dulbecco's phosphate-buffered saline without calcium or magnesium (DPBS; GIBCO). The cell suspensions were centrifuged at 200 g for 10 min at 4°C and the platelet-rich supernatant was aspirated and discarded. The cell pellets were resuspended in 25 ml of DPBS and washed once by centrifugation as above. The final cell pellets were resuspended in 25 ml of DPBS at room temperature. These suspensions were layered over 10 ml of LSM in 50-ml polypropylene tubes and were centrifuged at 400 g for 25 min at room temperature. The mononuclear cell layers at the gradient interface were aspirated and pooled in two 50-ml polypropylene tubes. The cells were diluted to 50 ml with DPBS at room temperature and centrifuged at 200 g for 10 min at room temperature. The cell pellets were resuspended with 8 ml of Tris-buffered red cell lysing buffer (2.05 g of Tris-HCl/liter, 7.47 g of NH_4Cl/liter, adjusted to pH 7.2) and incubated at 37°C for 10 min to lyse the remaining red blood cells. The treated cells were centrifuged and washed twice with 50 ml of DPBS at 4°C by centrifugation at 200 g, followed by resuspension. The pooled HPBMC pellets were resuspended at 8 × 10^6 cells/ml in serum-free RPMI-1640 medium at 4°C.

For mononuclear cell cultures, HPBMCs prepared by either of the above methods were placed in tissue culture flasks [e.g., Corning (Corning, NY) T-150] or wells of tissue culture plates (e.g., Costar 6-, 24-, or 96-well plates) at a density of 2×10^6 cells/cm^2 for 1 hr at 37°C in a 5% CO_2 atmosphere to promote cell adherence. An equal volume of $2\times$ culture medium was then added, with or without various stimulatory agents, and the cultures were maintained at 37°C in a 5% CO_2 atmosphere for 1–7 days. Culture medium ($2\times$) was RPMI-1640 medium supplemented with 2% fetal bovine serum (Hyclone), 40 mM N-2-hydroxyethylpiperazine-N'-2-ethanesulfonic acid (HEPES) buffer (GIBCO), and gentamicin (100 μg/ml) (GIBCO). For monocyte cultures, the nonadherent cells were removed from the culture vessels and discarded after the 1-hr adherence step by aspiration and three successive rinses with HBSS at room temperature. Culture medium ($1\times$) was then added, with or without various stimulatory agents, to the adherent cells (mostly monocytes) at the same volume as the initial cell inoculum in the culture vessel and the cultures were incubated for 1–7 days at 37°C in a 5% CO_2 atmosphere. Supernatants were removed from the cultures and were centrifuged at 400 g for 10 min to remove cells and debris. The cell-free supernatants were then sterile filtered through low protein-binding 0.22-μm pore size cellulose acetate filters (e.g., Cat. No. 25942; Corning) and frozen at -70°C until further use.

Bioassays for IL-1 Antagonist Activity

The detection and quantification of IRAP in the cell culture supernatants was accomplished in several different ways. Because IRAP competes for IL-1 binding to IL-1 receptors, a radioligand receptor-binding assay (24) could be used. Various dilutions of culture supernatants were mixed with a constant amount of ^{125}I-labeled recombinant human IL-1α (rhIL-1α) (Du Pont-New England Nuclear, Boston, MA) and added to IL-1 receptor-bearing cells, such as human YT cells, and incubated for 1–2 hr at room temperature. Competition for radioligand binding to the cells was measured as a reduction in cell-bound radiolabel. This assay is reasonably sensitive for IRAP [the 50% inhibitory concentration (IC_{50}) for rhIRAP was 2–8 ng/ml], but cannot distinguish IRAP from IL-1, which often is present in the mononuclear cell supernatants. Two bioassays were also used to detect IRAP as IL-1 antagonist activity in the culture supernatants: the murine thymocyte costimulator assay (43) and the murine LBRM-33-1A5/HT-2 ("1A5") assay (44, 45). Although the 1A5 assay is about 30-fold more sensitive to IL-1 than the thymocyte assay, these 2 assays are equally sensitive to inhibition by IRAP (IC_{50} for rhIRAP was 0.3–0.6 ng/ml). Briefly, the thymocyte assay for IRAP employed C3H/HeJ mouse thymocytes cultured for 72 hr at 37°C in the presence of a half-maximal amount of rhIL-1β (1 U/ml, 50 fg/ml; Upjohn, Kalamazoo, MI) and phytohemagglutinin (PHA, lot HA-17; Burroughs-Well-come, Research Triangle Park, NC) (2 μg/ml) with or without various dilutions of mononuclear cell culture supernatants. Interleukin activity was measured as incorporation of [^{3}H]thymidine into thymocyte DNA following addition of the radiolabel for the final 4 hr of the culture period.

The primary bioassay used for the detection of IRAP in culture supernatants was the 1A5 assay. This assay measures IL-2 production by the murine 1A5 thymoma cell line stimulated with IL-1 and PHA. A half-maximal amount of rhIL-1β (0.04 U/ml, 2 fg/ml) was added to a mixture of 1 × 10^5 LBRM-33-1A5 cells (ATCC) PHA (2 μg/ml), and aliquots of culture supernatants in quadruplicate in wells of V-bottomed microtiter plates (NUNC-96V; GIBCO). Each component in the assay was prepared in RPMI-1640 medium supplemented with 5% fetal bovine serum, gentamicin (50 μg/ml), and 20 mM HEPES buffer. The plates were incubated at 37°C for 16 hr in a 5% CO_2 atmosphere, centrifuged at 300 g for 6 min, and 100 μl of the cell supernatants were transferred to the wells of flat-bottomed microtiter plates (NUNC-96F) with an Octapette (Costar, Cambridge, MA). To these wells were added 50 μl of HT-2 cells (ATCC) at 2 × 10^5 cells/ml diluted in RPMI-1640 medium supplemented with 2% fetal bovine serum, gentamicin (50 μg/ml), 20 mM HEPES buffer, and 5 × 10^{-5} M 2-mercaptoethanol. The HT-2 cells were previously grown and maintained in the presence of 10% Rat T-Stim (ConA-stimulated rat spleen cell supernatant; Collaborative Research, Waltham, MA) and were washed free of IL-2 prior to use in the assay. The HT-2 cell cultures were incubated for 20 hr at 37°C in a 5% CO_2 atmosphere and 50 μl of [^{3}H]thymidine (2 Ci/mmol; Amersham) at 10 μCi/ml was added for an additional 4 hr. The contents of each well were transferred to glass fiber filters with a Skatron cell harvester (Skatron, Sterling, VA). The radiolabel on each filter disk was measured in a liquid scintillation counter. The proliferation of HT-2 cells is IL-2 dependent and the degree of incorporation of [^{3}H]thymidine into HT-2 cells is proportional to the IL-2 concentration in the medium, which in turn is proportional to the effective IL-1 concentration in the 1A5 cell cultures. A standard curve of IL-1 activity was plotted as a weighted linear regression analysis of the log IL-1 concentration vs a logit transformation of the percentage of maximum [^{3}H]thymidine incorporation.

IRAP Production by Human Mononuclear Cells

The ability of human mononuclear cells or the adherent monocytic cells from HPBMCs to produce IRAP with or without stimulation by various cytokines or other agents was assessed. Cells prepared as described above were cultured for 1–10 days in culture medium (1×) without deliberate stimulation and supernatants were assayed for IL-1 antagonist activity in the 1A5 assay. As shown in Fig. 3, no significant IL-1 antagonist activity (i.e., IRAP) was detected during the first 5 days of culture, but activity was detected from days 6 through 10. Because other studies in our laboratories showed that the IRAP-producing cells in human mononuclear cell cultures were monocytes, we investigated whether cytokines known to act on the monocyte/macrophage lineage could enhance IRAP production. Addition of rhGM-CSF (100 U/ml) to the cultures on day 0 resulted in the rapid appearance of IRAP in the supernatants as early as day 1 (Fig. 3). The level of IL-1 antagonist activity induced by rhGM-CSF reached a plateau by day 4 that was greater than the level in unstimulated cultures. Absorption of the supernatants from unstimulated or rhGM-CSF-stimulated cells from most donors with anti-IL-1α and anti-IL-1β antibodies on Sepharose beads did not appreciably increase IL-1 antagonist activity, suggesting that the supernatants

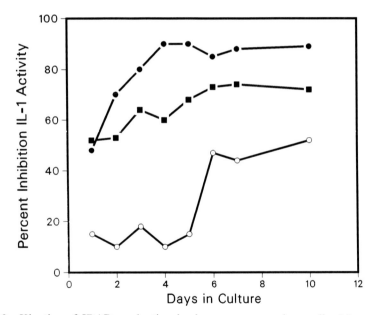

FIG. 3   Kinetics of IRAP production by human mononuclear cells. Mononuclear cells from a single donor were cultured for 10 days in the presence of plain culture medium (○), in culture medium containing rhGM-CSF (100 U/ml) (●), or in rhIL-3 (100 U/ml) (■). Cell-free supernatants were harvested at the various times shown and the supernatants were assayed at a 1 : 20 dilution for IL-1 inhibitory activity in the 1A5 assay.

contained little or no IL-1. Another monocyte stimulant, rhIL-3, at 100 U/ml also rapidly induced IRAP production to comparable levels as seen with rhGM-CSF stimulation (Fig. 3).

The studies with rhGM-CSF and rhIL-3 were extended to evaluate the IRAP-inducing potential of these and other cytokines and immobilized immunoglobulin, using cells from a number of different donors. The two additional cytokines tested were recombinant human tumor necrosis factor α (rhTNF-α) and rhIL-4, both at 100 U/ml. The immobilized immunoglobulin stimulation of cells was achieved by first pretreating the culture vessels with 5 μg of purified human IgG/ml (Sigma) in DPBS for 1 hr at 37°C, followed by three washes with DPBS. Cells were then added to the IgG-coated vessels in culture medium. Cells from 3 to 11 donors per stimulus were incubated with the various stimuli for 7 days and the supernatants were assayed for IL-1 antagonist activity. The results with unstimulated cultures, shown in Fig. 4, clearly show a wide variation in the levels of IL-1 inhibitory activity among the donors tested. In fact, about half the cultures contained, on balance, IL-1-like activity (although a −50% inhibition of IL-1 activity corresponds to only 25 fg of IL-1/ml). Cultures stimulated with rhGM-CSF, rhIL-3, rhIL-4, and IgG also produced variable levels of IL-1 antagonist activity, but the mean levels were significantly higher than those for unstimulated cultures (Fig. 4). In contrast, no difference from control IL-1 antagonist activity was seen with supernatants from rhTNF-α-stimulated cultures (Fig. 4).

In a large number of experiments with human mononuclear cells and human monocytes comparing IRAP levels induced by IgG or rhGM-CSF, IgG was clearly more efficacious than rhGM-CSF, rhIL-3, or rhIL-4. With regard to the levels of IRAP from cultures of different cell populations, we detected slightly higher IRAP levels from mononuclear cell cultures than from adherent monocyte cultures. Furthermore, the combination of IgG and rhGM-CSF gave rise to much higher IRAP levels than rhGM-CSF alone. That the IL-1 antagonist activity was truly due to IRAP in these cultures was verified by isolation and sequence analysis of purified IRAP from human mononuclear cell supernatants (24).

Other investigators have also observed IRAP (= IL-1i, IL-1 INH, and IL-1ra) induction in human monocytes by several of these agents. Arend *et al.* (31, 42) carefully studied the induction of IRAP and IL-1 mRNAs and proteins in human monocytes stimulated with immobilized IgG. Immobilized IgG induced high levels of IRAP and the IRAP mRNA was quite stable (31). In contrast, no IL-1 was induced by immobilized IgG. Roux-Lombard *et al.* (46) confirmed our findings of IRAP production in "unstimulated" monocyte cultures and enhancement by rhGM-CSF. In long-term monocyte cultures, they found that the immature monocytes produced IL-1 early in the culture period and that IRAP was produced later in the culture period by mature macrophages (46). The enhancement of IRAP production by rhGM-CSF may either be due to the cell differentiation induced by this cytokine or to its direct stimulatory effect on monocytes. These results were also confirmed by Janson et al. (47) in shorter term cultures of human monocytes. It is of interest that these results parallel the observations discussed above that U937 cells also respond to rhGM-CSF with enhanced IRAP production. Similarly, rhIL-4 induced IRAP production in both U937 cells and human monocytes.

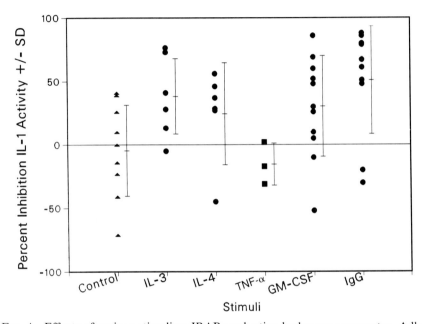

FIG. 4   Effects of various stimuli on IRAP production by human monocytes. Adherent monocytes from many different human donors were cultured for 3–7 days in plain culture medium (control), in culture medium containing rhIL-3 (100 U/ml), rhIL-4 (100 U/ml), rhTNF-α (100 U/ml), or rhGM-CSF (100 U/ml), or in plates precoated with human IgG (5 μg/ml). Cell-free supernatants were harvested at the end of the culture period and were assayed at a 1:40 dilution for IL-1 inhibitory activity in the 1A5 assay. Each point represents the activity of a supernatant from each donor in a separate experiment. The vertical bars show the means ± one standard deviation of the percentage inhibition of IL-1 activity. The data with stimuli that gave mean IL-1 inhibitory activities that were statistically different ($p < 0.05$) from the control supernatants are shown as filled circles, whereas stimuli (only TNF-α) that gave mean IL-1 inhibitory activities that were not statistically different ($p > 0.05$) from the control supernatants are shown as filled squares. Statistical significance was determined by a two-tailed Student's t test.

In contrast, rhIL-3 was active in enhancing IRAP production in human monocytes, but not in U937 cells. It is possible that the U937 cell line does not express IL-3 receptors or that the signal transduction pathways linking IL-3 receptors with IRAP induction are different in U937 cells and human monocytes. Besides the stimulatory agents just discussed, other investigators have shown IRAP induction in human monocytes by LPS (31, 47) and transforming growth factor-β1 (TGF-β1) (48). Because both GM-CSF and TGF-β1 are produced in inflammatory diseases such as rheumatoid arthritis, these cytokines may be partially responsible for the induction of high levels of IRAP seen in rheumatoid synovium (49).

REFERENCES

1. C. A. Dinarello, *Rev. Infect. Dis.* **6,** 51 (1984).
2. H. Besedovsky, A. Del Rey, E. Sorkin, and C. A. Dinarello, *Science* **233,** 652 (1986).
3. J. D. Sipe, S. N. Vogel, M. B. Sztein, M. Skinner, and A. S. Cohen, *Ann. N.Y. Acad. Sci.* **389,** 137 (1982).
4. R. D. Granstein, R. Margolis, S. B. Mizel, and D. N. Sauder, *J. Clin. Invest.* **77,** 1020 (1986).
5. R. P. Schleimer and B. K. Rutledge, *J. Immunol.* **136,** 649 (1985).
6. M. Dukovich, J. M. Severin, S. J. White, S. Yamazaki, and S. B. Mizel, *Clin. Immunol. Immunopathol.* **38,** 381 (1986).
7. F. S. di Giovine and G. W. Duff, *Immunol. Today* **11,** 13 (1990).
8. S. K. Dower, S. R. Kronheim, C. J, March, P. J. Conlon, T. P. Hopp, S. Gillis, and D. L. Urdal, *J. Exp. Med.* **162,** 501 (1985).
9. S. W. Lee, *Proc. Natl. Acad. Sci. U.S.A.* **85,** 1204 (1988); W. Lew, *J. Immunol.* **140,** 1895 (1988).
10. S. M. Wahl, L. C. Altman, and D. L. Rosenstreich, *J. Immunol.* **115,** 476 (1975); S. Gillis, G. R. Crabtreek, and K. Smith, *ibid.* **123,** 1624 (1979); D. S. Snyder and E. R. Unanue, *ibid.* **129,** 1803 (1982).
11. M. Turner, D. Chantry, G. Buchan, K. Barrett, and M. Feldmann, *J. Immunol.* **143,** 3556 (1989).
12. S. Demczuk, C. Baumberger, B. Mach, and J.-M. Dayer, *J. Mol. Cell. Immunol.* **3,** 255 (1987).
13. P. J. Knudson, C. A. Dinarello, and T. B. Strom, *J. Immunol.* **137,** 3189 (1986).
14. R. Schindler, B. D. Clark, and C. A. Dinarello, *J. Biol. Chem.* **265,** 10232 (1990).
15. R. Schindler, J. A. Gelfand, and D. A. Dinarello, *Blood* **76,** 1631 (1990).
16. R. Schindler, G. Lonnemann, S. Shaldon, K.-M. Koch, and C. A. Dinarello, *Kidney Int.* **37,** 85 (1990).
17. H. Mizutani, R. Black, and T. S. Kupper, *J. Clin. Invest.* **87,** 1066 (1991).
18. S. B. Mizel, *Immunol. Today* **10,** 390 (1990).
19. T. A. Bird, P. R. Sleath, P. C. deRoos, S. K. Dower, and G. D. Virca, *J. Biol. Chem.* **266,** 22661 (1991).

20. S. Grenfell, N. Smithers, K. Miller, and R. Solari, *Biochem. J.* **264**, 813 (1989).
21. E. E. Qwarnstrom, R. C. Page, S. Gillis, and S. K. Dower, *J. Biol. Chem.* **263**, 8261 (1988).
22. J. A. M. Maier, P. Voulalas, D. Roeder, and T. Maciag, *Science* **24**, 1570 (1990).
23. P. Seckinger, J. W. Lowenthal, K. Williamson, J.-M. Dayer, and H. R. MacDonald, *J. Immunol.* **139**, 1546 (1987).
24. D. B. Carter, M. R. Deibel, C. J. Dunn, C.-S. Tomich, A. L. Laborde, J. L. Slightom, A. E. Berger, M. J. Bienkowski, F. F. Sun, R. N. McEwan, P. K. W. Harris, A. W. Yem, G. A. Waszak, J. G. Chosay, L. C. Sieu, M. M. Hardee, H. A. Zurcher-Neely, I. M. Reardon, R. L. Heinrikson, S. E. Truesdell, J. A. Shelly, T. E. Eessalu, B. M. Taylor, and D. E. Tracey, *Nature (London)* **344**, 633 (1990).
25. C. H. Hannum, C. J. Wilcox, W. P. Arend, F. G. Joslin, P. L. Dripps, P. L. Heimdal, L. G. Armes, A. Sommer, S. P. Eisenberg, and R. C. Thompson, *Nature (London)* **343**, 336 (1990).
26. M. J. Bienkowski, T. E. Eessalu, A. E. Berger, S. E. Truesdell, J. A. Shelly, A. L. Laborde, H. A. Zurcher-Neely, I. M. Reardon, R. L. Heinrikson, J. G. Chosay, and D. E. Tracey, *J. Biol. Chem.* **265**, 14505 (1990).
27. G. J. Mazzei, L. M. Bernasconi, C. Lewis, J.-J. Mermod, V. Kindler, and A. R. Shaw, *J. Immunol.* **145**, 585 (1990).
28. S. J. Haskill, G. Martin, L. Van Le, J. Morris, A. Peace, D. G. Bigler, G. J. Jaffe, C. Hammerberg, S. A. Sporn, S. Fong, W. P. Arend, and P. Ralph, *Proc. Natl. Acad. Sci. U.S.A.* **88**, 3681 (1991).
29. P. Roux-Lombard, C. Modous, and J.-M. Dayer, *Cytokine* **1**, 45 (1989).
30. R. W. Janson, K. R. Hance, and W. P. Arend, *J. Immunol.* **147**, 4218 (1991).
31. W. P. Arend, M. F. Smith, R. W. Janson, and F. G. Joslin, *J. Immunol.* **147**, 1530 (1991).
32. M. Turner, M. D. Chantry, P. Datsikis, A. Berger, F. M. Brennan, and M. Feldmann, *Eur. J. Immunol.* **21**, 1635 (1991).
33. W. L. Farrar, P. L. Killian, M. R. Ruff, J. M. Hill, and C. B. Pert, *J. Immunol.* **139**, 459 (1987).
34. G. Katsuura, P. E. Gottschall, and A. Arimura, *Biochem. Biophys. Res. Commun.* **156**, 61 (1988).
35. E. B. De Souza, E. L. Webster, E. D. Grigoriadis, and D. E. Tracey, *Psychopharmacol. Bull.* **25**, 299 (1989).
36. F. Haour, E. Ban, G. Milon, D. Baman, and G. Fillion, *Prog. NeuroEndocrinImmunol.* **3**, 196 (1990).
37. E. T. Cunningham, E. Wada, D. B. Carter, D. E. Tracey, J. F. Battey, and E. B. De Souza, *J. Neurosci.* **12**, 1101 (1992).
38. P. Chomczynski and N. Sacchi, *Anal. Biochem.* **162**, 156 (1987).
39. J. Sambrook, E. F. Fritsch, and T. Maniatis, "Molecular Cloning," 2nd ed., p. 7.40. Cold Spring Harbor Lab. Press, Cold Spring Harbor, New York, 1989.
40. G. M. Church and W. Gilbert, *Proc. Natl. Acad. Sci. U.S.A.* **81**, 1991 (1984).
41. L. E. Maquat, R. Chilcote, and P. M. Ryan, *J. Biol. Chem.* **260**, 3748 (1985).
42. W. P. Arend, F. G. Joslin, and R. J. Massoni, *J. Immunol.* **134**, 3868 (1985).
43. I. Gery, R. K. Gershon, and B. H. Waksman, *J. Exp. Med.* **136**, 128 (1972).

44. S. Gillis and S. Mizel, *Proc. Natl. Acad. Sci. U.S.A.* **78,** 1133 (1981).

45. D. E. Tracey, M. M. Hardee, K. A. Richard, and J. W. Paslay, *Immunopharmacology* **15,** 47 (1988).

46. P. Roux-Lombard, C. Modoux, and J.-M. Dayer, *Cytokine* **1,** 45 (1989).

47. R. W. Janson, K. R. Hance, and W. P. Arend, *J. Immunol.* **147,** 4218 (1991).

48. M. Turner, D. Chantry, P. Katsikis, A. Berger, F. M. Brennan, and M. Feldmann, *Eur. J. Immunol.* **21,** 1635 (1991).

49. G. S. Firestein, A. E. Berger, D. L. Chapman, D. E. Tracey, J. G. Chosay, and N. J. Zvaifler, *Clin. Res.* **39,** 291A (1991).

[3] Identification of Intracellular Mediators of the Actions of Cytokines: Identifying Proteins Involved in Kinase Signaling Pathways

Gerald A. Evans, Hallgeir Rui, and William L. Farrar

Introduction

In the field of cellular biology, much research has been devoted to deducing the mechanisms by which hormones and growth factors control cellular physiology. A key event in signal transduction of membrane receptors is the regulation of intracellular effector proteins through alterations in their phosphorylation state. This can be achieved by regulation of protein kinases or protein phosphatases. In many cases, ligand-induced alterations of the levels of second messenger molecules such as cyclic nucleotides, inositol phosphates, and Ca^{2+} alter the activity of key protein kinases. In other cases, the receptors themselves posess intrinsic catalytic activity, for example, receptors for insulin, epidermal growth factor, and platelet-derived growth factor. Another class of receptors for hematopoietic cytokines and growth factors, termed the hematopoietin receptor superfamily (1), has been found by our group and others to rapidly activate tyrosine kinase activity (2, 3). These receptors mediate the effects of a growing number of ligands, including several of the interleukins (IL-2 through IL-7), colony-stimulating factors [granulocyte–macrophage colony-stimulating factor (GM-CSF) and granulocyte colony-stimulating factor (G-CSF)], erythropoietin, growth hormone, prolactin, and ciliary neurotrophic factor. Many of these cytokines have been implicated in the regulation of neuroendocrine cells or to have direct neurotrophic effects (4). The present work describes methodology that has proved useful in the elucidation of signal transduction mechanisms mediating the effects of some of these cytokines. Our approach has focused both on immediate protein phosphorylation at the level of receptor-associated proteins as well as phosphorylation events further downstream.

In general, before initiating signal transduction studies, it is worthwhile to consider several aspects of the design, which in many cases may mean the difference between success and failure. It is of considerable importance to select the best cellular model possible. In this regard, high numbers of specific receptors for the factor or cytokine that is being studied, as well as

Methods in Neurosciences, Volume 16

good and measurable physiological responses, are of the utmost importance. Another important consideration is the removal of factor from the cell medium prior to stimulation, both in the study of differentiation as well as of mitogenic signals. In cases of factor-dependent cell lines, that is, cell lines that are dependent on the specific factor for growth, best results are obtained if cells can be made quiescent by arrest in the G_0/G_1 phase of the cell cycle. This is most easily accomplished by removal or depletion of growth factor on which they are dependent on for growth. It should also be kept in mind that some cells produce and secrete factor in an autocrine fashion, and therefore a certain number of the receptors are constantly occupied. A quick pH reduction of the medium followed by washing of the cells may be used to dissociate bound ligands from their respective cell surface receptors, and thereby reduce background signal. After factor removal by low-pH washing or depletion by extended cell culture time, cells are usually allowed to "quiet" a further 12 to 24 hr in reduced serum medium to synchronize cells in G_0/G_1 phase and establish a cell population that is primed to respond vigorously to exogenous growth factor or cytokine. For each cell model studied, however, one must establish the optimum quieting procedure for signal generation as well as cell viability. With these considerations in mind, the following outlines several methods that have facilitated our studies of protein phosphorylation, with an emphasis on tyrosine kinase catalysis and its involvement in hematopoietin receptor signal transduction.

Identification of Protein Kinase Substrates Involved in Signal Transduction

Analysis of Protein Phosphorylation by $^{32}P_i$ Labeling and Immunoprecipitation

In our laboratory, a major focus has been on elucidating the kinase signaling pathways triggered by cytokines whose receptor belongs to the hematopoietin superfamily of transmembrane proteins. Receptors of this class have no known catalytic activity, but nevertheless have been shown to activate protein kinases and therefore stimulate the phosphorylation of specific substrates. A classic experimental design that attempts to identify proteins involved in cytokine-stimulated signal transduction involves radiolabeling the intracellular ATP pool with $^{32}P_i$, stimulating the cells with ligand, and analyzing phosphoproteins by electrophoresis and autoradiography. We have used this design to identify several proteins that were phosphorylated in response to phorbol myristate acetate (PMA), interleukin 3 (IL-3), and GM-CSF in human myeloid cell lines. The intracellular phosphate pool is radiolabeled by equilibrating with $^{32}P_i$. AML-193 cells, a human meyloid leukemic cell line, are recovered from log-phase cultures and washed twice with phosphate-free RPMI-1640 medium. Approximately 50×10^6 cells are labeled per treatment, but the optimal number may vary between cell types. After washing cells are resuspended at 50×10^6 cells/ml in phosphate-free RPMI-1640 supplemented with 5% fetal calf serum (dialyzed against phosphate-free RPMI), glutamine, antibiotics, and $^{32}P_i$ (0.2–0.5 mCi/ml) and incubated for 2 hr at 37°C in a shaking water bath. For cytokine stimulation, ^{32}P-labeled cells at 50×10^6 cells/ml are treated with an excess of cytokine (i.e., 10- to 100-fold above K_d), to rapidly activate as many receptor molecules as possible, or with PMA (100 ng/ml). After stimulation cells are recovered by rapid centrifugation and frozen for later lysis or lysed immediately with nonionic detergent.

For a standard cell lysis, freshly isolated cells or frozen pellets are adjusted to a final concentration of 10^8 cells/ml with lysis buffer [10 mM Tris-HCl (pH 7.6), 5 mM ethylenediaminetetraacetic acid (EDTA), 50 mM NaCl, 30 mM sodium pyrophosphate, 50 mM sodium fluoride, 100 μM sodium orthovanadate, 1% Triton X-100, 1 mM phenylmethylsulfonyl fluoride, aprotinin (5 μg/ml), pepstatin A (1 μg/ml), and leupeptin (2 μg/ml)] and incubated, rotating end over end, for 1 hr at 4°C. Cell lysates are clarified by centrifugation at 12,000 g for 30 min and radiolabeled phosphoproteins are analyzed by one-dimensional (5) or two-dimensional polyacrylamide gel electrophoresis (PAGE) (6). For any given experimental design, care should be taken in choosing and using detergents for cell lysis. This is covered in detail elsewhere (7).

Using this methodology we have identified a 68-kDa protein from total cell lysates that is phosphorylated in response to a number of cytokines. Figure 1 shows autoradiographs of two-dimensional gels showing p68 phosphorylation within 15 min in response to GM-CSF, IL-3, and PMA in the human myeloid cell line AML-193.

In addition to the analysis of total cell lysates, much information regarding ligand-stimulated phosphorylation of specific substrates can be obtained from the analysis of radiolabeled cell lysates by precipitation with anti-phosphotyrosine antibodies followed by electrophoresis and autoradiographic analysis. Using this approach, clarified cell lysates, prepared as described above, are incubated with anti-phosphotyrosine antibody (5 μg/ml) [available from many manufacturers; we use PY20, available from ICN (Costa Mesa, CA), or monoclonal anti-phosphotyrosine from UBI, Lake Placid, NY] and a 20-μl pellet volume of protein A-conjugated Sepharose (Pharmacia, Piscataway, NJ) for 2 to 4 hr. Immune precipitates are washed three times with extraction buffer containing 0.1% bovine serum albumin (BSA) and three times with

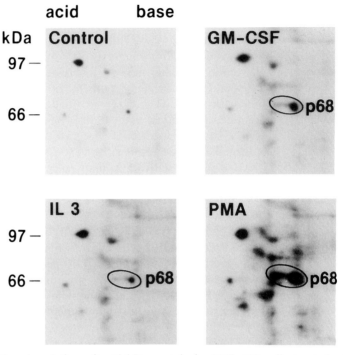

FIG. 1   Phosphorylation of a 68-kDa protein in AML-193 cells treated with GM-CSF, IL-3, or PMA. AML-193 cells were recovered from log-phase culture labeled with ^{32}P; (0.5 mCi/ml) at a cell density of 40×10^6 cells/ml for 2 hr at 37°C. Approximately 40×10^6 cells in 1 ml were stimulated with the indicated cytokine or PMA for 10 min. Cells were pelleted, lysed in extraction buffer, and equal aliquots were subjected to two-dimensional electrophoresis (isoelectrofocusing followed by SDS-PAGE). Ligand-modulated phosphoproteins were visualized by autoradiography. [Data were adapted from D. Linnekin and W. L. Farrar, *Biochem. J.* **271**, 317 (1990).]

extraction buffer without BSA. Proteins are eluted with 50 μl of 2× sodium dodecyl sulfate (SDS)-PAGE sample buffer for SDS-PAGE or 50 μl of isoelectric focusing (IEF) sample buffer for two-dimensional electrophoresis. Proteins are then analyzed by electrophoresis and autoradiography. Phosphotyrosyl-containing proteins that are phosphorylated in response to IL-2 in human T lymphocytes are shown in Fig. 2.

By using these approaches one can easily observe the phosphoproteins, both autophosphorylating protein kinases as well as protein kinase substrates, that are involved in ligand-dependent signal transduction. Although these methods identify phosphoproteins they give us no information as to the specific amino acid that is phosphorylated in response to stimulation by

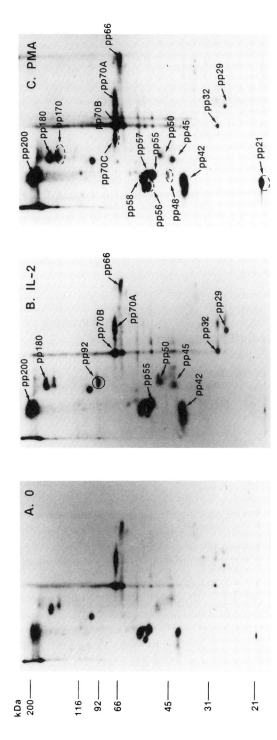

Fig. 2 Interleukin-stimulated phosphorylation of T lymphocyte proteins isolated by anti-phosphotyrosine immune precipitation. Human T lymphocytes were isolated by counterflow centrifugal elutriation from normal donors. T cells (1 × 10⁶ cells/ml) were activated by treatment with phytohemagglutinin (1 μg/ml) and cultured in RPMI-1640 medium supplemented with 10% fetal calf serum, glutamine, and antibiotics for 72 hr. Cells were recovered, washed free of growth factor, and quieted for 24 hr in RPMI-1640 supplemented with 1% fetal calf serum. Quieted cells were recovered, labeled with ³²P, for 2 hr at 50 × 10⁶ cells/ml, and stimulated with or without IL-2 (1 μg/ml) or PMA (50 ng/ml) for 15 min. Cells were washed, lysed in extraction buffer, and subjected to anti-phosphotyrosine immunoprecipitation. Immunoprecipitates were analyzed by two-dimensional electrophoresis and autoradiography. Specific proteins that show reproducible, increased phosphorylation in response to IL-2 or PMA are indicated.

cytokine. Even in the case of anti-phosphotyrosine immunoprecipitation, there is no direct evidence that ligand-dependent phosphorylation occurred on tyrosine residues. To determine which residue is phosphorylated, resolved proteins are subjected to phosphoamino acid analysis.

Determining Phosphoamino Acids by Protein Hydrolysis and Thin-Layer Electrophoresis

Many methods currently exist for determining phosphoamino acids. The method that has been most used in our laboratory involves acid hydrolysis followed by resolving amino acids by thin-layer electrophoresis. To identify phosphorylated amino acids, specific proteins, identified by one- or two-dimensional electrophoresis and autoradiography, are excised from the gels and rapidly rehydrated with 3–5 drops of distilled water. Gels are separated from the drying support (usually paper) and placed in a solution containing 20 mM sodium bicarbonate, 0.1% SDS, and 5% (v/v) 2-mercaptoethanol. Enough buffer is used to cover the gel, usually 0.5 ml, and the gel is boiled for 5 min and incubated for 24–48 hr at 37°C. The gel slice is discarded and proteins are precipitated by adjusting to 10–20% trichloroacetic acid (TCA) and BSA (2–5 μg/ml) as carrier protein, and incubating on ice for 4–18 hr. Proteins are recovered by centrifugation at 12,000 g for 30 min at 4°C. The precipitate is washed three times in a solution of ethanol–ether (3:1) and air dried. Proteins are hydrolyzed in 200 μl of 5.7 N HCl for 60–90 min at 110°C and dried under vacuum (SpeedVac; Savant, Hicksville, NY). Dried hydrolysate is resuspended in 7–10 μl of a solution containing 2 mg/ml each of phosphoserine, phosphothreonine, and phosphotyrosine standards (Sigma, St. Louis, MO) in distilled water and carefully spotted on cellulose-coated plates. Spotted samples are allowed to dry and then subjected to thin-layer electrophoresis, using an electrophoresis plate cooled to 4°C (LKB, Bromma, Sweden) with anode and cathode buffer containing water–acetic acid–pyridine at a 189:10:1 ratio. Samples are electrophoresed for 60 min at 1500 V and the plate is dried at 100°C. Phosphoamino acid standards are visualized by staining with a ninhydrin solution prepared by mixing 1 vol of 0.33% ninhydrin in t-butanol with 1 vol of acetic acid–pyridine–water (1:5:5). Radiolabeled phosphoamino acids are determined by autoradiography and comparing to ninhydrin-stained standards.

Analysis of several proteins identified in Figs. 1 and 2 revealed that the ligand-modulated phosphorylation of p68 by IL-3, GM-CSF, and PMA was on serine and that most of the proteins identified by anti-phosphotyrosine immunoprecipitation are phosphorylated on tyrosine as well as serine–threonine (Fig. 3). From the results of these experiments, along with time course analysis of protein phosphorylation after ligand stimulation, we can formulate a general model of signal transduction involving protein phosphorylation for several cytokines. This model implicates tyrosine kinase activation as an initial signaling event, based on the observation of rapid tyrosine phosphorylation of specific proteins, followed by serine kinase activation. Because of these observations, much of the interest in our laboratory has focused on identifying the kinases and substrates involved in propagating phosphotyrosyl signal triggered by ligand binding to the appropriate receptor. Further, because the hematopoietin class of receptors does not contain intrinsic protein kinase catalytic activity we have become interested in identifying the protein kinase associated with receptors of this family that is responsible for transducing signal.

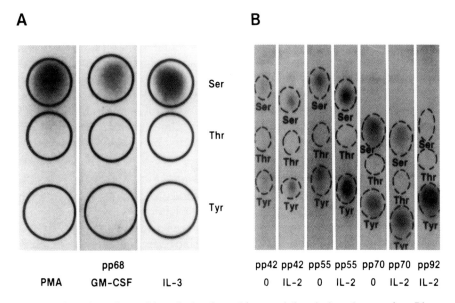

FIG. 3 Phosphoamino acid analysis of ctyokine-modulated phosphoproteins. Phosphoproteins were identified by autoradiography, excised from the gels, and subjected to acid hydrolysis and thin-layer electrophoresis. Radiolabeled phosphoamino acids were identified by autoradiography and comparison to ninhydrin-stained phosphoamino acid standards. (A) phosphoamino acid analysis of p68, from AML-193 cells (Fig. 1), phosphorylated in response to PMA, GM-CSF, and IL-3. (B) Phosphoamino acid analysis of selected proteins (Fig. 2) from human T cells modulated by IL-2 and isolated by anti-phosphotyrosine immune precipitation. [Data were adapted from W. L. Farrar and Ferris, *J. Biol. Chem.* **264**, 12562 (1989).]

Analysis of Protein Tyrosine Phosphorylation by Immunoprecipitation and Immunoblot with Anti-Phosphotyrosine Antibodies

The most direct method for analyzing protein tyrosine kinase activation and substrate phosphorylation in response to ligand stimulation is immunoblotting electrophoretically resolved proteins with anti-phosphotyrosine antibodies. This eliminates the necessity for phosphoamino acid analysis and further eliminates the detection of serine–threonine phosphorylation, which, in many experimental designs with radiolabeled protein, will constitute much of the observed phosphorylation.

In this approach, aliquots of total cell lysate or anti-phosphotyrosine immune precipitates are subjected to SDS-PAGE and Western transfer (8) to Immobilon polyvinylidene difluoride (PVDF) paper (Millipore, Bedford, MA). The paper is blocked with 1% high-grade dephosphorylated BSA (ICN) in TBS [Tris-buffered saline, 20 mM Tris (pH 7.4), 130 mM NaCl, 0.01% sodium azide] for 1 hr at room temperature or overnight at 4°C. Several blocking agents have been used for immunoblotting and many of these contain phosphorylated proteins that give rise to high background in anti-phosphotyrosyl immunoblots (i.e., dry milk). After blocking, blots are incubated for 2 to 6 hr with anti-phosphotyrosine monoclonal antibody (from UBI or PY20 from ICN) at a concentration of 1 μg/ml in TBS containing 0.05% Tween-20 (TBST). Blots are washed three times (10 min each) with TBST and anti-phosphotyrosine antibody is detected by one of several methods.

Colorimetric Development of Immunoblots

An exhaustive discussion of methods for the development of immunoblots can be found elsewhere (9). In our laboratory, we routinely use an alkaline phosphatase-based system for colorimetric development. After primary antibody incubation and washing, the blot is incubated with alkaline phosphatase-conjugated anti-mouse IgG at a concentration of 0.1–1 μg/ml in TBST for 1 to 2 hr at room temperature. Blots are washed three times (10 min each) with TBST and developed by incubating in phosphatase buffer [100 mM Tris (pH 9.5), 100 mM NaCl, 5 mM MgCl$_2$] containing nitroblue tetrazolium chloride (NBT) (3.3 μg/ml) and 5-bromo-4-chloro-3-indolyphosphate (BCIP) (1.65 μg/ml) until band visualization.

Chemiluminescent Development of Immunoblots

A much more sensitive method for the development of immunoblots incorporates the use of chemiluminescent technology coupled to substrate utilization within either an alkaline phosphatase- or horseradish peroxidase-based system. Several kits are available that use these systems and we have obtained equivalent results from several manufacturers. For the purposes here we will discuss the use of peroxidase-based chemiluminescent development. Blots are blocked, incubated with anti-phosphotyrosine monoclonal antibody, and washed as described above. Blots are then incubated with biotinylated anti-mouse IgG at 0.1–0.5 μg/ml in TBST for 1 hr at room temperature. Immunoblots are then washed three times (10 min each) with TBST and incubated for 30 min with horseradish peroxidase-conjugated streptavidin (10–50 ng/ml in TBST). Blots are washed three times (5 min each) and incubated with ECL chemiluminescence substrate (Amersham, Arlington Heights, IL) for 1 to 2 min. Substrate-soaked blots are then sealed in plastic bags and excess substrate mix is thoroughly drained from the blot. Immunoreactive proteins are visualized by exposure to X-ray film for 1 to 60 min.

Because of the growing interest in tyrosine-specific phosphorylation, its involvement in ligand-stimulated signal transduction, and the availability of a fast, nonradioactive, and specific method to identify tyrosine phosphorylation, many researchers have chosen antiphosphotyrosine immunoblots followed by chemiluminescence development as the method of choice to study receptor signaling. Figure 4 presents results from several experiments that utilize this approach to identify substrates involved in tyrosine kinase signal transduction stimulated by prolactin and IL-2.

Analysis of Receptor-Associated Phosphotyrosyl Proteins

Tyrosine kinase activation has been demonstrated to be a first signal generated by many hematopoietic cytokines, and tyrosine kinase activity can be copurified with cytokine receptors, which themselves do not contain intrinsic domains homologous to the tyrosine kinases. Because all tyrosine kinases possess a certain level of autophosphorylating activity, a good initial design that attempts to identify candidate receptor-associated tyrosine kinases is one that looks for receptor-associated, ligand-modulated, phosphotyrosyl proteins. This design couples antiphosphotyrosine immunoblotting with specific receptor purification strategies to characterize these proteins.

We have employed three different methods to obtain partially purified hematopoietin receptor complexes. The most feasible method involves using receptor-specific antibodies to immune precipitate receptor and associated signal-transducing proteins. If the goal is to purify activated or ligand-bound receptor, it is important that the antibodies recognize epitopes outside the ligand-binding site. Because of this, monoclonal antibodies that block ligand binding will generally not work. They can, however, be used to immunoprecipitate unoccupied receptor. Polyclonal antibodies normally work well, despite the potential ability to block ligand binding when preincubated with the

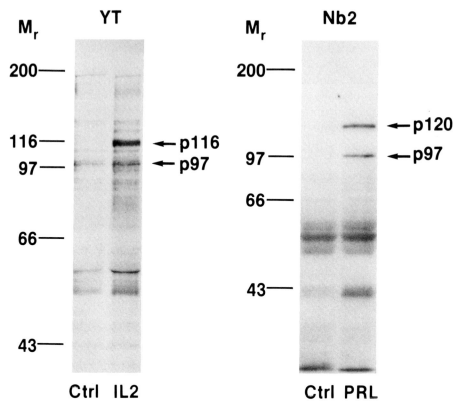

FIG. 4   Tyrosine phosphorylation of specific proteins in human YT cells treated with IL-2 and rat Nb2 cells treated with prolactin and detected with anti-phosphotyrosine immunoblotting. YT cells treated with or without IL-2 and Nb2 cells treated with or without prolactin were lysed and subjected to anti-phosphotyrosine immune precipitation. Precipitated proteins were subjected to SDS-PAGE, Western Transfer, and immunoblotting with anti-phosphotyrosine antibody followed by colorimetric development (YT) or chemiluminescent development (Nb2). Distinct tyrosine phosphorylation of proteins of 116 and 97 kDa by IL-2 and 120 and 97 kDa by prolactin can be seen.

receptor preparation. This is because of the presence within the polyclonal mixture of antibody molecules that react with many different epitopes, both within and outside the ligand-binding domain. An alternative approach that we have used utilizes anti-ligand antibody to isolate ligand-bound receptor complexes. This approach is made possible because of the characteristically low dissociation rate of ligand from hematopoietin receptors after initial binding. In theory, the best antibodies for this purpose are monoclonal antibodies directed against exposed epitopes on receptor-bound ligand so that competition between antibody, receptor, and ligand does not occur. In practice, however, polyclonal antibodies also work well as long as incubation times are kept relatively short to minimize dissociation of ligand and receptor. Short incubation periods also seem beneficial because of dissociation of receptor and receptor-associated proteins. Such dissociation will be dependent on the nature of the detergent used as well as salt concentration and pH of the lysis buffer. A variant of this method, which can be used when anti-ligand antibodies are not available, employs biotinylated ligand and streptavidin–agarose affinity purification to isolate receptor complex (10). Of these methods, anti-receptor or anti-ligand antibodies, in our hands, has yielded the most consistent results with minimal background binding of nonspecific proteins. As an example, we have identified a 120-kDa phosphotyrosyl protein that is specifically associated with the prolactin receptor and is modulated by ligand (Fig. 5). By using these methods we have now identified a candidate catalytic protein involved in prolactin-triggered signal transduction that is involved at the receptor level. Further analysis is necessary, however, to determine whether this protein is in fact an autophosphorylating protein kinase or simply a receptor-associated substrate that is phosphorylated by a distal tyrosine kinase.

Identification of Protein Kinases Involved in Signal Transduction

Analysis of Receptor-Associated Kinases by an in Vitro Kinase Assay

Within the hematopoietic cytokines, much of the work that has been devoted to identifying protein kinases involved in signal transduction has been focused on identifying those protein kinases specifically associated with receptor that are modulated in activity on ligand binding. In isolating and identifying known kinases that act at, or distal to, the receptor the most useful tools are specific antibodies, monoclonal or polyclonal, that can immune precipitate the kinase of interest and determine the relative *in vitro* activity following ligand stimulation. This approach, along with the use of specific protein kinase substrates and inhibitors, has been used extensively to show the involvement of both serine–threonine and tyrosine kinases in cytokine signaling. A much more difficult approach, and one that we will discuss here, is attempting to identify unknown protein kinases, especially those associated with receptor, that propagate the initial signal or are involved distally but early in cytokine signaling.

On having identified one or more receptor-associated phosphoproteins, a next step is to determine whether any of these proteins can be phosphorylated *in vitro* in affinity-purified receptor complexes. There are in principle several

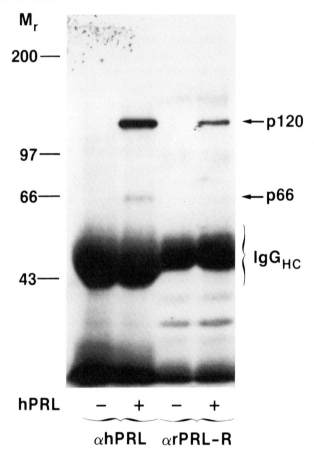

FIG. 5 The association of the prolactin-stimulated phosphoprotein, p120, with the prolactin receptor. Immunoblot of solubilized, affinity-purified PRL receptor complexes separated by SDS-PAGE under reducing conditions and probed with anti-phosphotyrosine antibodies. Both polyclonal anti-hPRL antiserum and monoclonal anti-rPRL receptor antibodies (U6) were capable of immunoprecipitating a p120 strongly phosphorylated on tyrosine residues from lysates of Nb2 cells stimulated with 100 nM hPRL for 3 min at 37°C (lanes 2 and 4, respectively), but not from unstimulated cells (lanes 1 and 3). Relative molecular weight ($M_r \times 10^{-3}$) of protein markers are indicated. Arrows identify phosphotyrosyl proteins p120 and p66, and brace marks immunoglobulin heavy chains (IgG$_{HC}$).

ways of assaying receptor-associated kinase activity following receptor purification, using any one of the methods previously discussed. One way is to incubate the partially purified receptor complex with [γ-^{32}P]ATP and protein kinase substrate in a kinase assay buffer and analyze, by comparison to control immune precipitates, the ability of receptor-specific immune precipitates to phosphorylate substrate and/or endogenous receptor-associated proteins (11). Exogenous substrate can be any of a number of proteins; however, for tyrosine kinase assays we prefer enolase (usually from rabbit skeletal muscle) or synthetic tyrosine kinase substrates, for example, poly(Glu : Tyr) (4 : 1) (E4Y). For this assay, receptor and control immunoprecipitates are incubated with and without substrate (enolase or E4Y) at a concentration of 1 mg/ml in 100 μl of kinase assay buffer [25 mM N-2-hydroxyethylpiperazine-N'-2-ethanesulfonic acid (HEPES) (pH 7.4), 10 mM MgCl$_2$, 10 mM MnCl$_2$] with the addition of 10 μM ATP containing [γ-^{32}P]ATP (100 μCi/ml). Immune precipitates are assayed for 10 min at 30°C and stopped by adding 100 μl of a solution containing 4% SDS and 5 mM EDTA. Twenty microliters of this material is then spotted on Whatman (Clifton, NJ) 3MM filter paper (2 × 2 cm squares) and dropped into ice-cold 10% TCA. Filters are washed five to eight times with 10% TCA until no detectable counts are found in the wash solution. Filters are then washed twice in 100% ethanol, air dried, dropped in scintillation fluid, and counted. The presence of receptor-specific kinase activity is determined by analyzing substrate-specific phosphorylation and comparing this to that seen in the control precipitates. Alternatively, when using enolase as a substrate, reactions can be stopped with 2× SDS sample buffer and the reaction mix subjected to SDS-PAGE. Autoradiography will reveal the relative and specific phosphorylation of enolase as well as the *in vitro* phosphorylation of endogenous receptor-associated proteins. It is important to consider that when using this approach, unless the substrate used contains only one phosphorylatable residue (i.e., E4Y), phosphoamino acid analysis is necessary to determine the type of protein kinase activity detected in this assay. Additionally, the components of the kinase assay mix can greatly influence the ability to detect certain kinase activities. It has been argued, for example, that 15 μM ATP and 3 mM MnCl$_2$ (no MgCl$_2$) favors tyrosine-specific phosphorylation (12).

A more specific approach that identifies receptor-associated tyrosine kinase activity is to incubate partially purified receptor complexes with and without unlabeled ATP and analyze the complex for the appearance of *in vitro* tyrosine-phosphorylated proteins, using anti-phosphotyrosine immunoblotting and chemiluminescent development. Although this approach can readily identify tyrosine kinase activity, it also has the advantage of potentially identifying receptor-associated, autophosphorylating tyrosine kinases. In the prolactin receptor system we showed the presence of one receptor-associated phosphotyrosyl protein, p120 (Fig. 5). Because of its minimal complexity, this system was ideally suited for analysis by *in vitro* ATP incubation and antiphosphotyrosine immunoblotting. Using this, we clearly show that p120 is tyrosine phosphorylated *in vitro* (Fig. 6) and, further, that this most likely represents tyrosine kinase autophosphorylation because it is the only protein found in the complex that is phosphorylated *in vitro* by this assay.

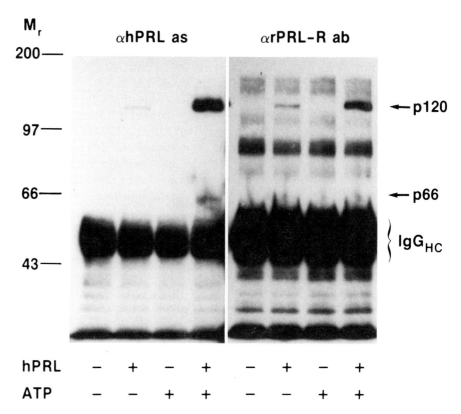

FIG. 6 *In vitro* phosphorylation of prolactin receptor-associated p120 as determined by an *in vitro* kinase assay incorporating anti-phosphotyrosine immunoblotting. Immunoblot from PRL–receptor immune complex tyrosine kinase assay. PRL–receptor complexes immunoprecipitated with either polyclonal anti-hPRL antiserum (left) or monoclonal anti-rPRL receptor antibodies (U6; right) from stimulated and unstimulated Nb2 cells (10 nM hPRL for 30 min at 22°C) were incubated with 15 μM ATP in the presence of 3 mM Mn^{2+} at room temperature for 30 min. Middle panel indicates whether cells corresponding to the individual lanes had been stimulated with PRL or not, and whether the same immunoprecipitates had been incubated in the presence or absence of ATP. Relative molecular weights ($M_r \times 10^{-3}$) of protein markers are indicated. Arrows indicate p120 and p66, and brace marks immunoglobulin heavy chains.

Identifying Protein Kinases by Azido-ATP Binding

All protein kinases share certain basal characteristics, including the ability to bind and utilize ribonucleotide triphosphates, predominantly ATP and to a lesser extent GTP. We have used this characteristic to identify ligand-modulated phosphoproteins as potential protein kinases based on their ability to specifically bind ATP at physiological concentrations. This design uses a modified nucleotide (8-azido-ATP) that, on exposure to ultraviolet light, covalently binds to amino acid residues within the nucleotide-binding domain of the protein. The use of radiolabeled nucleotides for this experiment provides an efficient means of detecting nucleotide-binding domains. Several approaches exist that employ nucleotide photoaffinity labeling and are reviewed in Haley (13).

In general, the following should be considered when designing a photoaffinity labeling experiment: (1) the concentration of 8-azido-ATP should be close to the K_d of ATP binding for the enzyme studied; (2) the use of appropriate metal ions, Mg^{2+} or Mn^{2+}, at the optimum concentration for enzyme activity and therefore ATP binding should be used for initial studies; however, in certain instances, changing the metal ion may result in good ATP binding with minimal hydrolysis, leading to increased overall labelling (Ref. 13); (3) dithiothreitol (DTT) or other reducing agents should be eliminated from the reaction mix; (4) care should be taken in choosing the buffer constituents to minimize the use of reagents that absorb light in the ultraviolet range; and (5) any observed radiolabeled ATP cross-linking must be competitively inhibited by an excess of unlabeled ATP. With these considerations in mind we have effectively labeled a number of proteins, isolated by any of the methods described above, with 8-azido-ATP. Our principal procedure involves immune precipitation of the protein or protein complex containing the protein to be labeled followed by incubation with a reaction mix containing 8-azidoadenosine $5'-[\alpha-^{32}P]$triphosphate (ICN) in the presence of low-intensity UV light with or without an excess of unlabeled ATP, followed by electrophoretic analysis.

For this procedure, growing cells are lysed and immune precipitated as described above. The immunoprecipitate is washed free of nonspecific protein as described above and resuspended in 50 μl of a buffer containing 40 mM HEPES (pH 7.5), 1 mM $MgCl_2$, and 2 μCi of 8-azido-$[\alpha-^{32}P]$ATP (2–10 Ci/mmol; ICN) yielding a 5 μM final concentration of azido-ATP, in the presence or absence of 1 mM unlabeled ATP. The immune precipitates are placed on ice and exposed to low-intensity (1000 μW), low-wavelength (254 nm) ultraviolet light for 1 to 2 min. The immune precipitates are washed several times in lysis buffer (above) and eluted with SDS sample buffer and subjected to SDS-PAGE. When performing a photoaffinity-labeling experiment it is always important, as mentioned above, to eliminate or minimize as much as possible the presence of UV-absorbing material during photoaffinity labeling. We have found that the presence of large amounts of Sepharose from the immunoprecipitation may interfere with photoaffinity labeling by blocking UV light. Because of this we perform a series of exposures and minimize the amount of protein A-conjugated Sepharose used in the initial immune precipitation.

Identifying Protein Kinases by a Protein Kinase Renaturation Assay

The most direct and powerful of the methods used to specifically identify a phosphoprotein as a protein kinase is a kinase renaturation assay. Total cell lysates or immunoprecipitates are subjected to SDS-PAGE. By separating the mixture electrophoretically we effectively isolate protein kinase from soluble substrate, eliminating substrate phosphorylation to a large degree and allowing the observation of specific kinase autophosphorylation. Because protein kinases in this mixture have been denatured in the presence of SDS, they must be renatured to restore catalytic activity. This is most easily done by transferring the proteins to a solid support (PVDF paper), thoroughly denaturing the proteins, and removing SDS with $7 M$ guanidine and allowing their slow renaturation by removal of guanidine in the presence of low concentrations of reducing agent and nonionic detergent. Renatured kinases are then assayed by incubation with radiolabeled ATP and cofactors, exhaustive washing, and autoradiography. The method of assay that we have used with most success is a modification of the procedure of Ferrell and Martin (14).

Ten to 50 μg of protein from whole-cell lysate or immunoprecipitated protein from approximately 10^8 cells is subjected to SDS-PAGE and transferred to Immobilon PVDF paper (Millipore) by the method of Towbin *et al.* (8), in buffer without methanol. Blotted samples are incubated for 1 hr at room temperature with gentle rocking in a solution containing $7 M$ guanidine-HCl, 50 mM Tris (pH 8.3), 2 mM EDTA, and 50 mM DTT. Membranes are then washed briefly in renaturation buffer [50 mM Tris (pH 7.5), 100 mM NaCl, 2 mM DTT, 2 mM EDTA, 1% BSA, 0.1% Nonidet P-40] until the blot regains a white opaque color and then are incubated at 4°C in fresh renaturation buffer for 12–16 hr with gentle rocking. Blots are blocked for 1 hr at room temperature with 5% BSA in 30 mM Tris (pH 7.5) and 120 mM NaCl. Kinases are then assayed by incubating with [γ-^{32}P]ATP (50 μCi/ml) in 25 mM HEPES (pH 7.5), 10 mM MgCl$_2$, and 10 mM MnCl$_2$ for 30 min at room temperature. Blots are washed three times in a solution containing 30 mM Tris (pH 7.5), 120 mM NaCl, and 0.05% Tween-20. Each wash is for 10 min and is carried out at room temperature. Blots are then treated with a 1 *M* solution of KOH for 20 min at room temperature and washed with water three times, 10 min/wash, followed by 10% acetic acid for 10 min and two final washes with water. The blots are air dried and autophosphorylating protein kinases are identified by autoradiography.

To determine the type of autophosphorylating protein kinase, phosphoamino acid analysis is necessary. Phosphoamino acid analysis of renatured protein kinases is performed essentially as described above except that excised protein bands on the PVDF paper are hydrolyzed directly by dropping into 5 *N* HCl. Recovery of hydrolysate and thin-layer electrophoresis are performed as described above. With this procedure we have identified several protein serine–threonine kinases that are modulated in response to T cell receptor triggering (15). The identification of tyrosine kinase activity, however, is much more difficult than identifying serine–threonine kinase activity. This may be due to a number of factors, most importantly the potential inability of the tyrosine kinase catalytic domain to completely renature using this procedure. In spite of this we have successfully renatured purified c-*abl* tyrosine kinase as well as several unidentified tyrosine kinases, but the relative protein load required to visualize this is on the order of 10 to 100 times that required to detect a representative serine kinase, such as cAMP-dependent protein kinase.

Acknowledgments

This project has been funded at least in part with federal funds from the Department of Health and Human Services under Contract Number NO1-CO-74102 with Program Resources, Inc./DynCorp. The content of this publication does not necessarily reflect the views or policies of the Department of Health and Human Services, nor does mention of trade names, commercial products, or organizations imply endorsement by the U.S. Government.

References

1. J. F. Bazan, *Proc. Natl. Acad. Sci. U.S.A.* **87**, 6934 (1990).
2. E. M. Saltzman, R. R. Thom, and J. E. Casnellie, *J. Biol. Chem.* **263**, 6956 (1988).
3. P. H. B. Sorenson, A. Mui, S. Murthy, and G. Krystal, *Blood* **13**, 406 (1989).
4. D. A. Weigent, D. J. J. Carr, and J. E. Blalock, *Ann. N. Y. Acad. Sci.* **579**, 17 (1990).
5. U. K. Laemmli, *Nature (London)* **277**, 680 (1970).
6. D. Linnekin and W. L. Farrar, *J. Biol. Chem.* **264**, 317 (1990).
7. J. D. Neugebauer, *in* "Methods in Enzymology" (M. P. Deutscher, ed.), Vol. 182, p. 239. Academic Press, San Diego, 1990.

8. H. Towbin, T. Staehelin, and J. Gordon, *Proc. Natl. Acad. Sci. U.S.A.* **76**, 4350 (1979).

9. T. M. Timmons and B. S. Dunbar, *in* "Methods in Enzymology" (M. P. Deutscher, ed.), Vol. 182, p. 679. Academic Press, San Diego, 1990.

10. D. F. Michiel, G. G. Garcia, G. A. Evans, and W. L. Farrar, *Cytokine* **3**(5), 428 (1991).

11. E. Racker, *in* "Methods in Enzymology" (T. Hunter and B. M. Sefton, eds.), Vol. 200, p. 107. Academic Press, San Diego, 1991.

12. L. C. Mahadevan and J. C. Bell, *in* "Receptor-Effector Coupling" (E. C. Hulme, ed.), p. 191. IRL Press, Oxford, UK, 1990.

13. B. A. Haley, *in* "Methods in Enzymology" (T. Hunter and B. M. Sefton, eds.), Vol. 200, p. 477. Academic Press, San Diego, 1991.

14. J. E. Ferrell and G. S. Martin, *J. Biol. Chem.* **264**, 20723 (1989).

15. G. A. Evans, D. Linnekin, S. Grove, and W. L. Farrar, *J. Biol. Chem.* **267**(15), 10313 (1992).

[4] Measurement of Transport of Cytokines across the Blood–Brain Barrier

William A. Banks and Abba J. Kastin

Introduction

Cytokines exert powerful effects on the central nervous system (CNS) either after peripheral administration or when given directly into the CNS. How cytokines administered peripherally or circulating in the blood can affect the CNS is problematic because it generally has been assumed that the blood–brain barrier (BBB) would prevent them from entering the brain. Most work, therefore, has focused on mechanisms by which cytokines could circumvent the BBB or indirectly relay messages across the BBB. By contrast, we have examined the ability of cytokines to cross the BBB and so to interact with brain tissue directly. Our work has shown that cytokines can be transported across the BBB by saturable transport systems in amounts sufficient to produce effects on the CNS. We will review here the methods used to address the major questions that arise with regard to the measurement of such transport.

Brief History of the Passage of Regulatory Substances across the Blood–Brain Barrier

The view of the BBB as an interface regulating the flow of information between the CNS and the peripheral circulation is a new one. The BBB typically has been regarded as a restrictive membrane responsible for maintaining the homeostatic and nutritive environment of the brain. It has been known for years that steroids cross the BBB and so influence the function of the CNS (1). However, this passage occurs because of the ability of the lipid-soluble steroids to diffuse across cell membranes and so the BBB is usually considered to play a passive role. The passage of larger, water-soluble peptides and proteins was generally thought to be insignificant (2).

An understanding of the morphology of the BBB supported this view. The BBB can be thought of as existing in two forms: the endothelial barrier and the ependymal barrier (3). The capillaries that make up the vascular bed of the brain are fused together by tight junctions to form the endothelial barrier; the term *blood–brain barrier* is often used in a more selective sense to refer

Methods in Neurosciences, Volume 16

to this barrier. Tight junctions between ependymal cells form the blood–cerebrospinal fluid (CSF) barrier of the choroid plexus and delimit the circumventricular organs, areas of the brain where the endothelial barrier is deficient. These barriers present to circulating substances a continuous cell membrane. This prevents the formation of a plasma ultrafiltrate and, thus, the entry of circulating materials, including peptides and proteins, as well as glucose, amino acids, electrolytes, minerals, and others, into the brain by this route.

Substances enter the brain by one of three mechanisms. First, a residual leakiness of the BBB is demonstrated by the fact that a small amount of albumin does enter the CNS. The concentration of albumin in the CSF is only 0.5% of that found in serum and the entry rate of albumin into the brain is about 10^{-5} to 10^{-6} ml/g · min. This rate is about 100,000 times less than that of water, which easily permeates the BBB. Although leakage may occur because the endothelial and ependymal barriers are not absolute, evidence has shown that a major site of entry for circulating proteins into the CNS occurs through blood vessels at the pial surface (4). As will be discussed below, the rate of entry of peptides and at least some cytokines is too great to be accounted for only by leakage.

Second, substances may diffuse across the cell membranes that comprise the BBB. Some substances may be able to diffuse across the tight junctions, behind the tight junction by way of the inner leaflet, or from the lumenal membrane through the cytoplasm to the ablumenal leaflet and so into the CSF/interstitial fluid. Lipid solubility is a key determinant in passage by this route, but other characteristics of the compound, such as ionization, molecular weight, the tendency to form electroneutral complexes, and structure (5), also affect permeability. Many peptides appear to cross the BBB primarily by this route, which will be referred to here as transmembrane diffusion (6).

Third, substances may be transported across the BBB by saturable transport or carrier systems. As in other cell membranes, the systems in the BBB are highly selective for their ligands and may be uni- or bidirectional. Transport systems for amino acids and glucose are classic examples, but systems for electrolytes, minerals, nucleic acids, anions, vitamins, organic acids, and many other substances have been described. In general, substances for which transport systems exist are water-soluble compounds needed by the brain for homeostasis and metabolism. Some substances are transported into the CNS, others out of the CNS into the circulation, and still others bidirectionally. The discovery of transport systems for regulatory peptides and proteins that are modified by physiological, pathological, and pharmacological events suggests that the BBB may also play a role in brain–body communication (7). The finding of a saturable transport system for the interleukins (8, 9) suggests that they may participate in this form of interaction.

Despite low lipid solubility, moderately high molecular weights, and rapid degradation by circulating enzymes, some regulatory peptides have been shown to cross the BBB by transmembrane diffusion and some by saturable transport systems. Although entry rates are modest, about 10^{-2} to 10^{-3} those of glucose and amino acids and 10^2 faster than albumin, numerous examples now exist that show that a specific effect on the CNS of a peripherally administered peptide is due to its action directly on the brain after its passage across the BBB (7). This has served as a reminder that both potency and permeability must be considered in deciding whether the degree to which a substance crosses the BBB is relevant. In comparison with peptides, cytokines generally are potent substances, have a similar lipid solubility, higher molecular weights, and less susceptibility to enzymatic degradation. It is reasonable, therefore, to investigate the possibility that they might cross the BBB to a significant extent.

Questions Relevant to Passage of Cytokines across the Blood–Brain Barrier

Our laboratory has used several methods to address the following specific questions relevant to the passage of cytokines across the BBB. Do cytokines cross the BBB in the direction of the blood to CNS or the direction of CNS to blood? Is entry by leakage, transmembrane diffusion, or saturable transport? Is the amount of cytokine crossing the BBB large enough to be biologically relevant? What regions of the brain are accessible to peripherally administered cytokines? Do cytokines enter as intact molecules? Do cytokines disrupt the BBB? We will describe specific methods used in our laboratory to address these questions regarding the interleukins.

Passage across the Blood–Brain Barrier

The method used to study the brain-to-blood passage of cytokines was developed for peptides, but it has been applied to other compounds. It is an easily performed method that quantifies the amount of substance entering the circulation from the CNS. Because it has been previously reviewed in a related series (10), it will not be further discussed here. Its application to human interleukin 1α (IL-1α), murine IL-1α, and murine IL-1β shows that these cytokines all exit the CNS after intraventricular administration (9, 11). However, no saturable component has been detected (11). This suggests that the CNS-to-blood passage of these compounds occurs with the reabsorption of CSF.

Several methods now exist that are sensitive enough to detect low rates of passage from the blood into the CNS. As with any menu of techniques, they each have relative advantages and disadvantages. The techniques developed by Takasato et al. (12) and Zlokovič et al. (13) involve perfusion of the brain through the carotid artery. They therefore allow the investigator to deliver to the brain a known concentration of substance in a defined medium. They obviate the need for considerations of such variables as volume of distribution, half-time disappearance from the blood, degradation by blood and peripheral tissues, binding by serum proteins, and the effect of endogenous ligand on estimates of transport kinetics. This allows a relatively pure investigation of the BBB–ligand interaction.

Another procedure is the multiple time regression analysis method, as developed by Patlak et al. (14) and others (15–17) and as applied by Blasberg (18), that measures the unidirectional influx constant after intravenous injection. The relative stability of cytokines in the circulation makes this an ideal method for these substances. This much easier technique does not require a great deal of surgical preparation and, as an *in vivo* rather than an *in situ* method, can be used to study a wider range of altered physiological states. The method has been widely applied to various substances, tissues, and species, including humans (in a variation of the technique that relies on external detection of signal rather than removal of brain tissue).

The rationale of this method is straightforward. If a new substance were introduced into the blood and maintained at a constant concentration, its rate of accumulation by brain tissue would be linear with regard to time until equilibrium between brain and blood was approached. This unidirectional influx could be quantified by measuring the change in the brain-to-blood ratio over time. Unfortunately, it is difficult both to instantly achieve and to subsequently maintain constant concentrations of exogenous substances in the blood. After being injected intravenously, for example, most substances show continuously decreasing concentrations in the blood.

Multiple time regression analysis relies on a mathematical procedure that is also straightforward. This procedure corrects for the change in the concentration of the substance in blood over time, thus effectively reexpressing the data as if a steady state in blood existed. This new expression, termed exposure time, is calculated for each actual experimental time (t) in a two-step process. First, for the relationship of concentration in blood vs experimental time, the area under the curve is found for the period from time 0 to time t. Second, this value is divided by the concentration in blood for time t. For substances for which the relationship between the log(blood concentra-

tion) vs experimental time is linear,

$$\text{Exposure time} = (t)10^{(-at/2)} \tag{1}$$

where t is experimental time and a is the slope of the line for the relationship between log(blood concentration) and experimental time:

$$\text{log(blood concentration)} = a(t) + y \text{ intercept} \tag{2}$$

The brain-to-blood ratio is calculated for each experimental time, and this is plotted against its exposure time. The slope of the linear portion of this curve is taken as a measure of K_i, the unidirectional influx constant for that compound. Deviation from this linearity toward a flatter curve at later times indicates that brain and blood are approaching equilibrium. This area, therefore, no longer represents a relatively pure influx phase and so is excluded from analysis.

The experimental design for this method, as we have applied it to cytokines, is also straightforward. Anesthetized mice or rats are injected intravenously with radioactively labeled material. Arterial whole blood and brain samples are collected at various times, and the levels of radioactivity are measured for a known volume of serum and a known weight of whole brain or brain part. The times of collection will vary as a function of the rate of entry, the duration of the unidirectional influx phase, and the stability of the material in the circulation. For cytokines, a typical time course for collection of samples might be 2, 5, 10, 20, 30, 45, and 60 min after intravenous injection, with as few as one or two animals being studied per time point. For human IL-1α, a relatively pure unidirectional influx phase has been measured to just over 150 min of exposure time (11), or about 90 min of experimental time. The K_i (when expressed in ml/g · min), has been in the $0.2–1.3 \times 10^{-3}$ range for the cytokines measured so far. A literal interpretation of a rate of 10^{-3} ml/g · min would state that the equivalent amount of cytokine found in 1.0 μl of arterial serum enters each gram of brain every minute.

We express the brain-to-blood ratio in units of milliliters per gram instead of grams per milliliter, for reasons outlined below.

Brain-to-blood ratio
        = (cpm/g of brain)/(cpm/ml of blood)   (rearrange)
        = (cpm)(ml of blood)/(cpm)(g of brain)   (cpm units cancel)
        = ml/g

This method has many advantages, but there are some prerequisites for its appropriate application (14). The substance being measured must have a period when influx is dominant, as evidenced by a linear phase of the relationship of the brain-to-blood ratio vs exposure time. The substance should undergo minimal metabolic change in the blood during the study period. It is assumed that the physiological status of the animal, at least as regards those factors relevant to the permeability of the material across the BBB, does not change during the course of study. This method does not address differences in cerebral blood flow. However, the rate of entry of cytokines is so low as to not be dependent on flow rate, so that changes in cerebral blood flow are unlikely to affect the results. Most other requirements for the use of this method are easily met when tracer amounts of radioactive materials are used.

This method offers many advantages. Because ratios are used, the results are not overly sensitive to small variations in the amount of material injected, and much intraindividual variability in distribution volumes is obviated. Regression coefficients often exceed 0.9, making the method sensitive to the detection of changes among treatment groups. Because regression curves are calculated over a linear area, flexibility in the choice of time points can be exercised. Data collected over a series of times, unlike data from a single time point, can distinguish between actual passage across the BBB and vascular trapping (18). For data from a single time point, the radioactivity in a unit of brain represents both the material trapped in the vascular space and material found in brain tissue. For data from a series of times, the linear portion of the curve can be extrapolated back to time 0. This line does not pass through the origin, but intercepts the ordinate. This intercept, termed V_i, is an estimate of those spaces that rapidly and reversibly come into equilibrium with the circulation. This includes, but is not limited to, the vascular space of the brain. The V_i also reflects those nonvascular components that are in rapid and reversible equilibrium with the vascular space and may include sequestration by the endothelial or ependymal cells, association with the pia–glial vessels, or binding to endothelial receptors. This leaves the slope, or K_i, largely representing material that has completely crossed the BBB to enter actual brain tissue.

The K_i measured for human IL-1α by this method has ranged from $2.36–4.27 \times 10^{-4}$ ml/g · min (8, 9, 11), about 20 times higher than the K_i simultaneously measured for albumin ($0.9–2.5 \times 10^{-5}$ ml/g · min). Both IL-1α and IL-1β are each about one-fourth the molecular weight of albumin and, because permeability is related to the inverse square of molecular weight, the IL-1s would be predicted to cross the BBB only about twice as fast as albumin. The much higher entry rate, therefore, suggests that human IL-1α does not cross by leakage or by transmembrane diffusion. This is further

supported by the finding that despite similar molecular weights, murine IL-1β crosses about 40% faster and murine IL-1α about 4.5 times faster than human IL-1α.

Measurement of Saturability

The question of saturability can be addressed directly by inclusion of various doses of unlabeled cytokine with the radioactively labeled material. Dose-inhibition curves have shown that a dose of 29.7 μg of human IL-1α/kg is needed to inhibit the K_i of radioactively iodinated human IL-1α, whereas only 63.7 ng of murine IL-1α/kg is needed to produce a 50% self-inhibition, and 43.8 ng/kg is needed to self-inhibit the K_i of murine IL-1β by 50% (9). This shows that these three compounds all enter the CNS by saturable transport. Cross-inhibition can also be tested by this method. It was found that a 10-μg/kg dose of any one of these three cytokines will inhibit the entry rate of either of the other two (9). This shows that these cytokines either share a single transport system or a family of systems with overlapping affinities rather than having three totally separate transport systems.

Amount of Cytokine Entering the Brain

The percentage of the intravenous injection that actually enters the CNS can be calculated by correction of brain-to-blood ratios for vascular content. Correction for the vascular space may be accomplished either by measurement of the space with a vascular marker, such as albumin, or by use of the V_i for the compound. Because the V_i is usually higher than the albumin space, this represents a more conservative estimate. For example, correction by use of the albumin space shows that about 0.08% of the dose of radioactively iodinated human IL-1α injected intravenously enters the brain; correction with the V_i places the estimate closer to 0.05%. Because only about 1/1000 to 1/3000 of the intravenous (iv) dose of IL-1α or IL-1β is needed when given intracerebroventricularly (icv) to elicit temperature and gastric acid secretion responses (19, 20), the calculated amount of entry is sufficient to explain these central actions after peripheral administration. This suggests that these effects of peripherally administered interleukins occur because of a direct effect on the CNS induced by cytokines that have crossed the BBB.

Calculation of the K_i and of the percentage of injection entering the brain are complementary. The K_i, derived from the brain-to-blood ratios and exposure times, is independent of half-time disappearance from the blood and volume of distribution. By contrast, the calculation of the percentage of injection

entering the brain is affected by both of these factors. For two compounds with identical K_i values, a larger percentage of the injected dose of the compound with the longer half-time disappearance and smaller volume of distribution will enter the brain. The K_i, therefore, may be more useful in physiological studies, in which one wishes to calculate the amount of endogenous circulating cytokine available to the brain. The percentage entering the brain may be more useful in pharmacological studies, in which the experimental design involves peripheral injection of a known dose.

Brain Distribution of Peripherally Administered Cytokines

The K_i values for brain regions may also be determined by dissecting the brain into the regions that need to be assessed, weighing them, and plotting the brain-to-blood ratio against the exposure time (11). We found that the K_i values for human IL-1α ranged from 0.69×10^{-4} ml/g·min for midbrain to 1.28×10^{-4} ml/g·min for the hypothalamus in the rat. However, the hypothalamus accounted for only about 2% of the total amount of human IL-1α entering the brain, whereas the cortex accounted for about 40%. The widespread appearance of human IL-1α during a short period of time suggests that cytokines derived from the circulation may be able to directly affect brain function at multiple sites. It also shows that entry does not occur exclusively at the circumventricular organs (CVOs) or at any other single site, because material entering there would be confined to that region by the ependymal barrier delimiting it and by limitations in the rate of diffusion within the CNS.

Entry of Intact Material

Peptides and proteins, including cytokines, are susceptible to enzymatic degradation. Therefore, it must be determined whether the radioactive material entering the brain after intravenous injection represents the cytokine that was injected rather than a degradation product.

An initial indication of the integrity of the injected cytokine can be assessed by extraction of the radioactive material from the brain and determination of whether it can still be precipitated with acid. More than 95% of radioactively labeled human IL-1α can be precipitated with acid and a decrease from this level indicates degradation to nonprecipitable or less precipitable forms. Precipitation by acid does not assure that the radioactively labeled material is still attached to the intact cytokine, only that it is still attached to a protein large enough to be precipitated.

Therefore more sophisticated methods, such as high-performance liquid chromatography (HPLC), are usually needed. Brains are first cleared of the contents of their vascular space by clamping of the abdominal aorta and perfusion of the left ventricle with lactated Ringer's solution for about 1 min. This removes well over 90% of the blood from the brain, so that the remaining radioactivity is almost exclusively in the brain. We usually have extracted radioactivity from homogenized brains or blood with ammonium acetate or with sodium hydroxide (8, 9). Much of the degradation occurring in brain tissues takes place during homogenization, when intracellular enzymes are released. Therefore tissue controls consisting of the *in vitro* addition of radioactive cytokine to brain tissue before homogenization should also be analyzed and results expressed relative to these. The results with radioiodinated human IL-1α indicate that 10 min after intravenous injection, 100% of the radioactivity in the brain elutes by HPLC as intact interleukin. Thirty minutes after intravenous injection, about 30–40% of the radioactivity found in the brain and about 100% of the radioactivity circulating in the blood elutes as intact cytokine.

Cytokines and Disruption of the Blood–Brain Barrier

Several reports have indicated that cytokines can disrupt the BBB. Interleukin 2 has been found to disrupt the BBB as early as 1 hr after a single intravenous injection of 100,000 units/kg (21). Other studies examining longer periods or multiple doses have tended to confirm these results (22, 23). However, in each of these studies detecting disruption of the BBB after administration of IL-2, disruption was also found in control animals that received vehicle devoid of IL-2. Because any disruption of the BBB would be abnormal in the control animals, it is probable that some contaminant in the vehicle was responsible for the disruption. All studies that have found disruption relied on a single supply that included the biological detergent sodium dodecyl sulfate (SDS) in the IL-2 and vehicle. Kobiler *et al.* (24) have shown that SDS in doses one-fourth of that found in the vehicle of the above studies causes disruption of the BBB in amounts large enough to allow the passage of viral particles into the brain.

The above studies usually relied on methods that could not quantify the degree of BBB disruption, such as the detection by electron microscopy of particles of horseradish peroxidase. We reexamined this question, using IL-2 that was free of SDS and measuring brain-to-blood ratios of the vascular marker albumin, a substance traditionally used to measure disruption of the BBB. In addition, these brain-to-blood ratios were expressed relative to exposure time with the multiple time regression analysis method described above. Because the previous studies had indicated that disruption occurred at least as early as 1 hr after injection and was long lasting, increased sensitivity to any disruption as well as its quantification might be achieved by time series analysis. However, no disruption was caused by IL-2, IL-1α, or IL-1β in doses equal to or higher than those previously tested (8, 9, 25). Interleukin 2 was also given icv, but still no disruption was detected in either the direction of brain to blood or blood to brain. The BBB was then reversibly disrupted with intravenous epinephrine by a standardized method, but IL-2 was not shown either to enhance or prolong this damage (25). These results supported the conclusion of Kobiler *et al.* (24) that SDS, not IL-2, was the cause of the disruption of the BBB.

Conclusions

Simple, but powerful and highly sensitive, techniques exist for the examination of the ability of cytokines to cross the BBB. A method for quantifying brain-to-blood passage, previously reviewed, has been applied to cytokines. We have concentrated here on describing a versatile technique that can be applied to the study of the blood-to-brain passage of cytokines and have illustrated it with our work with human IL-1α, murine IL-1α, murine IL-1β, and human IL-2. Application of variations of this method combined with HPLC and administration of vascular markers has shown that IL-1α and IL-1β cross the BBB by a saturable transport system as intact molecules in amounts sufficient to induce effects on the CNS. The two cytokines each inhibit the entry of the other and so are not transported by two completely distinct systems, but either by a single system or systems with overlapping affinities. Human IL-1α enters all regions of the brain examined, with less than a twofold variation in the transport rate. Contrary to earlier studies, IL-1α, IL-1β, or IL-2 did not disrupt the BBB or enhance epinephrine-induced damage to the BBB.

These methods should be generally applicable to cytokines. The resulting information should facilitate further understanding of the interactions between the immune and central nervous systems.

References

1. H. Davson, K. Welch, and M. B. Segal, "The Physiology and Pathophysiology of the Cerebrospinal Fluid." Churchill-Livingstone, London, 1987.
2. W. M. Pardridge and L. J. Mietus, *Endocrinology (Baltimore)* **109,** 1138 (1981).

3. M. Bradbury, "The Concept of a Blood–Brain Barrier." Wiley, New York, 1979.

4. R. D. Broadwell, *Acta Neuropathol.* **79,** 117 (1989).

5. S. I. Rapoport, "Blood–Brain Barrier in Physiology and Medicine." Raven Press, New York, 1976.

6. W. A. Banks and A. J. Kastin, *Psychoneuroendocrinology* **10,** 385 (1985).

7. W. A. Banks and A. J. Kastin, *Am. J. Physiol.* **259,** E1 (1990).

8. W. A. Banks and A. J. Kastin, *Life Sci.* **48,** PL117 (1991).

9. W. A. Banks, L. Ortiz, S. R. Plotkin, and A. J. Kastin, *J. Pharmacol. Exp. Ther.* **259,** 988 (1991).

10. W. A. Banks and A. J. Kastin, *in* "Methods in Enzymology" (P. Conn, ed.), Vol. 168, p. 652. Academic Press, San Diego.

11. W. A. Banks, A. J. Kastin, and D. A. Durham, *Brain Res. Bull.* **23,** 433 (1989).

12. Y. Takasato, S. I. Rapoport, and Q. R. Smith, *Am. J. Physiol.* **247,** H484 (1984).

13. B. V. Zlokovič, D. J. Begley, B. M. Djuricič, and D. M. Mitrovič, *J. Neurochem.* **46,** 1444 (1986).

14. C. S. Patlak, R. G. Blasberg, and J. D. Fenstermacher, *J. Cereb. Blood Flow Metab.* **3,** 1 (1983).

15. A. Gjedde and M. Rasmussen, *J. Neurochem.* **35,** 1463 (1981).

16. K. Go and J. J. Pratt, *Brain Res.* **93,** 329 (1975).

17. M. W. B. Bradbury and C. R. Kleeman, *Am. J. Physiol.* **213,** 519 (1967).

18. R. G. Blasberg, J. D. Fenstermacher, and C. S. Patlak, *J. Cereb. Blood Flow Metab.* **3,** 8 (1983).

19. M. Hashimoto, T. Bando, M. Iriki, and K. Hashimoto, *Am. J. Physiol.* **255,** R527 (1988).

20. E. S. Saperas, H. Yang, C. Rivier, and Y. Tache, *Gastroenterology* **99,** 1599 (1990).

21. M. D. Ellison, J. T. Povlishock, and R. E. Merchant, *Cancer Res.* **47,** 5765 (1987).

22. R. G. Watts, J. L. Wright, L. L. Atkinson, and R. E. Merchant, *Neurosurgery* **25,** 202 (1989).

23. M. D. Ellison, R. J. Krieg, and J. T. Povlishock, *J. Neuroimmunol.* **28,** 249 (1990).

24. D. Kobiler, S. Lustig, Y. Gozes, D. Ben-Nathan, and Y. Akov, *Brain Res.* **496,** 314 (1989).

25. W. A. Banks and A. J. Kastin, *Int. J. Immunopharmacol.* **14,** 629 (1992).

Section II

Anatomical Localization Studies

[5] *In Situ* Hybridization Techniques for Localization of Interleukin 1 and Interleukin 1 Receptor Antagonist mRNA in Brain

Ma-Li Wong, Philip W. Gold, and Júlio Licinio

Introduction

The method of choice for studying the distribution and density of particular messenger RNA (mRNA) in small anatomical and heterogeneous tissues is *in situ* hybridization histochemistry (ISHH) (1–4). The brain is anatomically complex, and adjacent brain regions can express many different genes; therefore the ISHH approach is a powerful tool for the localization of interleukin mRNA in the brain, because single-cell resolution can easily be obtained. Single-cell resolution is not possible with solution or Northern blot hybridization (5). In ISHH labeled complementary DNA (cDNA) or RNA (cRNA) probes form hybrids with a specific cellular mRNA, and the hybrids are visualized by autoradiography. High sensitivity and unique resolution are the advantages of the ISHH technique. It is also important to note the limitations of this technique: the careful user is alert for changes in hybridization specificity and in accessibility to hybridization probes to target tissue due to nonconstant diffusion in tissue sections (2, 6).

Interleukin 1 (IL-1) is an inflammatory peptide hormone with potent neuroendocrine effects. Interleukin 1 acts centrally to stimulate the release of growth hormone, thyroid-stimulating hormone (TSH) (7), and somatostatin (8). Interleukin 1 inhibits the secretion of prolactin (7) and luteinizing hormone (9). Because of the important role of IL-1 in inflammatory processes, there has been an interest in compounds that antagonize IL-1 action (10–12). Two new interleukin 1 receptor antagonists have been purified, characterized, and cloned. Interleukin 1 receptor antagonist (IL-1ra) is a pure endogenous antagonist of IL-1 (13, 14).

Three main classes of probe are in current use: complementary DNA (cDNA), RNA probes (riboprobes or cRNA), and oligonucleotide probes. Probes may be synthesized by vector systems, chemically, or with a combination of synthetic and enzymatic approaches (6, 15). Probes are generally selected because of high specificity to the target mRNA, and low homology to ribosomal RNA to reduce nonspecific binding. Table I lists some of the characteristics of each type of probe (16). Oligonucleotide probes have been used in ISHH studies to localize IL-1 (cRNA) (17) and IL-1ra (cDNA) (18).

Several protocols can be successfully used for ISHH. Interestingly, the protocols used in localizing IL-1 and IL-1ra present several differences that are detailed in the following paragraphs.

General Considerations about *in Situ* Hybridization Histochemistry

1. Special care should be taken to avoid RNase contamination of tissues and reagents.

2. Gloves should be worn throughout the procedures to prevent contamination by ribonucleases from fingertips.

3. Diethylpyrocarbonate-treated water (DEPC-H_2O) (0.1%) is used to make most of the solutions for ISHH:

DEPC (Sigma, St. Louis, MO)   1 ml
Distilled H_2O 1000 ml

The solution is mixed vigorously, allowed to stand in a fume hood overnight, and autoclaved to inactivate the remaining DEPC. Solutions used for ISHH are made up in DEPC-H_2O and autoclaved or filtered. The DEPC inhibits RNases.

TABLE I   Types of *in Situ* Hybridization Probes[a]

Probe type	Advantages	Disadvantages
cDNA	Ease of use High specific activity	Reannealing in solution Double stranded Familiarity with molecular biology required Vector sequences might be present
cRNA	Single stranded Stable hybrids High specific activity	Probe "stickiness" Familiarity with molecular biology required Presence of vector sequences
Oligonucleotide	Single stranded Ease of use Good tissue penetration Customized probes	Less stable hybrids Access to DNA synthesizer required for continued supply of the probe

[a] Table modified from Ref. 16 [In Situ *Hybridization, Applications to Neurobiology* (K. L. Valentino, J. H. Eberwine, and J. D. Barchas, eds.). © Oxford Univ. Press, 1987].

In Situ Hybridization Histochemistry Study on the Localization of IL-1

Bandtlow *et al.* (17) have localized IL-1β by a technique that requires brain perfusion and postfixation treatments, and radiolabeled oligonucleotide cRNA probes (Figs. 1–3). They have applied a variation of the protocols detailed below.

Brain Removal, Sectioning, and Tissue Preparation

Animals are intracardiacally perfused with a combined paraformaldehyde and phosphate buffer. Although fixation by perfusion provides better preservation of morphological integrity, it may increase background signal present in tissue (19).

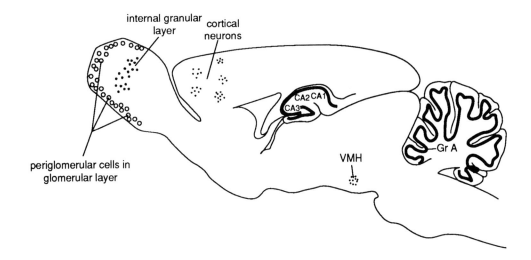

FIG. 1   Schematic presentation of the localization of IL-1β mRNA in the adult rat brain. The sites of synthesis are dotted and represent the hippocampus (CA1–CA3), cerebellar granule cells (GrA), granule and periglomerular cells of the olfactory bulb, neurons in the frontal cortex, and neurons of the ventromedial hypothalamus (VMH). Not shown are hybridizations of IL-1β mRNA in the striatum and septum. Abbreviations and drawings after Pellegrino *et al.* (1979). [Reproduced from Ref. 17 (*Journal of Cell Biology*, 1990, **111**, 1701–1711) by Copyright permission of the Rockefeller University Press.]

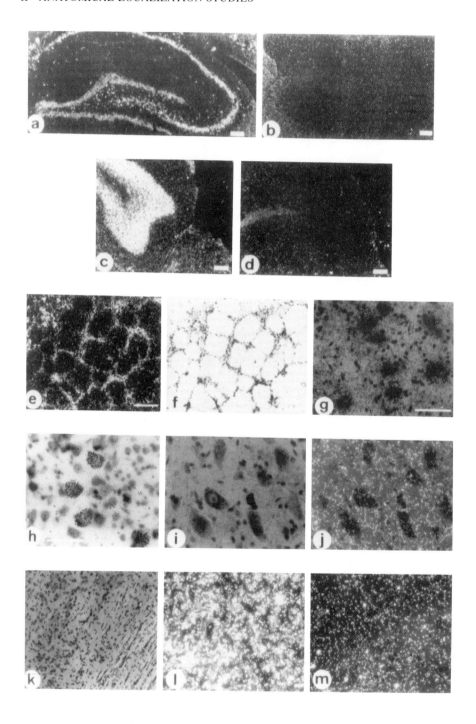

Solutions for Perfusion and Postfixation

   Depolymerized paraformaldehyde (4%) for perfusion: Combine 40 g of
      paraformaldehyde powder, 22.6 g of NaH_2PO_4, and 25.2 g of NaOH;
      adjust final volume to 1000 ml with distilled H_2O, and adjust pH to
      7.3; heat solution to 65°C and add drops of 10 N NaOH until solution
      clears. Let solution cool before use
   Phosphate-buffered saline (PBS) (10×): Combine 90 g of NaCl, 1.22 g
      of KH_2PO_4, and 8.15 g of Na_2PO_4; adjust final volume to 1000 ml
      with distilled H_2O, and adjust pH to 7.4. (To make 1× PBS, dilute
      100 ml of 10× PBS in 900 ml of distilled H_2O)
   Sucrose medium: Combine the following:

Sucrose (0.32 M)	75 ml
Na_2HPO_4 (0.2 M)	23.1 ml
NaH_2PO_4 (0.2 M)	6.9 ml
Distilled H_2O	20 ml

Perfusion

   1. Anesthesia: Ether or pentobarbital [50–60 mg/kg, intraperitoneal (ip)]
is commonly used.
   2. Rapidly expose the heart. Make a small incision in the left ventricle
near the apex with iris scissors. Thread a 15-gauge cannula through the left
ventricle to the aortic root, taking care not to rupture the intraventricular
septum. Cut the right atrium. Perfuse with PBS for about 20 sec and perfuse
with paraformaldehyde to ~1 cm^3/g body weight.

FIG. 2 Results from *in situ* hybridization of rat brain sagittal sections to IL-1/40
riboprobes. Positive IL-1β hybridizations are shown for the hippocampus (a), the
granule cells of the cerebellum (c), periglomerular cells of the olfactory bulb (e) with
corresponding phase-contrast photomicrograph (f), neurons of the hypothalamus (g),
and neurons of the frontal cortex (h). No specific labeling is seen on sections hybridized with the sense IL-1/40⁻ probe (b and d). Positive labeling is also shown over
glial cells in the septum (j) and striatum (l), with corresponding phase-contrast pictures
(i and k). Background labeling is shown of a section through the striatum hybridized
with the sense IL-1/40⁻ riboprobe (m). All sections were counterstained with cresyl
violet. Exposure time was 5.5 weeks at 4°C. Bars: 1 mm (a–d); 50 μm (e–m). [Repro-
duced from Ref. 17 (*Journal of Cell Biology*, 1990, **111**, 1701–1711) by Copyright
permission of the Rockefeller University Press.]

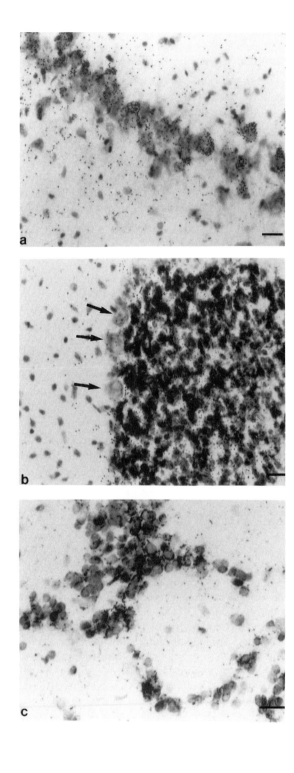

Postfixation/Cryoprotection

Clearing of residual fixative from tissue and some protection against ice artifact formation that occurs during tissue freezing is accomplished in this part of the protocol.

Brains are immersed in fixative (paraformaldehyde solution could be used) for 2 hr at 4°C. Brains are then transferred to sucrose medium for 30 min at 4°C for cryoprotection. Tissues are rapidly frozen in powdered dry ice, and stored at $-70°C$ until use.

Glass Slide Coating: Poly-L-lysine (20)

This coating can also be used in immunohistochemistry studies.

1. Acid clean (Chromerge PGC Scientific, Gaithersburg, MD) microscopic slides for 2–4 hr. This can be done in coplin jars in which slides are placed diagonally and then washed under running water for 4 hr. Rinse the slides well in distilled H_2O.

2. Prepare a poly-D-lysine (Sigma) working solution (0.01%) for coating the slides. This can be made by diluting 1 ml of a stock solution of 100 mg/ml (add 5 ml of distilled H_2O to 500 mg of poly-D-lysine) in 1 liter of distilled H_2O. Stock and working solutions should be stored at $-20°C$.

3. Soak the slides in the working polylysine solution for 30–60 min, then rinse well in distilled H_2O and dry the slides at 37°C overnight.

Sectioning

Frozen tissues can be mounted in cryostat chucks and frozen sectioned.

1. Cryostat sectioning: Section tissue at $-20°C$ (10–20 μm in thickness) and thaw-mount sections on slides. Slides may be dried on a slide warmer at 37–40°C for a few minutes. Store the tissue sections at $-70°C$ until use.

2. Slides can be pretreated to minimize nonspecific "sticking" of probes to the slides, and maximize section retention on the slides through the rigorous treatments involved in ISHH.

FIG. 3   Higher magnifications of the positive IL-1β mRNA hybridization signals found over granule cells of the dentate gyrus (a), the cerebellum (b), and the periglomerular cells of the olfactory bulb (c), indicating a differential expression of the IL-1β mRNA. Note that Purkinje cells (arrows) in the cerebellum are not labeled (b). Exposure time was 4 weeks at 4°C. Bar: 100 μm. [Reproduced from Ref. 17 (*Journal of Cell Biology*, 1990, **111,** 1701–1711) by Copyright permission of the Rockefeller University Press.]

3. Solutions for pretreatment of slides are as follows:

Denhardt's solution (20×): Combine 4 g of Ficoll, 4 g of polyvinylpyrroli-
done, and 4 g of bovine serum albumin (BSA); adjust the final volume
to 1000 ml with distilled H_2O, heat and stir the solution until dissolved,
and store at $-20°C$ in aliquots. (To make 1× Denhardt's, dilute 50
ml of 20× Denhardt's solution in 950 ml of DEPC-H_2O)
Fix solution

| Ethanol (95%) | 300 ml |
| Glacial acetic acid | 100 ml |

Acetylation solution (0.1 M triethanolamine): To 74.26 ml of triethanolamine, add DEPC-H_2O to a final volume of 4000 ml; adjust pH
to 8.0; immediately before use add 10 ml of acetic anhydride and
mix vigorously
Ethanol solutions (50, 70, 90, 95, and 100%): Make with DEPC-H_2O
Hydrochloric acid (0.2 M): To 16.6 ml of concentrated HCl, add DEPC-
H_2O to a final volume of 1000 ml

4. Proteinase K working solution: Prepare the following three solutions:

Proteinase K stock solution: Combine 2.5 mg of proteinase K; add 1 ml
of 10 mM Tris solution, pH 7.7 (see below); store in 1-ml aliquots at
$-20°C$. Prior to use incubate for 30 min at 37°C to predigest RNase
Tris (10 mM): Dissolve Tris (1.476 g/liter); adjust pH to 7.7
$CaCl_2$ (2 mM): Dissolve 0.294 g/liter

Proteinase K working solution is prepared by combining stock proteinase K
(400 μg/liter; final concentration, 1 μg/ml), 10 mM Tris (82 ml/liter), and 2
mM $CaCl_2$. This solution should have a pH of 7.4 at 37°C.
  5. Slice pretreatment: Place the slides in glass staining trays, add a solution
of 1× Denhardt's, and incubate 1–3 hr at 65°C. Dip the slides in DEPC-
H_2O once and incubate in fix solution for 20 min at room temperature. Air
dry thoroughly.
  6. Acetylation of slides following Denhardt's treatment: Place the slides
in glass staining trays, add acetylation solution, and incubate for 10 min at
room temperature. Dehydrate the slides by dipping them consecutively for
5 min in solutions of 50, 70, 95, and 100% ethanol. Air dry thoroughly.
  7. Optional tissue pretreatments can also be used to enhance probe access
to mRNA, because of the increased ability of the probe to penetrate through
deproteinized membranes, and reduced interference with hybridization from

nascent polypeptide chains that were being translated. Hydrochloric acid and proteinase K pretreatments can be employed.

a. Hydrochloric acid (HCl) (21): Sections are dried at room temperature; slides are then washed in 0.2 *M* HCl (16.6 ml of concentrated HCl per liter) for 20 min at room temperature and washed in DEPC-H$_2$O.

b. Proteinase K pretreatment (21): Sections are dipped in a working proteinase K solution and incubated for 15 min at 37°C. Dehydrate the sections by dipping them twice in DEPC-H$_2$O and then washing them consecutively for 5 min in solutions of 70, 70, and 90% ethanol. Air dry thoroughly.

Probe Synthesis

Bandtlow *et al.* (17) subcloned a synthetic 40-base oligonucleotide specific for IL-1β in the Bluescript vector (Stratagene, La Jolla, CA). *In vitro* single-stranded cRNA ^{35}S-labeled antisense and sense probes were made. For transcription of the antisense and sense probes, the vector was linearized with appropriated restriction enzymes and transcribed from the T7 and T3 promoters with the riboprobe system (Promega Biotech, Madison, WI) according to the instructions of the manufacturer. Detailed protocols can also be found in molecular biology manuals (22, 23). Following digestion of the DNA template with DNase 1 (1 unit/μg DNA), carrier tRNA (0.25 μg/ml) is added. The cRNa probes can be then purified with phenol–chloroform–isoamyl alcohol (50 : 49 : 1) and precipitated with ammonium acetate–ethanol (24). The labeled probes are then resuspended in 100 μl of 10 m*M* Tris-HCl (pH 7.4), 0.1 m*M* ethylenediaminetetraacetic acid (EDTA), and 10 m*M* dithiothreitol (DTT).

Hybridization

Hybridization incubations can be carried out in covered, clear, polystyrene boxes (tissue culture dishes, 245 × 245 × 20 mm; VSA/Scientific Plastics, Ocala, FL), with a sheet of Whatman (Clifton, NJ) 3MM filter paper saturated with 4× sodium chloride, sodium citrate (SSC) (1× SSC is 0.15 *M* NaCl and 15 m*M* sodium citrate, pH 7.2)/50% formamide in the bottom of the box (25, 26). An optional prehybridization step with 1× hybridization buffer can be performed if desired.

1. Hybridization buffer (26, 27): Stock solution of 2× hybridization buffer can be stored frozen until use. Ingredients listed in tabulation below are sterile stock solutions, amount of stock solution for 5 ml of 2× hybridization buffer, and reagent concentration in 2× buffer, respectively.

Sterile stock solution	Amount[a]	Final concentration
NaCl (5 M)	1.2 ml	1.2 M
Tris-HCl, pH 7.5 (1 M)	100 μl	20 mM
Ficoll (6%)	33 μl	0.04%
BSA (fraction V) (6%)	33 μl	0.04%
Polyvinylpyrrolidone (6%)	33 μl	0.04%
EDTA, pH 8.0 (0.5 M)	20 μl	2 mM
Denatured DNA (10 mg/ml)	100 μl	0.02%
Total yeast RNA (20 mg/ml)	250 μl	0.10% (type XI; Sigma)
Yeast RNA (50 mg/ml)	10 μl	0.01%
Dextran sulfate (50%)	2 ml	20% (M_r 500,000)

[a] Adjust final volume to 5 ml with DEPC-H$_2$O.

Working 1× hybridization buffer is made by thawing, briefly heat denaturing at 85°C for 5–10 min, and mixing the stock solution in 5 ml of formamide, 0.1% sodium dodecyl sulfate (SDS) (10% stock solution), 0.1% sodium thiosulfate (10% stock solution), and 100 mM DTT (5 M stock solution).

2. Radiolabeled probe (3–5 × 10^5 cpm/25 μl of hybridization buffer) should be used. The probe is then heat denatured. Approximately 50 μl of hybridization buffer is applied around each section with a Pipetman, taking care not to introduce bubbles. A glass coverslip (24 × 50 mm) is placed on the tissue section. Each hybridization box is then covered and incubated overnight at 50°C; incubation should be carried out in a humidified chamber, which could be achieved by placing a container with water together with the hybridization boxes.

RNase Treatment

1. Prepare the following solutions.

Stock solution of 20× sodium chloride, sodium citrate (SSC): Dissolve 175.3 g of NaCl and 88.2 g of sodium citrate in 800 ml of distilled H$_2$O; adjust pH to 7.0 with 1 M HCl; adjust final volume to 1000 ml with distilled H$_2$O, and autoclave. Working SSC solutions are made by diluting the stock solution with DEPC-H$_2$O
RNase buffer:

NaCl (5 M)	100 ml (final concentration, 0.5 M)
Tris-HCl, pH 8.0 (1 M)	10 ml (final concentration, 10 mM)
EDTA, pH 8.0 (0.5 M)	2 ml (final concentration, 1 mM)

adjust final volume to 1000 ml with distilled H$_2$O

RNase A stock solution: Stock solution of RNase A (10 mg/ml) in RNase buffer is prepared, aliquoted, and stored frozen until use (22). The stock solution is diluted to 20 μg/ml in RNase buffer prior to use

2. After hybridization, coverslips are float off by dipping the slides several times into a 2× SSC solution. Most of the remaining radioactive hybridization buffer is removed by dipping the slide succcessively through four 50-ml conical tubes containing 2× SSC. Slides are placed in a slide rack in glass staining dishes filled with 2× SSC, and then rinsed twice in 2× SSC at room temperature.

3. RNase treatment: Slides are incubated in the RNase A solution for 30 min at room temperature, and then incubated in the RNase buffer without RNase for 30 min.

Washing and Dehydration

1. Washing: Slides are rinsed twice in 2× SSC at room temperature, and then washed consecutively with 2× SSC/50% formamide (preequilibrated at 50°C) at 50°C (two washes, 15 min each), and 2× SSC (2 washes, 5 min each) at room temperature.

2. Dehydration: Slides are washed sequentially for 1 min each in ascending ethanol solutions of 50, 70, 90, and 95% ethanol (containing 300 m*M* ammonium acetate) and 100% ethanol. Air dry thoroughly.

Autoradiography and Tissue Staining

Autoradiography and tissue staining are detailed in the following study.

In Situ Hybridization Histochemistry Study on the Localization of IL-1 Receptor Antagonist

Licinio *et al.* (18) have localized IL-1ra by a technique described by Young (28), which is briefly described below (Fig. 4a and b and Fig. 5).

Brain Removal, Sectioning, and Tissue Preparation

Tissue preparation was performed by a method developed by Herkenham and Pert (29), using slide-mounted, frozen, unfixed tissue sections. Adult

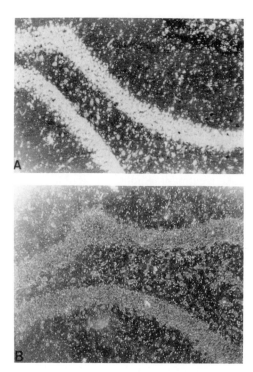

FIG. 4   (A) Dark-field photomicrograph of IL-1ra mRNA hybridized in dentate gyrus of hippocampus. (B) Dark-field photomicrograph of sense probe hybridized in dentate gyrus of hippocampus. [Reproduced from Ref. 18 (J. Licinio, M.-L. Wong, and P. W. Gold, Localization of Interleukin 1 Receptor Antagonist mRNA in Rat Brain, *Endocrinology*, 1991, **129**, 562–564) with permission. © The Endocrine Society.]

rats were sacrificed by decapitation, brains were rapidly removed and frozen by immersion in isopentane (2-methyl butane) on dry ice, and mounted onto cryostat chucks and frozen sectioned.

1. Glass slide coating ("subbing" or gelatin coating): This is a classic immunohistochemical and receptor autoradiographic slide coating for section retention.

a. Clean the microscope slides with soap, rinse them in running water to remove the detergent, place them in 80% ethanol for 1 hr, and rinse them again in distilled H_2O while preparing the gelatin solution.

b. Prepare 0.5% gelatin solution (type 1, 300 bloom from porcine skin; Sigma) and 0.05% chromium potassium sulfate (Fisher, Pittsburgh, PA).

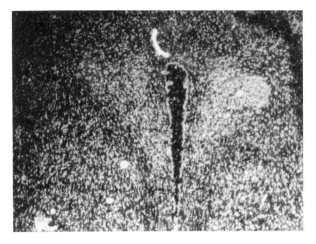

FIG. 5   Dark-field photomicrograph of IL-1ra mRNA hybridized in paraventricular nucleus. [Reproduced from Ref. 18 (J. Licinio, M.-L. Wong, and P. W. Gold, Localization of Interleukin 1 Receptor Antagonist mRNA in Rat Brain, *Endocrinology,* 1991, **129,** 562–564) with permission. © The Endocrine Society.]

Combine 3 g of gelatin with 150 ml of distilled H₂O at 50°C; stir on a hot plate until the gelatin is dissolved. Add 450 ml of distilled H₂O at room temperature to cool the solution to 30°C

Then add 0.3 g of chromium potassium sulfate and stir until it is dissolved; filter the solution through Whatman 1MM paper into a glass staining dish to remove air bubbles

Dip the cleaned slides into the gelatin solution, and let the slides dry in an 80°C oven overnight.

2. Cryostat sectioning: Section the tissue at -20°C (10–20 μm), thaw-mount the sections onto gelatin-coated slides, and dry on a slide warmer. Sections are stored at -70°C until use.

3. Tissue preparation: Prepare the following solutions.

Formaldehyde (4% in PBS)

Formaldehyde solution (100%)	106.4 ml
PBS (10×) (see below)	100 ml

adjust final volume to 1000 ml with DEPC-H₂O

Phosphate-buffered saline (PBS) ($10\times$): Combine 90 g of NaCl, 1.22 g of KH_2PO_4, and 8.15 g of Na_2PO_4; adjust the final volume to 1000 ml of distilled H_2O, pH to 7.4 and autoclave. To make $1\times$ PBS, dilute 100 ml of $10\times$ PBS in 900 ml of DEPC-H_2O

Triethanolamine-HCl (TEA-HCl), pH 8.0 (0.1 M)/NaCl (0.9%)

Stock TEA solution (7.5 M) (Sigma)	13.3 ml
HCl (6 N) (brings pH to 8.0)	6 ml
NaCl (5 M)	31 ml

adjust final volume to 1000 ml with DEPC-H_2O. This solution should be prepared fresh just prior to use

Ethanol solutions (50, 70, 95, and 100%): make with DEPC-H_2O

4. Sections are fixed in 4% formaldehyde in $1\times$ PBS (5 min), rinsed in $1\times$ PBS, rinsed in 0.1 M TEA-HCl, and treated with fresh 0.25% acetic anhydride in 0.1 M TEA-HCl solution (10 min). The slides are then rinsed twice in $2\times$ SSC.

5. Tissue dehydration and delipidation: Sections are rinsed in 70% (1 min), 80% (1 min), 95% (2 min), and 100% ethanol (1 min); they are then rinsed in 100% chloroform (5 min), and then in 100% (1 min) and 95% ethanol (1 min). Air dry thoroughly.

Probe

A 30-base antisense synthetic oligodeoxynucleotide probe for IL-1ra mRNA (14), and a sense probe were 3′ end labeled with [^{35}S]dATP ($>$1000 Ci/mmol; New England Nuclear, Boston, MA) with terminal deoxytransferase (TdT) (25 units/μl; Boehringer, Mannheim, Germany): specific activities of $4–10 \times 10^3$ Ci/mmol were obtained.

Solutions

TE (pH 8.0): Make a solution containing 10 mM Tris-HCl (pH 8.0) and 1 mM EDTA (pH 8.0)

Dithiothreitol (DTT) (1 M): Combine 3.09 g of DTT and 20 ml of 0.01 M sodium acetate (pH 5.2); sterilize by filtration and store in 1-ml aliquots at $-20°C$

Reaction

Perform the following reaction in 50 μl:

Distilled H$_2$O	30 μl
Oligodeoxynucleotide (0.1 μM)	1 μl
Tailing buffer (5$\times$)	10 μl
[^{35}S]dATP (New England Nuclear)	5 μl
TdT (Boehringer)	4 μl

Incubate the reaction for 30 min at 37°C and then add 400 μl of TE plus 2 μl of tRNA (25 mg/ml), extract with 400 μl of phenol–chloroform–IAA (50:49:1), spin in a microfuge at 15,000 rpm at room temperature for 2 min. Extract aqueous phase (top layer, which is transferred to another tube) with 400 μl of chloroform–IAA (24:1), spin for 1 min and transfer the top (aqueous) phase to a new tube. Precipitate by adding a 1/20 vol of 5 M NaCl (20 μl) plus 1 ml of ethanol, incubate on dry ice with ethanol for 30 min, and spin at 15,000 rpm at 4°C for 30 min. Discard the supernatant and wash the pellet with 1 ml of 70% ethanol (cold), redissolve the pellet in 100 μl of TE plus 1 μl of 1 M DTT, and count 1 μl (cpm/μl): 500,000 cpm/μl should be obtained.

Hybridization

Hybridization incubations are carried out in covered, clear, polystyrene boxes.

1. Prepare 1$\times$ hybridization buffer:

SSC (20$\times$)	2 ml
Formamide (100%)	5 ml
Denhardt's (20%)	0.5 ml
Ficoll (to 0.02%)	
Polyvinylpyrrolidone 360K (to 0.02%)	
BSA (to 0.02%)	
Yeast tRNA (250 mg/ml)	0.1 ml
Herring testes DNA (10 mg/ml)	0.5 ml
Dextran 500K (50%)	2 ml

2. Sections are hybridized overnight at 37°C with 2 × 10^6 cpm of probe and 2 μl of 5 M DTT/100 μl of hybridization buffer at 37°C. Approximately 25 μl (500,000 cpm) of hybridization buffer is applied to each section, taking

care not to introduce bubbles. Slides should be covered with glass coverslips or Parafilm. The hybridization box is covered and incubated in a humidified chamber.

Washing and Dehydration

Coverslips or pieces of Parafilm are floated off by dipping the slides several times in $1 \times$ SSC. The remaining radioactive buffer is removed by dipping the slides successively through four 50-ml conical tubes containing $1 \times$ SSC. The slides are placed in glass staining dishes filled with $1 \times$ SSC. The sections are then washed sequentially in $2 \times$ SSC/50% formamide (four washes of 15 min) at 40°C and $1 \times$ SSC (two washes of 30 min) at room temperature. Rinse briefly in H_2O. Rinse in 70% ethanol. Air dry thoroughly.

Autoradiography

Hybridized sections can be apposed to film [Hyperfilm-βMax (Amersham, Arlington Heights, IL) is used with ^{35}S- or ^{3}H-labeled probes] or can be dipped into Kodak (Rochester, NY) NTB2 or NTB3 nuclear track emulsion (diluted 1:1 with distilled H_2O). Anatomical localization of probe at the cellular level was performed for IL-1ra by dipping the slides in NTB-2 nuclear emulsion, exposing for 40 days, developing in Kodak D19 for 2 min at 16°C, and counterstaining. The localization of grains can be studied with a light microscope.

Preparation of Emulsion

1. All emulsion must be handled in a dark room under a Kodak 2 safe light.
2. Warm the NTB emulsion in a water bath at 45°C until liquid (approximately 1 hr).
3. Dilute the emulsion 1:1 in distilled H_2O, in a 50-ml conical tube. Let the tube sit in a 45°C water bath until all bubbles are removed (approximately 1 hr).
4. Several clean glass slides are then dipped into the emulsion to remove remaining bubbles.
5. Dip the *in situ* slides in emulsion (1 sec) and dry on a rack in the dark for 4–6 hr until dry.
6. Place slides in a small black box, close the box with light-safe tape, and store the box at 4°C during exposure.

Tissue Staining

Several standard histological stains may be used with ISHH, such as Congo red, cresyl violet, or toluidine blue.

Cresyl Violet staining solution

Acetic acid   60 ml
Cresyl violet   2 g
Water   940 ml

sonicate until dissolved and filter prior to use

Acid alcohol solution: Add 7 drops of 10% acetic acid to 95% ethanol in staining dish.

Rinse the slides in distilled H_2O, stain for up to 2 min in cresyl violet, and rinse the slides once in distilled H_2O. Rinse in acid alcohol (30 sec), 95% (30 sec), 95% (30 sec), 100% (60 sec), and 100% (60 sec) ethanol. Clear in Histoclear (National Diagnostics, Atlanta, GA) for 1 min.

Concluding Remarks

In situ hybridization can be used successfully to localize mRNA encoding cytokines of the interleukin 1 family. In this article we provide detailed protocols for the utilization of either cDNA or cRNA oligonucleotide probes in ISHH applied to the detection of IL-1β (Figs. 1–3) and IL-1ra (Figs. 4 and 5). The initial localization studies reveal that IL-1-family cytokines are localized in brain areas such as the hypothalamus and hippocampus, that control the stress response. The biological effects of IL-1 are similar to elements of the stress response, such as increase in temperature, increase in hypothalamic–pituitary–adrenocortical activity, decrease in appetite, and suppression of reproductive function. Molecular neuroanatomical studies, localizing this family of cytokines to specific brain areas that regulate the biological response to stress, help corroborate the idea that interleukin 1 cytokines may be an important element in the modulation of the stress response. Two fundamental questions on the role of interleukin 1 in brain remain to be answered: (1) Does interleukin 1 have a role in normal brain physiology? (2) Is interleukin 1 involved in the pathophysiology of stress-related central nervous system disorders? Semiquantitative techniques to ascertain variations in the levels of mRNA expression detected by *in situ* hybridization may be applied to studies of the effects of physiological and pathophysiological variables, and of drugs on IL-1β and IL-1ra gene expression in brain. Future studies using semiquantitation of IL-1β and IL-1ra mRNA levels detected by ISHH will provide definitive answers to important questions in this field.

References

1. J. G. Gall and M. L. Pardue, *Proc. Natl. Acad. Sci. U.S.A.* **63,** 378 (1969).
2. G. R. Uhl, "*In situ* Hybridization in Brain." Plenum, New York, 1986.
3. W. S. Young, *Trends Neurosci.* **9,** 549 (1986).
4. N. Barden, *Biotechnol. Update* **2,** 1 (1988).
5. R. J. Milner, G. A. Higgins, H. Schmale, and F. E. Bloom, *in* "*In situ* Hybridization: Applications to Neurobiology" (K. L. Valentino, J. H. Eberwine, and J. D. Barchas, eds.). Oxford Univ. Press, New York, 1987.
6. G. R. Uhl, *in* "Techniques in the Behavioral and Neural Sciences" (J. P. Huston, ed.), Vol. 3, p. 25. Elsevier, Amsterdam, 1988.
7. E. W. Bernton, J. E. Beach, J. W. Holaday, R. C. Smallridge, and H. G. Fein, *Science* **238,** 519 (1987).
8. D. E. Scarborough, S. L. Lee, C. A. Dinarello, and S. Reichlin, *Endocrinology (Baltimore)* **124,** 549 (1989).
9. C. Rivier and W. Vale, *Endocrinology (Baltimore)* **127,** 849 (1990).
10. J. E. Gershenwald, Y. Fong, T. J. Fahey, III, S. E. Calvano, R. Chizzonite, P. L. Kilian, S. F. Lowry, and L. L. Moldawer, *Proc. Natl. Acad. Sci. U.S.A.* **87,** 4966 (1990).
11. K. Ohlsson, P. Björk, M. Bergenfeldt, R. Hageman, and R. C. Thompson, *Nature (London)* **348,** 550 (1990).
12. H. R. Alexander, G. M. Doherty, C. M. Buresh, D. J. Venzon, and J. A. Norton, *J. Exp. Med.* **173,** 1029 (1991).
13. C. H. Hannun, C. J. Wilcox, W. P. Arend, F. G. Joslin, D. J. Dripps, P. L. Heimdal, L. G. Armes, A. Sommer, S. P. Eisenberg, and R. C. Thompson, *Nature (London)* **343,** 336 (1990).
14. S. P. Eisenberg, R. J. Evans, W. P. Arend, E. Verderber, M. T. Brewer, C. H. Hannun, and R. C. Thompson, *Nature (London)* **343,** 341 (1990).
15. K. H. Cox, D. V. De Leon, and L. M. Angerer, *Dev. Biol.* **101,** 485 (1984).
16. L. H. Tecott, J. H. Eberwine, J. D. Barchas, and K. L. Valentino, *in* "*In Situ* Hybridization: Applications to Neurobiology" (K. L. Valentino, J. H. Eberwine, and J. D. Barchas, eds.), p. 3. Oxford Univ. Press, New York, 1987.
17. C. E. Bandtlow, M. Meyer, D. Lindholm, M. Spranger, and R. Heumann, *J. Cell Biol.* **111,** 1701 (1990).
18. J. Licinio, M.-L. Wong, and P. W. Gold, *Endocrinology (Baltimore)* **129,** 562 (1991).
19. G. A. Higgings and M. C. Wilson, *in* "*In situ* Hybridization: Applications to Neurobiology" (K. L. Valentino, J. H. Eberwine, and J. D. Barchas, eds.), p. 146. Oxford Univ. Press, New York, 1987.

20. H. E. Gendelman, T. R. Moench, O. Narayan, and D. E. Griffin, *J. Immunol. Methods* **65,** 137 (1983).

21. M. Brahič and A. T. Haase, *Proc. Natl. Acad. Sci. U.S.A.* **75,** 6125 (1978).

22. J. Sambrook, E. F. Fritsch, and T. Maniatis, "Molecular Cloning: A Laboratory Manual." Cold Spring Harbor Lab. Press, Cold Spring Harbor, New York, 1989.

23. L. G. Davis, M. D. Dibner, and J. F. Battey, "Basic Methods in Molecular Biology." Elsevier, New York, 1986.

24. B. Perbal, "A Practical Guide to Molecular Cloning," 2nd ed. Wiley, New York, 1988.

25. B. S. Schachter, *in* "*In situ* Hybridization: Applications to Neurobiology" (K. L. Valentino, J. H. Eberwine, and J. D. Barchas, eds.), p. 111. Oxford Univ. Press, New York, 1987.

26. H. J. Whitfield, L. S. Brady, M. A. Smith, E. Mamalaki, R. J. Fox, and M. Herkenham, *Cell. Mol. Neurobiol.* **10,** 145 (1990).

27. J. E. Pintar and D. I. Lugo, *in* "*In situ* Hybridization: Applications to Neurobiology" (K. L. Valentino, J. H. Eberwine, and J. D. Barchas, eds.), p. 179. Oxford Univ. Press, New York, 1987.

28. W. S. Young, III, *in* "Methods in Enzymology" (P. Conn, ed.), Vol. 168, Part K, p. 702. Academic Press, San Diego, 1989.

29. M. Herkenham and C. B. Pert, *J. Neurosci.* **2,** 1129 (1982).

[6] Immunocytochemical Methods for Localization of Cytokines in Brain

John A. Olschowka

Introduction

Organisms respond to stresses of the immune system, for example, infection and inflammation, with complex and coordinated responses of the nervous, immune, and endocrine systems. Studies have begun to demonstrate the means by which these responses are elicited. The presence of interconnections between the nervous system and the immune organs is now quite well established. Less well understood is the ability of the immune system to affect the nervous system. The mechanism by which immune cells influence cells of the nervous system will presumably be by the release of cytokines, much the same as they communicate with each other. Although the cytokines may reach the nervous system via the vasculature, the demonstration of cytokine-secreting cells within the nervous system may be of great functional importance.

The presence of cytokines within the central nervous system (CNS) has been well established. What is not clear is whether these molecules are normally present in normal (noninjured/nonactivated) cells of the CNS. It should be remembered that normal, nonactivated immune cells do not express high levels of cytokines. Cytokine expression within immune cells necessitates activation of the cell, transcription of cytokine mRNA, translation of new protein, and its secretion or expression on the cell surface. Those examples of cytokine expression within the CNS have generally been in activated systems. Interleukin 2 (IL-2) activity has been described in injured rat brain (1), and has been localized immunocytochemically in multiple sclerosis brain (2). Interleukin 3 activity has been described in cultured astrocytes (3) and IL-3 mRNA has been described in CNS neurons and astrocytes (4). However, IL-3 has not been demonstrated immunocytochemically within the normal CNS. Interleukin 6 mRNA and IL-6 receptor mRNA have been described within normal rat brain (5), both in neurons and glia. Additionally, brain IL-6 or its mRNA appears to be activated following IL-1 (6, 7) or kainic acid (8) injection. Interleukin 6 has also been implicated in an acute-phase state in Alzheimer's disease and has been demonstrated immunocytochemically within senile plaques (9, 10). Finally, IL-6 has been described within the CNS of animals experiencing experimental autoimmune encepha-

Methods in Neurosciences, Volume 16

lomyelitis (EAE) (11) or viral diseases (12). Although IL-6 appears to be present in a number of activated states, it has been demonstrated immunocytochemically in very few instances (9, 10). Similarly, transforming growth factor β (TGF-β) has been described within cultured astrocytes and microglia (13), especially within astrocytes treated with IL-1 (14). Transforming growth factor β could be demonstrated immunocytochemically only in IL-1-treated astrocytes (14) or in human immunodeficiency virus (HIV)-infected microglia and astrocytes (15). In addition, a number of other cytokines have been demonstrated in inflammatory states in the CNS: tumor necrosis factor in EAE (16) and multiple sclerosis (MS) brain (17), macrophage colony-stimulating factor and granulocyte–macrophage colony-stimulating factor receptors in regenerating rat facial nucleus (18), and interferon-γ (IFN-γ) in MS brains (19). Together these studies suggest that a number of cytokines may be expressed within the CNS; however, it is not clear what cell types express each cytokine and under what circumstances. Immunocytochemical localization of the cytokines may lead to a much improved understanding of their role.

Of all cytokines examined, perhaps the greatest effort has surrounded the role of interleukin 1 (IL-1). Interleukin 1 has been implicated in various neuroendocrine functions, blood pressure regulation, fever, anorexia, induction of slow-wave sleep, and prostaglandin secretion (20). Immunocytochemically an IL-1 like protein has been demonstrated in neurons of human (21) and rat (22) brain. However, few studies have corroborated this localization to neurons. Our own work has failed to demonstrate IL-1 in nonactivated rat brain. Indeed, polymerase chain reaction (PCR) amplification was necessary to demonstrate IL-1 mRNA within normal brain (23, 24). However, following activation of the rat CNS with IFN-γ and/or lipopolysaccharide we could localize IL-1 mRNA with *in situ* hybridization or IL-1 protein immunocytochemically within microglia (23, 24). Although the final answer regarding IL-1 expression awaits further study, this situation demonstrates the possible problems in interpreting the immunocytochemical localization of a new cytokine to the CNS. The following manuscript attempts to describe a general (as well as a specific) method(s) for conducting immunocytochemistry for cytokines in the CNS.

Immunocytochemistry

As mentioned above, most cytokines are found in low quantities in normal inactivated cells and require activation and synthesis before they can be localized. Few studies have demonstrated cytokines within normal brain and, of these, the specificity of their staining may be questioned. Accordingly, immunocytochemical procedures must be quite sensitive to demonstrate low levels of the particular cytokine of interest. Additionally, appropriate controls are a necessity when localizing any new antigen within a particular tissue. Although all current labeling procedures (e.g., immunofluorescence, peroxidase–anti-peroxidase, avidin–biotin–peroxidase, and immunogold) may be appropriate, our experience has led us to develop a highly sensitive avidin–biotin–peroxidase method.

With any of the immunocytochemical procedures, the first problem to be considered is fixation of the tissue. Typically, an investigator must be concerned with (1) morphological preservation of the tissue, (2) retention of the antigen within the tissue, and (3) effects of the fixation on the antigenicity of the molecule of interest. Cold ethanol and/or acetone fixation has been successfully used by some investigators to localize CNS cytokines (25–27); however, these fixatives coagulate proteins in order to retain them within the tissue. They provide poor tissue preservation and may prove detrimental to the antigenicity of some proteins. In most cases cross-linking aldehyde fixatives are more useful. Paraformaldehyde provides adequate tissue preservation and antigen retention with little effect on most antigens. Alternatively, we have found acrolein to be a useful fixative, especially when rapid retention of the antigen is required. Acrolein, a monoaldehyde, is the most reactive of all aldehydes and retains up to 98% of all proteins within the tissue (28). This may be of use when little of the antigen is expected in the tissue. Typically, in our laboratory, animals are anesthetized and perfused via the ascending aorta with 0.15 M phosphate buffer, pH 7.3, containing 0.5% of the vasodilator sodium nitrite plus 2U of heparin/ml. This is then followed by 4% paraformaldehyde in 0.1 M phosphate buffer, pH 7.3 at 4°C. The brain and spleen are then removed, blocked into 2-mm slices, and postfixed 2–6 hr in the perfusate solution. The tissue is then placed in 20% sucrose in 0.15 M phosphate and infiltrated overnight at 4°C. Following infiltration, the tissue is frozen on dry ice. The freezing should be rapid enough to prevent formation of large ice crystals, which destroy tissue morphology. For large blocks, such as monkey brain, this may require freezing the brain in 2-methylbutane chilled with dry ice. The tissue is then sectioned at 30 μm on a sliding microtome. Sections are collected in a series of six wells containing phosphate buffer. Tissue to be stained immediately will be rinsed several more times in buffer. The remaining tissue is infiltrated with a cryoprotectant solution and the tissue stored at −25° until needed. The spleen tissue is used as a positive control when staining many new antigens in the CNS. For example, macrophages that stain for interleukin 1 may be observed in the marginal zone and scattered throughout the red pulp of the spleen.

Single-Label Immunocytochemistry

The light microscopic immunocytochemical procedure begins by preabsorbing the tissue in a solution of 10% normal serum (from the species in which the secondary antibody was generated) in 0.15 M phosphate buffer for 20–30 min. The tissue is then placed in appropriately diluted primary antibody in 0.15 M phosphate buffer plus 0.3% Triton plus 1% normal serum. The tissue is incubated for 48 hr at 4°C with gentle agitation. Although shorter incubation times may be possible, we have generally found better penetration of the antisera and more uniform staining with longer incubation periods. Following incubation in the primary antibody, the tissue is washed 10 times (5 min each) in 0.15 M phosphate buffer. The tissue is then incubated for 2 hr in biotinylated secondary antibody diluted in 0.15 M phosphate buffer with 1% normal serum. Following incubation in the secondary antibody, the tissue is washed six times (10 min each) in 0.15 M phosphate buffer. The tissue is then incubated for 2 hr at 25°C with agitation in an avidin–biotin–peroxidase complex (Elite-ABC kit, 2 μl of A plus 2 μl of B per milliliter; Vector Laboratories, Burlingame, CA) in 0.15 M phosphate buffer plus 0.25% bovine serum albumin (BSA). [*Note*: This is a 1:10 dilution of the Elite-ABC complex suggested in the kit. We have not found any loss in signal with dilutions of up to 1:15. With the nickel-enhanced diaminobenzidine (DAB) reaction described below, we found a specific set of rat neurons that stained nonspecifically with the Elite-ABC when used at the suggested concentration.] After incubation in the ABC solution, the tissue is processed with a nickel-enhanced DAB reaction. Briefly, the tissue is washed six times (5 min each) in a buffer consisting of 175 mM sodium acetate plus 10 mM imidazole, pH 7.0. After washing the tissue is reacted with the DAB solution, which consists of 0.09% DAB, 0.1 M nickel sulfate in 125 mM sodium acetate plus 10 mM imidazole buffer, pH 7.0, and 0.01% hydrogen peroxide. This solution contains nickel sulfate to enhance the reaction product, imidazole to act as an electron donor for the DAB reaction, and DAB and hydrogen peroxide in non-rate-limiting concentrations. After ≤10 min in the DAB solution the tissue is removed and washed in 0.15 M phosphate buffer. Under these conditions we have determined that the DAB reaction is linear over 12 min, after which the integrated optical density of the reaction product plateaus. Therefore, to ensure that the DAB reaction product indicating the level of antigen is comparable between animals, the reaction is stopped at or before 10 min. In addition all tissues for control and experimental animals are run identically. The reaction with nickel produces a permanent black-blue reaction product. See Fig. 1.

We have begun to use a new product, BLAST (Du Pont, Wilmington,

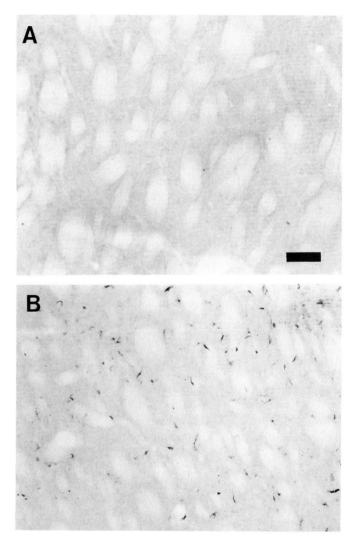

FIG. 1 Immunocytochemical localization of IL-1 in rat striatal microglial cells. The tissue sections were stained identically by the nickel-enhanced DAB method described in text. The antisera used was a rabbit anti-rat IL-1β (Cytokine Sciences, Inc.) diluted 1 : 1200. (A) Control striatum. The rat was injected with 150 nl of sterile saline into the striatum, perfused 3 days later, and processed for immunocytochemistry as described in text. (B) Striatum of rat injected with 150 nl of saline containing 30 units of murine IFN-γ and 300 ng of lipopolysaccharide (LPS), perfused 3 days later, and processed for immunocytochemistry. Note the marked induction of IL-1 staining within the striatal microglial cells. Magnification bar, (A) and (B): 100 μm.

DE), which greatly enhances the sensitivity of our immunocytochemistry. This Du Pont BLAST product is based on a catalyzed reporter deposition method published by Bobrow *et al.* (29, 30). The product relies on the ability of horseradish peroxidase (HRP) and hydrogen peroxide to catalyze the activation of a phenolic group to covalently bind to electron-rich moieties in the vicinity of the HRP. Following the normal avidin–biotin–peroxidase (Elite-ABC) incubation described above, a biotin–phenolic compound (bio-tinyl-tyramide) is incubated with the tissue. This results in the covalent binding of large numbers of biotin molecules at the site of the antigen. In practice, following the incubation in Elite-ABC, the tissue is washed six times (5 min each) with buffer and then incubated for 10 min in 10 μl of the biotinyl-tyramide solution per milliliter of 0.003% H_2O_2 in 0.1 M borate buffer, pH 8.5, all from the BLAST kit. The tissue is then washed, incubated a second time in the Elite-ABC solution, washed, and finally the DAB reaction is carried out. Although we have not completed a quantitative analysis of the BLAST method at this time, it has increased the sensitivity of our immunocytochemical method at least 50-fold. An anti-rat IL-1 antiserum (rabbit anti-rat IL-1β; Cytokine Science, Inc., Boston, MA), which we previously used at a 1 : 1000 dilution, can now be used at 1 : 50,000 dilution with superior results if the BLAST step is included. These early results suggest that the use of the catalyzed reporter deposition technology will greatly enhance the ability to localize cytokines found at low levels in the CNS. Additionally, the increased sensitivity accorded by the BLAST method allows (and/or demands) the dilution of the primary and secondary antisera, thus reducing the cost to the investigator.

Double-Label Immunocytochemistry

Often it may be of interest to label two antigens in the same tissue section. Many methods have been described (combined immunoperoxidase, dual immunofluorescence, immunogold methods with different-sized gold particles, etc.). In general the method will be determined by whether the two antigens are expected to be in the same or different cells. When the antigens are in different cell types, we prefer the combined immunoperoxidase method, because of its sensitivity and permanence of the label. Briefly, the first antigen is localized by the nickel-enhanced DAB method, and the tissue is washed and processed a second time, exactly as described above for the second antigen. The major difference in staining the second antigen is that a normal DAB reaction, without nickel, is employed. Briefly, after incubation in the Elite-ABC complex, the tissue is washed six times (5 min each) in a 0.05 M Tris plus 0.6% NaCl buffer, pH 7.2. After washing, the tissue is reacted with DAB in a solution containing 0.09% DAB and 0.01% hydrogen peroxide in a 0.05 M Tris plus 0.6% NaCl plus 10 mM imidazole buffer, pH 7.2. This will produce a brown reaction product. After 5–10 min the reaction is stopped by washing the tissue in 0.15 M phosphate buffer. The tissue is then mounted on gelatin-coated slides, dehydrated, and coverslipped.

An alternative double-labeling method is the use of fluorescent secondary antibodies, for example, Texas red and fluorescein isothiocyanate (FITC). The advantages of the fluorescent method are that (1) two antigens may be localized within a single cell and (2) the processing of the two antigens can be carried out simultaneously (if care is chosen in selecting primary antibodies from different species). This greatly decreases the time involved in processing of the tissue. Its one disadvantage is that it may not be as sensitive as the DAB method. With an appropriate fluorescent microscope one can perform the same image analysis as is proposed with the DAB method when a camera capable of imaging fluorescence is used. Briefly, the tissue is incubated in the primary antibody as described above. It is then washed and incubated for 1–2 hr in the Texas red- or FITC-labeled antisera diluted 1 : 500 in 0.15 M phosphate buffer at room temperature. The tissue is then washed, mounted on subbed slides, quickly dehydrated, and coverslipped in DPX mountant (Gallard-Schlesinger Chemical Mfg. Corp., Carle Place, NY). We have found sections coverslipped with DPX to have superior optical characteristics to PBS-glycerine cover-slipped sections. Additionally, the DPX appears to inhibit the photobleaching of the fluorescent dyes.

Electron Microscopy Immunocytochemistry

As at the light microscopic level, the ultrastructural localization of cytokines raises the questions of choice of fixation and immunocytochemical method. Although we have used both immunogold and immunoperoxidase methods, the immunoperoxidase method will be described here. First, animals are perfused with a solution containing 2.5% acrolein and 4% paraformaldehyde in 0.1 M phosphate buffer, pH 7.3. This fixative provides excellent ultrastructural preservation with little loss in antigenicity of tissue antigens. [Indeed, some antigens (e.g., Fos oncoprotein) are far easier to stain following acrolein fixation.] Following fixation the brain is removed and sectioned at 30 μm on a vibratome. The tissue is then incubated for 20 min in 0.1 M sodium periodate in 0.05 M Tris plus 0.6% NaCl buffer, pH 7.2, washed in phosphate buffer, and incubated for 30 min in 1% sodium borohydride. Again the tissue is washed and then transferred to the preabsorption solution as described above. The processing of the tissue is identical to that described above except that no detergent is used. Following completion of the final DAB reaction the tissue is postfixed in 1.0% osmium plus 1.5% potassium ferricyanide in 0.1 M sodium cacodylate buffer. The tissue is then dehydrated through an ascending series of methanol to 70%. The tissue is then block stained in 0.1% uranyl acetate in 70% methanol for 30 min. Afterward the dehydration is completed and the tissue infiltrated with an Epon–Araldite mixture. Without the use of Triton, the staining is limited to the outer 4–6 μm of the section and sectioning of the block surface is required. A method to flat embed the sections to allow easier thin sectioning has been previously described (31). Briefly, the tissue is placed between two glass slides previously coated with a liquid release agent (EM Sciences, Fort Washington, PA) and the resin polymerized overnight in a 60°C oven. One of the glass slides is removed and the tissue is then examined and photographed in the light microscope. Those sections demonstrating good staining are covered with a fresh drop of resin and a polymerized embedding capsule is placed on top. The tissue is again placed overnight in a 60°C oven. The tissue with attached embedding capsule is then removed from the second glass slide. The flat-embedded tissue is trimmed and thin sectioned. Thin sections (70 nm) are collected on copper thin-bar grids and are viewed without further staining.

Antisera and Controls

When localizing any new antigen within a tissue, careful characterization of the antiserum is required. Certainly a number of standard controls should be run. First, omission of the primary antibody should result in the complete loss of the signal. Similarly, preabsorption of the primary antisera with purified antigen should also result in the complete loss of staining. When antigens are known to exist that closely resemble the antigen of interest, it may prove useful to include preabsorption controls using these antigens. Perhaps the most important control is a Western blot of the tissue with the antiserum against the new antigen. The value of this control has been illustrated regarding the localization of interferon-γ (IFN-γ) within the rat CNS. A number of published reports all used the monoclonal DB1 against rat IFN-γ within the CNS (25–27). Although this antiserum has been characterized to localize IFN-γ within immune tissue, Kiefer *et al.* (32) have demonstrated in Western blot analysis that this antisera does not recognize true IFN-γ, but rather a IFN-γ-like antigen. This emphasizes the value of the Western blot analysis. An additional control we routinely use is the immunocytochemical localization of the antigen in a tissue with a known distribution of the antigen. For example, we use spleen sections as a positive control for our studies of IL-1 localization. Finally, because many of the cytokines have been cloned, we often corroborate our immunocytochemical localization by *in situ* hybridization for the mRNA of the antigen. Although this technique may not be available to all investigators, this control has proved quite important in our IL-1 studies (23, 24).

Computerized Image Analysis and Analysis of Data

In many instances the differences in cytokine staining between experimental and control animals will be analyzed using computerized image analysis. Tissue from experimental and control animals should be processed for immunocytochemistry together in order to minimize differences in staining intensity due to daily variations in the method, for example, antibody concentrations, length of DAB reactions and duration of washes. The stained tissues should then be matched to compare as closely as possible identical fields or nuclei in the brain. In our laboratory the fields are analyzed on a Leitz Orthoplan light microscope (E. Leitz Co., Rockleigh, NJ) to which is attached a Dage-MTI series 68 video camera (Michigan City, IN). If densitometric analysis of the reaction product is to be carried out, the microscope and camera should be provided with a constant-voltage power source. The microscope illumination should be optimal (e.g., clean optics, recollimated optics if the necessary, and Kohler illumination). With the Dage-MTI series 68 camera, a constant source of black is provided to the camera in order to allow the auto-black function to be used (this camera heats up internally if the auto-black is shut off for extended periods and thus may give erroneous readings). Charge-coupled device (CCD) cameras do not have this problem, but not all CCD cameras have the ability to shut off the auto-gain and auto-black controls necessary for densitometry. The output of the camera is sent to the image based analysis system (IBAS) image analysis computer (Carl Zeiss, Inc., Thornwood, NY). The computer consists of a dedicated host computer and array processor, a real-time board for real-time image processing, and a 20-Mbyte hard disk. The software allows sophisticated image enhancement and morphometric and densitometric analysis.

In an analysis of immunocytochemically stained material a number of parameters can be analyzed. Because most cytokines are in low levels normally and must be induced, it may be of interest to determine the level of cytokine per cell as an indication of cell activation. Although this can at best be called a semiquantitative method, a densitometric analysis of the reaction product may yield this information. However, a number of precautions must be considered in order for this technique to be valid. First, the linearity of the DAB reaction should be determined and the reaction stopped before the staining plateaus. As mentioned above, our protocol yields a reaction that is linear for 12 min and we stop all reactions by 10 min. Second, the tissue must be processed identically for all samples and the areas selected for analysis should be identical. Third, all antiserum concentrations must be optimized so that the only variable in the staining is the antigen density. This can be done on tissue sections as well as on simulated sections, for example, nitrocellulose. In our laboratory we blot known amounts of antigen to nitrocellulose paper and then perform the immunocytochemical procedure. For example, the peroxidase method described above yielded a linear relationship of integrated optical density vs IL-1 concentration when our IL-1 antisera concentration was optimized. Interestingly, this linear relationship remained the same after silver staining of the nickel–DAB reaction product. This suggests that for antigens that stain poorly, silver enhancement of the DAB reaction product may still allow densitometric analysis.

In addition to determining the staining intensity per cell, the number of cells that stain and their size may be of interest. Unfortunately, a number of laboratories continue to use biased estimates of these parameters. During the last decade, a number of new unbiased methods have been developed that more truly represent estimates of cell size, number, and volume (33, 34). These unbiased methods include the dissector, nucleator, fractionator, and selector. Although it is not the purpose of this article to summarize these methods, it should be pointed out that many laboratories and computer-based systems still continue to use biased methods. A useful and practical review of these unbiased methods has been published by Gundersen *et al.* (35).

Conclusion

The preceding comments were designed to illustrate many of the problems encountered in the immunocytochemical localization of cytokines. As mentioned previously, any number of immunocytochemical methods have been used successfully. There is no one "right" method, but each investigator must decide on the method that he/she is most comfortable with. Although we have provided the details for a sensitive immunoperoxidase method, it may not fulfill the needs of all investigators, and other methods may and should be considered. Regardless of the staining method chosen, the specificity of the staining should always be questioned. The immunocytochemical controls suggested have proved invaluable in our hands and may help in our interpretations of the CNS cytokine literature as it evolves. Additionally, we have briefly attempted to illustrate the correct methods for the analysis of the immunocytochemical data.

Acknowledgments

The author would like to thank Ms. Lee Trojanczyk for excellent technical assistance in the development of the described methods. Ms. D. Herrara is gratefully acknowledged for assistance in the photographic representations. Supported by PHS Grant NS 29400 to J.A.O.

References

1. M. Nieto-Sampedro and K. G. Chandy, *Neurochem. Res.* **12**, 723 (1987).
2. F. M. Hofman, R. I. von Hanwehr, C. A. Dinarello, S. B. Mizel, D. Hinton, and J. E. Merrill, *J. Immunol.* **136**, 3239 (1986).
3. K. Frei, S. Bodmer, C. Schwerdel, and A. Fontana, *J. Immunol.* **135**, 4044 (1985).
4. W. L. Farrar, M. Vinocour, and J. M. Hill, *Blood* **73**, 137 (1989).
5. B. Schöbitz, D. A. M. Voorhuis, and E. R. De Kloet, *Neuro. Sci. Lett.* **136**, 189 (1992).
6. B. L. Spangelo, W. D. Jarvis, A. M. Judd, and R. M. MacLeod, *Endocrinology (Baltimore)* **129**, 2886 (1991).
7. M. G. De Simoni, M. Sironi, A. De Luigi, A. Manfridi, A. Mantovani, and P. Ghezzi, *J. Exp. Med.* **171**, 1773 (1990).
8. M. Minami, Y. Kuraishi, and M. Satoh, *Biochem. Biophys. Res. Commun.* **176**, 593 (1991).
9. J. Bauer, S. Strauss, U. Schreiter-Gasser, U. Ganter, P. Schlegel, I. Witt, B. Yolk, and M. Berger, *FEBS Lett.* **285**, 111 (1991).
10. S. Strauss, J. Bauer, U. Ganter, U. Jonas, M. Berger, and B. Yolk, *Lab. Invest.* **66**, 223 (1992).
11. K. Gijbcls, J. Van Damme, P. Proost, W. Put, H. Carton, and A. Billiau, *Eur. J. Immunol.* **20**, 233 (1990).
12. K. Frei, U. V. Malipiero, T. P. Leist, R. M. Zinkernagel, M. E. Schwab, and A. Fontana, *Eur. J. Immunol.* **19**, 689 (1989).
13. A. Da Cunha and L.Vitkovič, *J. Neuroimmunol.* **36**, 157 (1992).
14. D. B. Constam, J. Philipp, UV. Malipiero, P. ten Dijke, M. Schachner, and A. Fontana, *J. Immunol.* **148**, 1404 (1992).
15. S. M. Wahl, J. B. Allen, N. McCartney-Francis, M. C. Morganti-Kossmann, T. Kossmann, L. Ellingsworth, U. E. H. Mai, S. E. Mergenhagen, and J. M. Orenstein, *J. Exp. Med.* **173**, 981 (1991).
16. I. Y. Chung, J. G. Norris, and E. N.Benveniste, *J. Exp. Med.* **173**, 801 (1991).
17. F. M. Hofman, D. R. Hinton, K. Johnson, and J. E. Merrill, *J. Exp. Med.* **170**, 607 (1989).
18. G. Raivich, J. Gehrmann, and G. W. Kreutzberg, *J. Neurosci. Res.* **30**, 682 (1991).
19. U. Traugott and P. Lebon, *J. Neurol. Sci.* **84**, 257 (1988).
20. C. A. Dinarello, *FASEB J.* **2**, 108 (1988).
21. C. D. Breder, C. A. Dinarello, and C. B. Saper, *Science* **240**, 321 (1988).

22. R. M. Lechan, R. Toni, B. D. Clark, J. G. Cannon, A. R. Shaw, C. A. Dinarello, and S. Reichlin, *Brain Res.* **514**, 135 (1990).
23. J. A. Olschowka, J. Dopp, and G. A. Higgins, *in* "Peripheral Signaling of the Brain: Neural-Immune and Cognitive Function" (R. C. A. Frederickson, J. L. McGaugh, and D. L. Felten, eds.), p. 117. Hogrefe & Huber Publishers, Toronto, 1991.
24. G. A. Higgins and J. A. Olschowka, *Mol. Brain Res.* **4**, 143 (1991).
25. T. Olsson, K. Kristensson, A. Ljungdahl, J. Maehlen, and R. Holmdahl, *J. Neurosci.* **9**, 3870 (1989).
26. A. Ljungdahl, T. Olsson, P. H. Van derMeide, R. Holmdahl, L. Klareskog, and B. Hojeberg, *J. Neurosci. Res.* **24**, 451 (1989).
27. A. Eneroth, K. Kristensson, A. Ljungdahl, and T. Olsson, *J. Neurocytol.* **20**, 225 (1991).
28. M. A. Hayat, "Fixation for Electron Microscopy." Academic Press, New York, 1981.
29. M. N. Bobrow, T. D. Harris, K. J. Shaughnessy, and G. J. Litt, *J. Immunol. Methods* **125**, 279 (1989).
30. M. N. Bobrow, K. J. Shaughnessy, and G. J. Litt, *J. Immunol. Methods* **137**, 103 (1991).
31. J. A. Olschowka, *J. Electron Microsc. Technol.* **10**, 373 (1989).
32. R. Kiefer, C. A. Haas, and G. W. Kreutzberg, *Neuroscience* **45**, 551 (1991).
33. D. C. Sterio, *J. Microsc. (Oxford)* **134**, 127 (1984).
34. M. J. West and H. J. G. Gundersen, *J. Comp. Neurol.* **296**, 1 (1990).
35. H. J. G. Gundersen, P. Bagger, T. F. Bendtsen, S. M. Evans, L. Korbo, N. Marcussen, A. Møller, K. Nielsen, J. R. Nyengaard, B. Pakkenberg, F. B. Sørensen, A. Vesterby, and M. J. West, *Acta Pathol. Microbiol. Immunol. Scand.* **96**, 857 (1988).

Localization of Type I Interleukin 1
Receptor mRNA in Brain and
Endocrine Tissues by *in Situ*
Hybridization Histochemistry

Emmett T. Cunningham, Jr., and Errol B. De Souza

Introduction

A number of techniques are now available for detection of tissue-derived messenger ribonucleic acid (mRNA) species, including Northern blot analysis, RNase protection, and *in situ* hybridization. Northern blot analysis was the first of these techniques to be developed, and offers the advantage of technical simplicity. It also provides information on the size and relative abundance of the mRNA species of interest. Northern analyses are limited, however, by the ability of the investigator to separate distinct populations of cells, and are, therefore, most useful to detect and compare mRNA species harvested from homogeneous tissues or pure cell lines. The technique of RNase protection after solution hybridization is more sensitive than Northern hybridization but suffers from the same anatomical limitations, and, unlike Northern analysis, does not provide information on mRNA size. *In situ* hybridization is unique in that it provides both sensitivity and high anatomical resolution, allowing cellular localization of low-abundance mRNA species in intact tissue sections. These advantages of the *in situ* methodology have been exploited to great gain for the localization of relatively low-abundance receptor mRNA species such as the type I interleukin 1 receptor (IL-1-R), particularly in anatomically complex tissue such as the brain and endocrine organs. Below, we present the protocol used in our studies on the distribution of IL-1-R mRNA in brain, pituitary, adrenal gland, and testis. For further details on the specific results of these studies and their interpretation, the reader is referred to the original papers (1–4).

In Situ Hybridization Histochemistry

Various *in situ* hybridization protocols have been published (5–10), and it is not our intention to compare and contrast these methods. For those inter-

Methods in Neurosciences, Volume 16

ested in attempting an *in situ* study, it is important to realize that any of these methods will produce excellent results given adequate message levels. However, for low-abundance message we have had the most success with the method developed by Simmons and colleagues (7), which makes use of ^{35}S-labeled RNA probes complementary to mRNA, known as cRNA or riboprobes. The reader is therefore referred to their original description for the details of the protocol outlined below. Those interested in the use of oligonucleotide probes for the detection of more abundant mRNA species are referred to an excellent review by Young (9).

Tissue Preparation

As with immunohistochemistry, proper tissue preparation for *in situ* hybridization histochemistry is essentially a balance between adequate fixation to preserve morphology and stabilize mRNA, on the one hand, and sufficient cellular membrane permeabilization to permit probe penetration, on the other. Although not studied systematically, there is a general consensus that formaldehyde-based fixatives perform better than other commonly used fixation techniques such as glutaraldehyde, alcohols, or organic acids (9). Methods of membrane permeabilization are presented below under Prehybridization.

Fixative

We routinely use either 4% paraformaldehyde or 10% formalin for tissue fixation for *in situ* hybridization studies. Whereas formalin may be diluted directly, paraformaldehyde should be dissolved in an alkaline solution heated to approximately 65°C. The final solution may then be cooled to 4°C and buffered for use. A protocol for preparing enough pH 9.5-buffered 4% paraformaldehyde to perfuse one adult rat (500 ml) would be as follows.

1. Heat 400 ml of distilled water to 65°C.
2. Dissolve 2 g of NaOH.
3. Dissolve 20 g of paraformaldehyde.
4. Dissolve 19.07 g of sodium tetraborate ($Na_2B_4O_7 \cdot 10H_2O$).
5. Add enough distilled H_2O to bring final volume to 500 ml.
6. Cool to 4°C.
7. Adjust the pH to 9.5 with concentrated NaOH or HCl as needed.

Acidic buffers, such as sodium acetate, or neutral buffers, such as potassium or sodium phosphate, may be used with comparably good results.

Perfusion

Optimal tissue preparation is best performed transcardially across the aortic valve, and should be preceded by a rinse with isotonic saline [0.9% (w/v) for rodents]. We use approximately 100 ml of isotonic saline for an adult rat weighing between 200 and 300 g, and one-tenth that volume for an adult mouse. The 400- to 500-ml volume of fixative used for rats, or 40- to 50-ml volume of fixative used for mice, may then be set to run over 20 to 30 min. If only the brain and pituitary are to be collected, the descending aorta may be clamped and the perfusate volume and time reduced by 25–50%. We rinse with saline at room temperature and perfuse with fixative at 4°C.

Postfixation, Sectioning, and Cryoprotection

In situ hybridization may be performed on tissue postfixed from 4 hr to more than 4 weeks. We have found, however, that with our protocol signal sensitivity tends to increase with longer postfixation times, and we now tend to postfix for at least 1 week. Once postfixed, sections may be cut on either a freezing microtome or cryostat, the choice depending largely on tissue friability. We use 20-μm thick sections, although we have used 5- to 40-μm thick sections with success. Thicker sections do, however, tend to produce higher background, whereas thinner sections are more fragile, and difficult to handle. Extra sections cut on a freezing microtome may be stored at -20°C in a solution of 30% ethylene glycol and 20% glycerol in neutral phosphate-buffered saline (PBS) (0.05 M, pH 7.3). One-liter aliquots of PBS (0.1 M, pH 7.3) may be prepared as follows.

> PBS: Combine
> 3.2 g of sodium phosphate, monobasic ($NaH_2PO_4 \cdot H_2O$), and 10.9 g of sodium phosphate, dibasic (Na_2HPO_4); bring to a 1-liter volume with distilled H_2O; adjust pH to 7.3 with NaOH or HCl as needed

Once cut, all materials that come in contact with tissue sections should be RNase free, and the person handling the material is best advised to wear gloves to prevent RNase contamination. Sections intended for *in situ* hybridization should be mounted onto slides serially coated with gelatin and poly-L-lysine to provide adequate adhesiveness to withstand the elevated temperatures and changes in salt concentrations required during subsequent steps in the protocol. In addition, slides should be well dried under vacuum at room temperature for 6–12 hr prior to prehybridization. Slides prepared in this manner may be stored for short periods at -70°C, although we have found that extended storage markedly decreases signal intensity.

Prehybridization

Slides dried at room temperature are ready for immediate use. Slides stored for short periods at $-70°C$ should be allowed to warm to room temperature prior to prehybridization. Once at room temperature, we have obtained improved morphology and minimized the separation of sections from the slides by dipping the mounted sections into a solution of 10% neutral-buffered formalin for 30–60 min prior to proceeding with the prehybridization. This should be followed immediately by a total of four washes in potassium phosphate-buffered saline (KPBS), 0.02 M, with each wash 5 min in duration. One-liter aliquots of KPBS may be prepared as follows.

> KPBS (0.1 M): For 1 liter, combine 9.0 g of NaCl, 0.45 g of potassium phosphate, monobasic (KH_2PO_4), and 3.56 g of potassium phosphate, dibasic ($K_2HPO_4 \cdot 3H_2O$); bring to 1 liter with distilled H_2O; adjust pH to 7.4 with NaOH or HCl

This minor modification notwithstanding, the prehybridization protocol we use is identical to that employed by Simmons and colleagues (7), and the reader is encouraged to consult their original paper for source of reagents and details of the preparation of the various solutions. In brief, mounted slides are dipped serially through the following solutions for the times indicated.

1. Proteinase K (0.01%) in 0.1 M Tris with 0.05 M ethylenediaminetetra-acetic acid (EDTA) for 15 to 30 min, which acts to permeabilize the cell membranes to allow probe penetration. When maintenance of morphology is critical, or the tissue is particularly friable, sections may go untreated or be permeabilized with the detergent Triton X-100. Sections not treated with proteinase K will, however, have markedly reduced signal
2. Distilled H_2O for 3 min without agitation
3. Triethanolamine (TEA) (0.1 M), pH 8.0, for 3 min
4. Acetic anhydride (0.25%) in 0.1 M TEA, pH 8.0, for 10 min to reduce nonspecific background
5. A 2× concentration of NaCl–sodium citrate (SSC) (two changes, 2 min each). The SSC should be prepared in 20× stock solutions as follows.

> SSC (20× stock): Combine 800 ml of distilled H_2O, 175.3 g of NaCl, and 88.2 g of sodium citrate; adjust pH to 7.0; bring volume to 1 liter and filter sterilize

6. Ascending concentrations of ethanol in distilled H_2O, as follows.

Ethanol (50%), 30 sec
Ethanol (70%), 30 sec
Ethanol (95%), 30 sec
Ethanol (100%), two changes, each 30 sec

The slides should then be allowed to dry with desiccant under vacuum at room temperature for 2 hr. Slides may then be stored at $-70°C$ prior to hybridization.

Probe Synthesis

We use a slight modification of the probe synthesis protocol presented by Simmons *et al.* (7), such that two radiolabeled nucleotides are incorporated into the cRNA probes rather than one. Once a cDNA of interest is subcloned into an appropriate transcription vector, it is a fairly routine matter to linearize and transcribe sense and antisense probes (Fig. 1). In general, longer

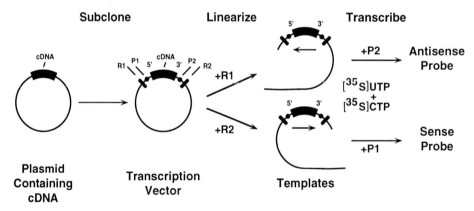

FIG. 1   A schematic summary of the techniques used to generate sense and antisense ^{35}S-labeled riboprobes from a plasmid containing a cDNA insert of interest. First, the cDNA must be subcloned into one of the many commercially available transcription vectors, such as those provided by Promega (pGEM) or Stratagene (La Jolla, CA) (pBS). These vectors contain "built-in" restriction (R1 and R2) and polymerase (P1 and P2) sites to allow for linearization and direction-specific transcription, respectively. These linearized templates can then be exposed to a mixture of polymerase and ^{35}S-labeled nucleotides, such as ^{35}S]UTP and ^{35}S]CTP, for transcription of the riboprobes.

probes incorporate more labeled nucleotide and, in theory, provide increased signal. However, larger probes have more difficulty penetrating the tissue, and so may require longer proteinase K treatments at the expense of morphology. Alternatively, full-length probes may be exposed to controlled alkaline hydrolysis to produce a collection of smaller probes, as originally described by Cox *et al.* (11). However, we have been able to obtain good results with probes 1–2 kilobases (kb) in length without having to resort to alkaline hydrolysis. The method is as follows.

1. Fifty to 100 μg of plasmid containing the coding region of interest should be linearized by restriction endonuclease digestion. The digestion should be monitored for completion by minigel electrophoresis of 0.25 to 0.5 μg of digested DNA. Once digested, the remaining DNA may be purified by serial phenol–chloroform extraction, chloroform extraction, and ethanol precipitation.

2. After thawing, 250 μCi of each radiolabeled nucleotide ([^{35}S]UTP and [^{35}S]CTP) should be aliquoted into a 1.5-ml microcentrifuge tube and dried by vacuum centrifugation. Once dry, each of the following should be added.

Component	Volume
Transcription buffer (5×): For T3 or T7 RNA polymerase this includes 200 mM Tris (pH 8.0), 125 mM NaCl, 40 mM MgCl$_2$, and 10 mM spermidine. For Sp6 RNA polymerase this includes 200 mM Tris (pH 8.0), 30 mM MgCl$_2$, and 10 mM spermidine	2 μl
GTP (5 mM), ATP (5 mM), UTP (0.25 mM), and CTP (0.25 mM)	1 μl each
Dithiothreitol (DTT) (0.1 M)	1 μl
Linearized DNA template (1 μg/μl)	1 μl
RNasin (30–50 units/μl)	0.5 μl
RNA polymerase (T3, T7, etc.), 20–50 units	1 μl
Sterile H$_2$O	To 10 μl (add 0.0–1.0 μl)

Incubate for 30 min at 42°C, then add 1 μl of additional RNA polymerase and incubate for an additional 30 min to complete incorporation of labeled nucleotides.

3. Add 1 μl of RQ1 DNase (1 μg/μl) and 0.5 μl of RNasin and incubate for 10 min at 37°C to digest the DNA template.

4. Purify the probe with serial organic extractions and ethanol precipitations as follows.

   a. After adding 70 μl of sterile H$_2$O, 5 μl of yeast tRNA (10 mg/ml),

10 μl of 5 M NaCl, 100 μl of phenol, and 100 μl of chloroform, mix by vortexing.

b. Separate phases of the above mixture by microcentrifugation for 3 min. Transfer the aqueous phase to a new tube. Add 150 μl of chloroform, mix by vortexing, and separate phases by microcentrifugation for 3 min. After transferring the aqueous phase to a new tube, add 300 μl of ethanol, incubate on ice for 10 min, and then microcentrifuge at 4°C for 10 min to collect precipitated nucleic acids.

c. Decant the supernatant and resuspend the nucleic acid pellet in 200 μl of a solution including 0.2% sodium dodecyl sulfate (SDS), 2 mM EDTA, 0.3 M ammonium acetate (pH 5.2), and 600 μl of ethanol. Vortex and incubate on ice for 15 min. Microcentrifuge for 10 min at 4°C, decant the supernatant, and repeat step c.

d. Wash the collected pellet with 500 μl of ethanol. Microcentrifuge for 1 min, decant the supernatant, and air dry.

e. Resuspend the pellet in 100 μl of a solution containing 10 mM Tris, pH 7.4, and 1 mM DTT. Apply 1 μl to a filter, air dry, and load into a scintillation counter. Good nucleotide incorporation will be reflected in counts of 1–5 $\times$ 10^6 cpm/μl. Probe may be stored at -70°C for up to 2 months, although signal intensity decreases significantly after the first 2 weeks.

Our experiments used a previously characterized murine full-length T cell IL-1 receptor cDNA just over 2 kb in length that had been cloned into a pGEM plasmid vector (Promega, Madison, WI) (12). ^{35}S-Labeled sense and antisense cRNA probes were prepared by transcription with Sp6 and T7 RNA polymerase, respectively (1–3).

Hybridization

We dilute and store all transcribed probes in hybridization buffer at a final concentration of 10^7 cpm/ml. Preparation of 10 ml of hybridization buffer with probe requires two steps.

1. Dilute probe as follows:
   a. Place 10^8 cpm of probe in a sterile, RNase-free vial.
   b. Add 500 μl of sterile yeast tRNA, 10 mg/ml.
   c. Add 100 μl of DTT, 1 M.
   d. Add RNase-free H$_2$O such that the total volume of H$_2$O plus probe is 680 μl. The amount of H$_2$O will vary depending on the radioactivity of the original probe preparation.

2. The total volume of this solution should be brought to 10 ml with an appropriate amount of the following solution, which may be made in aliquots of approximately 40 ml and stored at $-70°C$.

Component	Volume
Formamide, reagent grade (to lower the melting temperature of the RNA–RNA hybrids)	25 ml
NaCl (5 M)	3 ml
Tris (pH 8.0), 1 M	0.5 ml
EDTA (pH 8.0), 0.5 M	100 μl
Denhardt's solution (20×) (to lower nonspecific binding of probe)	2.5 ml
Dextran sulfate (50%)	10 ml

This final mixture of probe and hybridization buffer should be vortexed, and may be stored for use for 4–6 weeks. Buffer with probe added should be heated to 65°C for 5 min, and microcentrifuged at 4°C for 10 min prior to use. This solution may then be applied directly to flat slides, which are then coverslipped and allowed to incubate on a slide warmer at 55°C for 8–12 hr. Care must be taken at this step not to trap air bubbles under the coverslip, as these portions of the slide will not hybridize. The hybridization solution tends to evaporate near the edge of the coverslip even when sealed with DPX, and so sections should be mounted so as to provide a 3- to 4-mm margin at the edge of the slide.

Posthybridization

Posthybridization entails washing the mounted sections with RNase and then exposing them to a series of high-stringency washes, both of which are designed to minimize nonspecific binding. The procedure we use is virtually identical to that published by Simmons *et al.* (7), and will be presented in brief below.

1. Slides with the coverslips attached should be placed in 4× SSC for 10–20 min. This will loosen the coverslips, which may then be removed with little or no damage to the tissue.

2. Uncovered sections should be rinsed through a total of four washes with 4× SSC, each lasting 5 min. The first two of these washes will be radioactive, and should be disposed of appropriately.

3. Sections are then rinsed in RNase A solution at 37°C for 30 min. We prepare 250 ml of RNase A solution as follows.

> RNase A solution: For 250 ml, combine 500 μl of RNase A (10 mg/ml), pretreated by boiling for 10 min, 25 ml of 5 M NaCl, 2.5 ml of 1 M Tris (pH 8.0), 500 μl of EDTA (pH 8.0), 0.5 M; Bring to a final volume of 250 ml with distilled H$_2$O

This solution will also be radioactive, and should be disposed of appropriately.

4. Sections are then taken through a series of decreasing salt concentrations, each of which should have 1 mM DTT added to stabilize the ^{35}S attachments to the riboprobe. This reduces the possibility that nonspecifically hybridized probe will react with sulfides in the tissue, and thereby decreases background signal.

> SSC (2×) for 5 min
> SSC (2×) for 5 min
> SSC (1×) for 10 min
> SSC (0.5×) for 10 min
> SSC (0.1×) for 30 min at 55–75°C. Lower temperatures may be used during this step for probes that have intrinsically low background, whereas temperatures up to 75°C may be required for high background probes. We routinely run this step at 65°C and adjust the temperature as required to minimize background
> SSC (0.1×) for 3 min at room temperature

5. Sections should then be dehydrated quickly through ascending ethanol concentrations as follows.

> Ethanol (50%) for 30 sec
> Ethanol (70%) for 30 sec
> Ethanol (95%) for 30 sec
> Ethanol (100%) for 30 sec, three changes

All but the 95 and 100% ethanol solutions should have 1 mM DTT–0.1× SSC added.

6. Sections are then vacuum dried for 1 to 2 hr prior to placing them under autoradiographic film.

Autoradiography

We have found it useful to perform film detection of autoradiographic signal following all hybridization runs, because this provides inexpensive and rapid visualization of signal with adequate resolution to tell whether the time and cost required to dip the sections in autoradiographic emulsion will be well spent. Those unfamiliar with autoradiographic techniques should consult the text by Rogers (13).

Film Detection

Slides should be placed in X-ray cassettes with the tissue side facing up, and secured to minimize movement. We use adhesive tape applied gently to the labeled end of the slide. Various autoradiographic films may be used for initial visualization, depending largely on the desired resolution. In general, Cronex 4 (Du Pont, Wilmington, DE) provides the most, whereas Hypermax-MP and βMax (Amersham, Arlington Heights, IL), provide progressively less resolution. However, Cronex requires up to two times the exposure time of Hypermax-MP, and up to four times the exposure time of βMax. In addition, βMax requires at least some degree of hand-processing, whereas Hypermax-MP and Cronex may be developed and fixed quickly in an automated film processor. For these reasons, and because we rely heavily on the final emulsion autoradiograms for analysis, we tend to use Hypermax-MP almost exclusively. Exposure times for this film typically vary from 1 to 4 days, although extremely weak signals may require 1- to 2-week exposures.

Emulsion Detection

For those sections that demonstrate or suggest specific signal on autoradiographic film, emulsion autoradiography should be performed to optimize detection of low-abundance mRNA, and to allow for cellular resolution (Figs. 2–4). Prior to dipping, all sections should be redehydrated through 95% ethanol and three changes of 100% ethanol, each for 3 min. Sections should then be delipidized through xylene, two changes of 15 min each, and brought back to 100% ethanol for 5 min prior to a brief 30-min drying under vacuum. Sections may then be dipped, in a darkroom, in a 1:1 dilution of Kodak NTB-2 or NTB-3 emulsion in distilled H_2O at 42°C. Emulsion solution needs to be mixed by slow turning in a sealed container, to be allowed to stand for 30 min prior to dipping, and to have a few blank slides dipped prior to dipping sections. All of these precautions act to minimize streaking and bubble artifact. Sections can then be dipped and dried standing in a high-humidity chamber at 23°C for 2–4 hr, boxed in light-tight containers, and

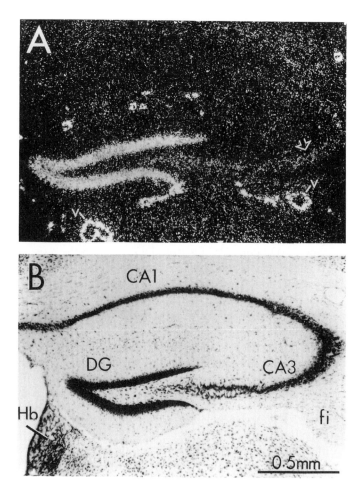

FIG. 2   A low-power dark-field photomicrograph of an emulsion autoradiogram of a coronal section through the murine hippocampus following *in situ* hybridization with an ^{35}S-labeled antisense cRNA probe for the type I IL-1 receptor (A). A Nissl-stained section is shown for reference (B). Dense signal is present over granule cells in the dentate gyrus (DG), and over endothelial cells of postcapillary venules (v). Less intense signal is present over pyramidal cells of the hilus and CA3 region (arrow). These sections illustrate one of the most important principles in identifying true signal, that is, an unmistakable increase in grain density observed in an anatomically or functionally defined, yet restricted, distribution, as seen here in the hippocampal fields. fi, Fimbria hippocampus; Hb, medial habenular nucleus. [Reproduced with permission from Cunningham *et al.* (1), Localization of interleukin-1 receptor messenger on RNA in murine hippocampus, *Endocrinology,* 1991, **128**(5), 2666–2668. © The Endocrine Society.]

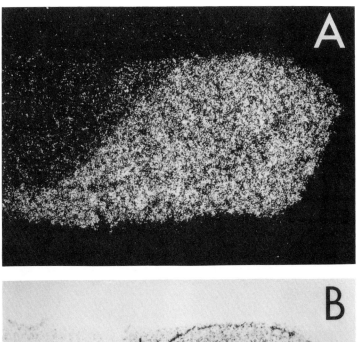

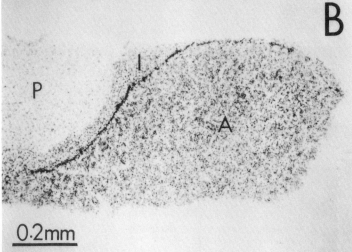

Fig. 3   A low-power dark-field photomicrograph of an emulsion autoradiogram of a coronal section through the murine pituitary gland following *in situ* hybridization with an ^{35}S-labeled antisense riboprobe for the type I IL-1 receptor (A). A bright-field photomicrograph of the same section stained with hematoxylin–eosin is shown for reference (B). Dense signal is present over the entire anterior lobe of the gland (A). The signal over the posterior (P) and intermediate (I) lobes is comparable to background. With pituitary, the best histology was obtained with cryostat cut sections. [Reproduced with permission from Cunningham *et al.* (2).]

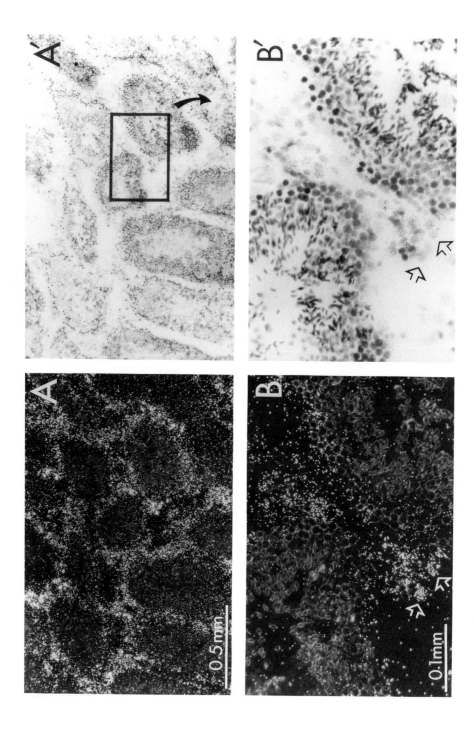

stored at 4°C for approximately four times the time required to obtain adequate signal on Hypermax-MP film. Last, slides are developed in Kodak (Rochester, NY) D-19 for 3 min, washed in a stop bath of distilled H_2O for 15 sec, and fixed with Kodak rapid fixer for 5 min. Slides should be washed under gently running tap water for 30 min prior to counterstaining and coverslipping.

Controls and Analysis

Prior to analysis, stringent controls should be run to assure that signal in fact represents endogenous levels of the mRNA species of interest. A number of controls are available, and not all need be run for every probe. In general, we like to control for general background signal by hybridizing an adjacent series from each animal with the sense strand labeled and hybridized alongside the antisense strand. Here, only those tissue regions that hybridize antisense but not sense probe would be considered specific signal. In those cases in which probe is hydrolyzed to optimize penetration as described by Cox *et al.* (11), the sense strand should also be hydrolyzed to fragments of comparable size prior to hybridization. Ideally, we then like to confirm signal specificity with a Northern blot analysis. Alternatives to this might be to use RNase protection after solution hybridization, or the use of two nonoverlapping portions of the coding region of interest. Some have advocated using sections previously treated with RNase A as a negative control, although we have found that this provides little additional information.

   Sections are most easily analyzed if lightly counterstained, either with a Nissl or hematoxylin–eosin technique. For brain, an adjacent series not exposed to either proteinase K or Triton X-100 should be Nissl stained to facilitate identification of cytoarchitectonic boundaries. Beyond this, perhaps the most useful indicators of true signal are (1) regional differences in signal distribution among or within structures of comparable cellular density, such

---

Fig. 4   Low-power (A) and high-power (B) dark-field photomicrographs of an emulsion autoradiogram of a section through the testis following *in situ* hybridization with an ^{35}S-labeled antisense riboprobe for the type I IL-1 receptor. Bright-field photomicrographs of the same section stained with hematoxylin–eosin are shown for reference (A' and B'). Intense signal is present over interstitial cells (arrowheads), the majority of which are known to be of the Leydig, or testosterone-producing, type. Note that the autoradiographic grains are concentrated over the cytoplasm of the Leydig cells. Like most endocrine tissues, the testis is somewhat friable and, as with the pituitary, the best histology was obtained with cryostat-cut sections. [Reproduced, with permission from S. Karger AG, Basel, from Cunningham *et al.* (3).]

as different cortical areas, distinct hippocampal fields (Fig. 2), or the various lobes of the pituitary gland (Fig. 3), and (2) preferential distribution of autoradiographic grains over cellular cytoplasm on high-power analysis (Fig. 4), as compared to nonspecific signal, which tends to accumulate at the edge of cells.

In our experiments in brain, an intense autoradiographic signal was observed over the granule cell layer of the dentate gyrus (Fig. 2), over the entire midline raphe system, over the choroid plexus, and over endothelial cells of postcapillary venules throughout the neuraxis (see Fig. 2). A weak to moderate signal was observed over the pyramidal cell layer of the hilus and CA3 region of the hippocampus (Fig. 2), over the anterodorsal thalamic nucleus, over sensory neurons of the mesencephalic trigeminal nucleus, over Purkinje cells of the cerebellar cortex, and in scattered clusters over the externalmost layer of the median eminence. In the pituitary gland, a dense and homogeneously distributed autoradiographic signal was observed over the entire anterior lobe (Fig. 3). No signal above background was observed over the posterior and intermediate lobes, or over the adrenal gland (1, 2). In the testis, an intense signal was observed over the interstitial cells, the majority of which are known to be of the Leydig type, and over the epithelial lining of epididymal ducts, most prominently in the head region. The signal over seminiferous tubule, and over sperm cells within tubules and epididymal ducts, was comparable to background (3). Together, these studies provide a substrate for the known effects of IL-1 on both the nervous and neuroendocrine systems, particularly its pronounced effects on the hypothalamic–pituitary–adrenal and –gonadal axes (4).

Acknowledgments

Our experiments described in this review were performed in collaboration with Drs. E. Wada, D. B. Carter, D. E. Tracey, and J. F. Battey. We thank Mr. C. M. Arias, and Drs. J. F. Battey, P. E. Sawchenko, and E. Wada for having thoughtfully read and commented on an early version of the manuscript.

References

1. E. T. Cunningham, Jr., E. Wada, D. B. Carter, D. E. Tracey, J. F. Battey, and E. B. De Souza, *Endocrinology (Baltimore)* **128**(5), 2666 (1991).
2. E. T. Cunningham, Jr., E. Wada, D. B. Carter, D. E. Tracey, J. F. Battey, and E. B. De Souza, *J. Neurosci.* **12**(3), 1101 (1992).
3. E. T. Cunningham, Jr., E. Wada, D. B. Carter, D. E. Tracey, J. F. Battey, and E. B. De Souza, *Neuroendocrinology* **56,** 94 (1992).

4. E. T. Cunningham, Jr. and E. B. De Souza, *Immunol. Today* (in press) (1993).

5. L. M. Angerer, M. H. Stoler, and R. C. Angerer, *in* "*In situ* Hybridization: Applications to Neurobiology" (K. L. Ventino, J. H. Eberwine, and J. D. Barchas, eds.), p. 42. Oxford Univ. Press, New York, 1987.

6. E. Wada, K. Wada, J. Boulter, E. Deneris, S. Heinemann, J. Patrick, and L. W. Swanson, *J. Comp. Neurol.* **284,** 314 (1989).

7. D. M. Simmons, J. L. Arriza, and L. W. Swanson, *J. Histotechnol.* **12**(3), 169 (1989).

8. P. C. Emson, *Comp. Biochem. Physiol. A* **93A** (1), 233 (1989).

9. W. S. Young, *in* "Handbook of Chemical Neuroanatomy" (A. Bjorklund, T. Hokfelt, F. G. Wouterlood, and A. N. van den Pol, eds.), Vol. 8, p. 481. Elsevier, New York, 1990.

10. M. E. Lewis and F. Baldino, Jr., *in* "*In situ* Hybridization: Histochemistry" (M.-F. Chesselet, ed.), p. 1. CRC Press, Boca Raton, FL, 1990.

11. K. H. Cox, D. V. DeLeon, L. M. Angerer, and R. C. Angerer, *Dev. Biol.* **101,** 485 (1984).

12. W. J. Chiou, P. D. Harris, P. K. W. Carter, and J. P. Singh, *J. Biol. Chem.* **264,** 21442 (1989).

13. A. W. Rogers, "Techniques of Autoradiography," 3rd ed. Elsevier, New York, 1979.

[8] Identification, Autoradiographic Localization, and Modulation of Interleukin 1 Receptors in Brain–Endocrine–Immune Axis: Methodology and Overview

Toshihiro Takao, Dimitri E. Grigoriadis, and Errol B. De Souza

Introduction

The cytokine interleukin 1 (IL-1) is one of the key mediators of immunological and pathological responses to stress, infection, and antigenic challenge (1–3). In addition to its immune effects, a role has been postulated for IL-1 as a neurotransmitter/neuromodulator/growth factor in the central nervous system (CNS). Interleukin 1 production has been reported in cultured brain astrocytes and microglia (4–6) and IL-1 has been detected in the brain following cerebral trauma (7, 8) and endotoxin treatment (9). Interleukin 1-like activity is also present in the cerebrospinal fluid (CSF) (10, 11), IL-1 mRNA is present in normal brain (12, 13), and immunohistological studies have identified neurons positive for IL-1β-like immunoreactivity in both hypothalamic (14, 15) and extrahypothalamic (15) sites in human brain. Central as well as peripheral administration of IL-1 has potent neuroendocrine actions, including stimulation of the hypothalamic–pituitary–adrenocortical axis (16–18) and inhibition of the hypothalamic–pituitary–gonadal axis (19). These effects of IL-1 are presumably mediated through actions of the cytokine at specific high-affinity receptors. Studies have identified at least two types of IL-1 receptors that are differentially expressed on the surface of certain types of immune cells and human- and murine-derived cell lines (20, 21) (Table I). Recombinant human IL-1α and IL-1β bind to both type I receptors on T-cells, fibroblasts, keratinocytes, endothelial cells, synovial lining cells, chondrocytes, and hepatocytes (21, 22) and type II receptors on various B cell lines, including the Raji human B cell lymphoma line (20, 23, 24). A newly described recombinant human IL-1 receptor antagonist (IL-1ra) was initially reported to label type I IL-1 receptors selectively and not to recognize type II receptors (25, 26). More recent studies have shown that IL-1ra competitively inhibits the binding to the type II IL-1 receptors albeit with a lower affinity (27, 28). The differential selectivity of IL-1 and IL-1ra for type I versus type II IL-1 receptors makes them useful ligands for

Methods in Neurosciences, Volume 16

TABLE I   Heterogeneity of IL-1 Receptors

Parameter	Receptor	
	Type I	Type II
Affinity	Low pM	Low nM
Pharmacology	IL-1α ≈ IL-1β ≈ IL-1ra	IL-1β > IL-1α ≥ IL-1ra
Molecular weight	~80,000	~68,000
Biochemical composition	Glycoprotein	Glycoprotein
Tissue	T cells, fibroblasts, kera-tinocytes, endothelial cells, synovial lining cells, chondrocytes, hepatocytes	B cell lines

determining further the characteristics of IL-1 receptors in the brain–endo-crine–immune axis. In this article, we summarize some of the data from our studies and elaborate on methods using ^{125}I-labeled recombinant human IL-1 (^{125}I-IL-1) and ^{125}I-labeled recombinant human IL-1 receptor antagonist (^{125}I-IL-1ra) to identify, characterize and localize IL-1 receptors in the mouse brain–endocrine–immune axis. In addition, we describe the *in vitro* and *in vivo* modulation of IL-1 receptors.

Methodology

Tissue Preparation

C57BL/6 mice (7–8 weeks) were sacrificed by cervical dislocation and brain and other tissues of interest were dissected (29), weighed, and placed in ice-cold preparation buffer [RPMI-1640, gentamicin (50 μg/ml), 20 mM N-2-hydroxyethylpiperazine-N'-2-ethanesulfonic acid (HEPES), sodium azide (1 mg/ml), aprotonin (100 KIU/ml), and 10^{-4} M bacitracin; pH 7.4]. Routine characterization assays in tissue homogenates were performed with freshly dissected tissue. Tissues were disrupted in buffer, using a Polytron tissue homogenizer (Brinkman Instruments, Westbury, NY) at setting 6 for 20 sec. The homogenate was centrifuged at 40,000 g for 12 min at 4°C and washed by resuspending in the same buffer and recentrifuging. After the wash, the tissues were resuspended in the same buffer, using a Polytron, to a final protein concentration of 50–80 mg original wet weight/ml (Fig. 1). The protein concentration of tissues was determined by a modification of the Lowry method (30), using bovine serum albumin (BSA) as the standard.

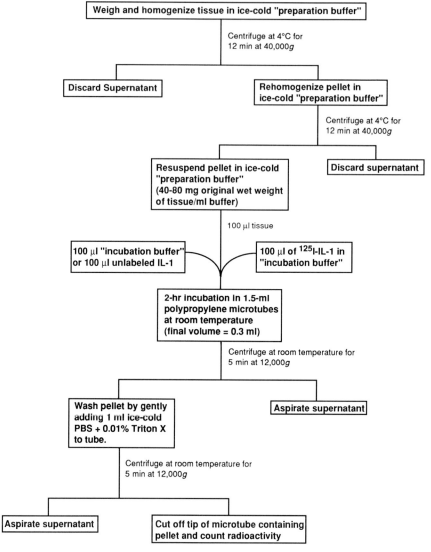

FIG. 1 The schematic flow chart of the ^{125}I-IL-1-binding assay. The preparation buffer contains RPMI-1640, including gentamicin (50 μg/ml), 20 mM HEPES, sodium azide (1 mg/ml), aprotinin (100 KIU/ml), and 10^{-4} M bacitracin; pH 7.4. The incubation buffer consists of tissue preparation buffer with 0.15% BSA.

IL-1 Receptor-Binding Assay

A schematic of the IL-1 receptor binding assay is shown in Fig. 1. One hundred microliters of the membrane suspension was added to a 1.5-ml polypropylene microtube containing 100 μl of an ^{125}I-IL-1 solution (final concentration range of approximately 30 to 100 pM in competition studies and 3 to 500 pM in saturation studies) and 100 μl of the incubation buffer (tissue preparation buffer with 0.15% BSA) or an appropriate concentration of unlabeled IL-1β or other competing peptide. Nonspecific binding was usually determined in the presence of 300 nM IL-1β. The reaction was allowed to proceed for 2 hr at room temperature (22°C), conditions found to be at equilibrium, that is, at the plateau of the association kinetics curve. The tissue was separated from the incubation medium by centrifugation in a Beckman (Fullerton, CA) microfuge for 5 min at 12,000 g at room temperature. The resulting pellet was washed with 1 ml of Dulbecco's phosphate-buffered saline (PBS) (GIBCO, Grand Island, NY) containing 0.01% Triton X-100, pH 7.2. The contents were recentrifuged for 5 min at 12,000 g. The supernatant was aspirated and the microtubes were cut just above the pellet. The radioactivity of the pellet was measured in an LKB (Gaithersburg, MD) γ counter at 80% efficiency.

Unlabeled recombinant human interleukin 1α (IL-1α), recombinant human interleukin-1β (IL-1β) and human recombinant tumor necrosis factor α (TNF-α) were cloned, expressed, and purified at the Upjohn Company (Kalamazoo, MI) (31) or the Du Pont-Merck Pharmaceutical Company (Wilmington, DE). An analog of IL-1β with three amino acids added to the carboxy terminal (IL-1β^{+}) was cloned, expressed, and purified at the Upjohn Company (31). Unlabeled recombinant human IL-1 receptor antagonist (IL-1ra), an analog of the clone 18 IL-1β with two substitutions at the amino terminus (from alanine–proline to threonine–methionine) (IL-1β^{c18}) were cloned, expressed, and purified at the Du Pont-Merck Pharmaceutical Company. Unlabeled rat/human corticotropin-releasing factor (CRF) was purchased from Peninsula Laboratories (Belmont, CA).

Chemical Affinity Cross-Linking of IL-1 to Receptors

Under equilibrium binding conditions (i.e., 120-min incubation; see above), 10 μl of disuccinimidyl suberate [DSS; final concentration, 1.5 mM in 100% dimethyl sulfoxide (DMSO)] was added to each tube and incubated for 20 min at 22°C. The chemical reaction was terminated by the addition of 1 ml of ice-cold 10 mM Tris-HCl and 1 mM ethylenediaminetetraacetic acid (EDTA) (pH 7.0) at 0–4°C and centrifugation at 12,000 rpm for 5 min in a

Beckman microfuge. The pellets were washed gently once with 1 ml of ice-cold 10 mM Tris-HCl and 1 mM EDTA and recentrifuged. Final pellets were solubilized in sodium dodecyl sulfate-polyacrylamide gel electrophoresis (SDS-PAGE) sample buffer containing 50 mM Tris-HCl, 10% glycerol, 2% SDS, and 5% 2-mercaptoethanol (pH 6.8 at 22°C) prior to electrophoresis on a discontinuous slab gel system [6% stacking and 12% separating; (32)] overnight. Prestained protein standards (Sigma, St. Louis, MO) were included on each gel and used to calculate a standard curve from their relative mobilities. Gels were then dried and autoradiograms generated by apposing gels to Kodac (Rochester, NY) X-AR film, using Lightning-Plus enhancing screens (Du Pont, Wilmington, DE) for approximately 10–20 days.

Autoradiography

Tissues were freshly dissected, flash frozen in isopentane (−50°C), and mounted with OCT compound (Miles, Elkhart, IN) for cryotomy. Frozen sections (10-μm thickness) were thaw-mounted onto chrome alum/gelatin-coated microscope slides, dried, and stored desiccated at −70°C. On the day of the assay, the slide-mounted tissue was brought to room temperature and incubated for 120 min in 100 pM ^{125}I-IL-1α or 40 pM ^{125}I-IL-1ra in the incubation buffer described above. Nonspecific binding was defined as binding in the presence of a 1000-fold excess (100 nM) of IL-1α or IL-1β. Following incubation, the slides were rinsed, washed for two 5-min periods at 4°C in PBS with 0.01% Triton X-100 at pH 7.4, and rinsed in distilled water at 4°C. The slides were then rapidly dried under a stream of cool, dry air. The dry, labeled slides and ^{125}I autoradiographic standards (Amersham, Arlington Heights, IL) were apposed to Ultrofilm (Cambridge, Nussloch, Germany) and exposed for 10–21 days. Following exposure, autoradiograms on Ultrofilm were tank developed for 5 min in GBX developer (Kodak), washed for 1 min in stop bath (Kodak), fixed in GBX fixer for 5 min (Kodak), washed in running water at 20°C for 20 min, and then air dried.

Data Analysis and Quantification of Autoradiograms

Data from saturation curves were analyzed by the nonlinear curve-fitting program LIGAND of Munson and Rodbard (33). The program provides parameters for the equilibrium dissociation constant (K_D) and maximum number of binding site (B_{max}) values along with statistics on the general fit of the estimated parameters to the raw data. Data from competition curves were also analyzed by the program LIGAND. For each competition curve, estimates of the affinity of radiolabeled ligand for IL-1 receptor was obtained in independent saturation experiments (as above), and these estimates were constrained during the analysis of the apparent inhibitory constant (K_i) values for the various related and unrelated peptides tested. For IL-1-related peptides, all data fit significantly to a single-site model.

In autoradiograms prepared with Ultrofilm, optical density readings, construction of standard curves, and rapid quantification were carried out with a personal computer-based digital image analysis system (Loats, Westminster, MD) (34). All regions of interest were sampled in quadruplicate from individual mice. Structures were identified at the end of the autoradiographic procedure on the same sections from which the autoradiograms were generated or when necessary on adjacent sections. The anatomical nomenclature used was derived from Slotnic and Leonard (35). Best fit standard curves of film optical density generated with the radioiodinated standards coexposed with labeled slides resulted when a third-order function was used to describe the relationship between radioactivity and optical density. By generating a standard curve concomitantly with the ^{125}I-IL-1 autoradiograms, the film optical density readings of the samples were related to the molar concentration of ^{125}I-IL-1 bound.

Quinolinic Acid Lesions of Hippocampus

The mice were anesthetized with epithesin [3 mg/kg intraperitoneal (ip)] and placed in a stereotaxic instrument (David Kopf, Tujunga, CA) to a flat skull position. After a sagittal incision was made, the skull was carefully cleaned of fascia and two holes (1 mm) were drilled bilaterally, using the following coordinates: -1.5 mm bregma, 1.5 mm lateral to midline (35). Two 30-gauge cannulas were placed 3 mm apart and were stereotaxically lowered 1.8 mm below the skull with the tips centered in the left and right hippocampus. PE-10 tubing was then connected to both cannulas and to a 50-μl syringe mounted on a microdrive. Accurate infusion amounts were calibrated by a predetermined amount of air space moving through a section of the PE-10 tubing. Quinolinic acid (300 nM, 0.5 μl) was infused over a 2-min period into the right hemisphere and isotonic saline (0.9%, 0.5 μl) was infused into the left hemisphere, simultaneously. The cannulas were then removed after a 1-min equilibration period. The head incision was then closed with autoclips and the animal was allowed to recover for 4 days, after which time the animal was sacrificed and the brain was removed and frozen with an isopentane slurry ($-50°$C). Frozen coronal sections (10-μm thickness) were taken from -3.2 to -0.9 bregma and thaw-mounted on chrome alum/gelatin-coated slides and processed for autoradiography as described above.

Choice of Radioligand

Two biochemically distinct forms of the cytokine, IL-1α and IL-1β, have been isolated (1–3). These polypeptides have been radioiodinated and used as radioligands to label the receptors in a variety of *in vitro* studies, including membrane homogenate and autoradiographic assays. Presently, we routinely use the commercially available preparations of ^{125}I-labeled recombinant human interleukin-1α (^{125}I-IL-1α) (specific activity, approximately 1500–2000 Ci/mmol) and interleukin-1β (^{125}I-IL-1β) (specific activity, approximately 2500–3000 Ci/mmol) from Du Pont-New England Nuclear (Boston, MA). A receptor antagonist to IL-1 produced from IgG-adherent human monocytes has been purified, sequenced, and cDNA for the 18-kDa protein expressed in *Escherichia coli* (25, 26, 36). Interleukin 1ra blocks several IL-1-stimulated responses *in vitro*, including prostaglandin E$_2$ (PGE$_2$) release, thymocyte proliferation, collagenase production, and leukocyte adherence (37, 38). *In vivo*, IL-1ra blocks IL-1-induced activation of the hypothalamic–pituitary–adrenal axis and reduces mortality from endotoxin shock (37, 38). Interleukin 1ra was radiolabeled with ^{125}I-labeled Bolton–Hunter reagent (^{125}I-IL-1ra) (specific activity, approximately 2300 Ci/mmol) at the Du Pont-Merck Pharmaceutical Co.. Although it has been reported that unlabeled IL-1α, IL-1β, and IL-1ra bind equally to type I IL-1 receptors (39), ^{125}I-IL-1α showed comparable to somewhat higher specific binding than ^{125}I-IL-1ra, which, in turn, showed much higher specific binding than ^{125}I-IL-1β in mouse tissues (Fig. 2). The lower level of ^{125}I-IL-1β binding in mouse hippocampus, spleen, and testis is probably a consequence of a structural modification in the molecule incurred during the radioiodination procedure, rendering the molecule less biologically active and therefore a poor radioligand to label the receptor. A loss of biological activity of recombinant human IL-1β but not IL-1α following radioiodination of the proteins has been reported (39). However, in view of reports demonstrating that IL-1α and IL-1β may have different effects on biological functions (40, 41) and the suggestion of multiple IL-1 receptors (20, 21), the detection of an ^{125}I-IL-1β-binding site in brain, endocrine, and immune tissues under different radioiodination or assay conditions cannot be excluded at the present time. On the basis of these experiments, all subsequent studies were performed with ^{125}I-IL-1α or ^{125}I-IL-1ra as the radioligand.

Choice of Species

[125]I-Labeled IL-1α or ^{125}I-IL-1ra binding were compared in mouse, rat, rabbit, and guinea pig tissues, including hippocampus, spleen, and testis (42, 43). In contrast to moderate to high levels of binding in mouse and rabbit tissues,

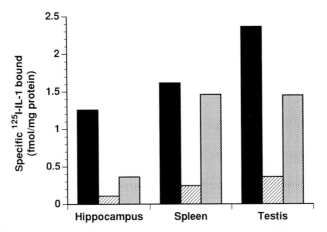

FIG. 2   Interleukin 1 binding in mouse tissues with different ^{125}I-IL-1 ligands (black bars, IL-1α; striped bars, IL-1β; gray bars, IL-1ra). Crude membrane preparations of hippocampus, spleen, or testis were incubated for 120 min at room temperature with ^{125}I-IL-1. A saturating concentration of ^{125}I-IL-1 (50–100 pM) was used in this study to detect primarily changes in receptor density. Nonspecific binding was determined in the presence of 300 nM IL-1β.

^{125}I-IL-1α and ^{125}I-IL-1ra binding to rat or guinea pig tissues were barely within the range of sensitivity of the assay. Representative data with ^{125}I-IL-1α binding in spleen are shown in Fig. 3. These lower levels of ^{125}I-IL-1α and ^{125}I-IL-1ra binding in rat tissues do not necessarily suggest a lack of IL-1 receptors, because recombinant human IL-1 in rats alters sleep (44), induces anorexia (45), induces adrenocorticotropic hormone (ACTH) release (46, 47), and modulates the acute release of growth hormone-releasing hormone and somatostatin (48). In addition, IL-1ra reduced the severity of experimental enterocolitis and lipopolysaccaride-induced pulmonary inflamation in rat (38). Furthermore, evidence suggests a multiplicity of IL-1 receptors (20, 21), and the possibility exists that the radioligands used in the present study (recombinant human ^{125}I-IL-1α and ^{125}I-IL-1ra) label only a subtype of these receptors that is present in some species, including mouse, rabbit, human, and monkey (unpublished data) but is absent in species such as rat and guinea pig. Additional studies using homologous ligands (i.e., rat IL-1 or IL-1ra) may be useful in resolving these species differences. Given the species differences, mouse tissues were used for the remainder of the studies.

Choice of Brain Regions

The regional distribution of binding sites for ^{125}I-IL-1α was examined in homogenates of discrete areas of mouse CNS in order to identify a brain

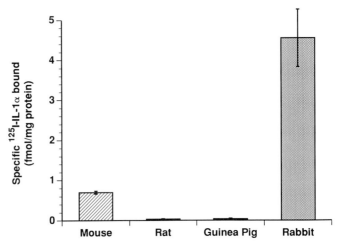

Fig. 3   Species differences in ^{125}I-IL-1α binding in mouse, rat, guinea pig, and rabbit spleen. Crude membrane preparations from frozen tissues were incubated for 120 min at room temperature with ^{125}I-IL-1α. A saturating concentration of ^{125}I-IL-1α (100 pM) was used in this study to detect primarily changes in receptor density. Nonspecific binding was determined in the presence of 300 nM IL-1β.

area(s) that may be ideally suited for subsequent characterization of the receptor. The highest density of binding sites in mouse CNS was present in the hippocampus (Fig. 4). Progressively lower, but significant densities of binding sites were detected in cerebral cortex, cerebellum, olfactory bulb, striatum, spinal cord, hypothalamus and medulla oblongata. Therefore, mouse hippocampus was used for the remainder of the characterization studies.

Characteristics of IL-1 Receptors

Effects of Tissue Protein Concentrations

Incubation of varying concentrations of membranes of mouse tissues with ^{125}I-IL-1α and ^{125}I-IL-1ra indicated that binding of the radioligand was linear over the protein concentration range examined (0–300 μg/tube) (42, 49, 50). On the basis of these studies, all subsequent assays were carried out with approximately 200–300 μg of protein/tube. Under these conditions, specific ^{125}I-IL-1α and ^{125}I-IL-1ra binding (i.e., 300 nM IL-1β displaceable) in mouse tissues was approximately 30–80% and 40–60% of the total binding, respectively (42, 49, 50).

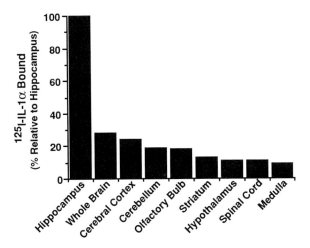

FIG. 4   Regional distribution of IL-1 receptors in mouse CNS. Crude membranes from each of the indicated regions were incubated for 120 min at room temperature in the presence of 50 pM ^{125}I-IL-1α. Nonspecific binding was determined in the presence of 50 nM IL-1β. Data are expressed as a percentage of specific ^{125}I-IL-1α binding to receptor densities (fmol/mg protein) in the hippocampus. Each bar represents the mean of a triplicate determination that varied by less than 10%. [Reproduced from Ref. 49 (T. Takao, D. E. Tracey, W.M. Mitchell, and E. B. De Souza, Interleukin-1 receptors in mouse brain: Characterization and neuronal localization, *Endocrinology*, 1990, **127**, 3070–3078) with permission. © The Endocrine Society.]

Binding Characteristics at Equilibrium

The concentration-dependent binding of ^{125}I-IL-1α and ^{125}I-IL-1ra to mouse tissues under equilibrium conditions was examined (42, 49, 50) and representative data of ^{125}I-IL-1ra are shown in Fig. 5. Specific ^{125}I-IL-1α or ^{125}I-IL-1ra (Fig. 5) binding was saturable and of high affinity. Scatchard analysis (Fig. 5, inset) of the saturation data showed comparable high affinity binding (K_D, 60–120 pM for ^{125}I-IL-1α and 20–30 pM for ^{125}I-IL-1ra) in mouse tissues. A summary of the affinity and density of ^{125}I-IL-1α and ^{125}I-IL-1ra binding is shown in Table II. The highest relative density of binding sites was present in the testis, using both ligands, with progressively lower densities evident in the spleen (^{125}I-IL-1ra), hippocampus, and kidney (^{125}I-IL-1α).

Characterization of Pharmacological Specificity

The pharmacological characteristics of the ^{125}I-IL-1α and ^{125}I-IL-1ra binding site were examined by determining the relative potencies of IL-1-related

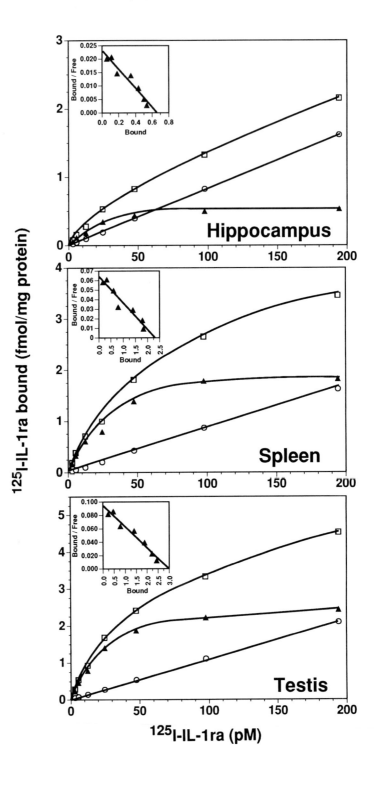

TABLE II   Affinity and Density of ^{125}I-IL-1α and ^{125}I-IL-1ra Binding in Mouse Tissues and AtT-20 Cells[a]

Tissue	K_D (pM)		B_{max} (fmol/mg protein)	
	^{125}I-IL-1α	^{125}I-IL-1ra	^{125}I-IL-1α	^{125}I-IL-1ra
Hippocampus	114 ± 35	28 ± 8	2.5 ± 0.4	0.9 ± 0.1
Spleen	ND	21 ± 6	ND	2.3 ± 0.2
Kidney	66 ± 10	ND	1.1 ± 0.2	ND
Testis	82 ± 4	23 ± 7	10.8 ± 1.5	3.3 ± 0.6
AtT-20	19 ± 2	ND	3.5 ± 1.8	ND

[a] Crude membrane preparations of mouse tissues were incubated for 120 min at room temperature with increasing concentrations of ^{125}I-IL-1α (10–500 pM) and 3–200 pM ^{125}I-IL-1ra. Nonspecific binding was determined in the presence of 300 nM IL-1β. The experiment was carried out three times and the equilibrium dissociation constant (K_D) and maximum number of binding site (B_{max}) values from saturation binding experiments were calculated by the nonlinear curve-fitting program LIGAND of Munson and Rodbard (33). ND, Not determined.

and -unrelated peptides in displacing specifically bound ^{125}I-IL-1α and ^{125}I-IL-1ra in homogenates of mouse tissues. The results of the homogenate studies with ^{125}I-IL-1α and ^{125}I-IL-1ra are summarized in Table III. Interleukin 1α and IL-1ra were more potent than IL-1β, which, in turn, was more potent than its weak analogs IL-1β^+ and IL-1β^{c18}. Corticotropin-releasing factor and TNF (at concentrations up to 100 nM) had no effect on ^{125}I-IL-1α or ^{125}I-IL-1ra binding. The relative inhibitory potencies of IL-1α, IL-1β, IL-1β^+, and IL-1β^{c18}, for the most part, paralleled their bioactivities in a murine thymocyte costimulation assay (51) (Table III).

Affinity Cross-Linking Studies

To determine the molecular weight of IL-1 receptors in various tissues, disuccinimidyl suberate (DSS), an irreversible amine-reactive homobifunctional cross-linking agent, was used to covalently attach ^{125}I-IL-1α to mem-

FIG. 5   The binding of ^{125}I-IL-1ra to mouse hippocampus, spleen, and testis as a function of increasing ligand concentration. Direct plot of data shows the total amount of ^{125}I-IL-1ra bound (□), binding in the presence of 300 nM IL-1α or β (○), and specific (total minus nonspecific) binding (▲). *Insets*: Scatchard plots of [^{125}I]IL-1ra-specific binding. Crude membrane preparations of mouse tissues were incubated for 120 min at room temperature with increasing concentrations of ^{125}I-IL-1ra. The data shown are from a representative experiment. [Reproduced with permission from Takao et al. (43).]

TABLE III Pharmacological Specificity of ^{125}I-IL-1α and ^{125}I-IL-1ra Binding to the Mouse Tissues[a]

Peptide	K_i(pM)						Biological activity (units/mg)
	Hippocampus		Spleen	Kidney	Testis		
	^{125}I-IL-1α	^{125}I-IL-1ra	(^{125}I-IL-1ra)	(^{125}I-IL-1α)	^{125}I-IL-1α	^{125}I-IL-1ra	
IL-1α	55 ± 18	70 ± 10	57 ± 9	28 ± 19	14 ± 2	46 ± 8	3.0×10^7
IL-1ra	ND	119 ± 63	104 ± 54	ND	ND	94 ± 49	No activity
IL-1β	76 ± 20	1,798 ± 234	3,138 ± 1,159	53 ± 23	89 ± 6	3,672 ± 1,317	2.0×10^{7b}
IL-1β$^+$	2,940 ± 742	ND	ND	5,560 ± 2,098	7,183 ± 604	ND	1.0×10^6
IL-1β^{c18}	ND	2,008 ± 350	2,780 ± 919	ND	ND	2.732 ± 474	ND
TNF	>100,000	>100,000	>100,000	>100,000	>100,000	>100,000	8.0×10^2
CRF	>100,000	>100,000	>100,000	>100,000	>100,000	>100,000	0.0

[a] Peptides at 3–10 concentrations were incubated with approximatey 100 pM ^{125}I-IL-1α and 40 pM ^{125}I-IL-1ra for 120 min at room temperature. All assays were conducted in triplicate in three separate experiments. The K_i (inhibitory binding affinity constant) values were obtained from competition curve data analyzed with the computer program LIGAND (33). Biological activity data were obtained in a murine thymocyte assay (51).

[b] Of note, IL-1β used in the ^{125}I-IL-1ra experiments had lower biological activity than IL-1β used in the ^{125}I-IL-1α experiments.

brane receptors. The reagent DSS has been widely used for the elucidation of the structural and biochemical characteristics of various peptidergic systems. For example, studies have been reported in which DSS was used to functionally couple ^{125}I-labeled human somatotropin (52), ^{125}I-labeled angiotensin II (53), vasoactive intestinal peptide (54), atrial natriuretic factor (55), and CRF (56, 57) to their respective receptors.

Figure 6 demonstrates the covalent attachment of IL-1α to EL-4 6.1 and AtT-20 cells as well as to mouse pituitary membrane homogenates. In the murine thymoma EL-4 6.1 cells and in the mouse AtT-20 pituitary tumor cells, ^{125}I-IL-1α was covalently linked to a membrane protein with an observed molecular weight of ~100,000 and a pharmacological profile that corresponded to that observed in membrane binding consistent with the labeling

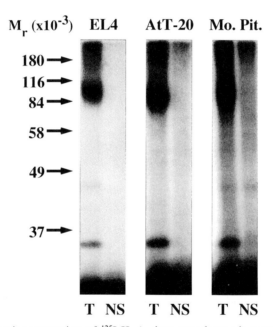

FIG. 6   Covalent incorporation of ^{125}I-IL-1α into membrane homogenates of EL-4 6.1 (EL4), AtT-20 cells, and mouse pituitary (Mo. Pit.). Membranes were incubated with ^{125}I-IL-1α (final concentration, 200 pM) for 2 hr at room temperature and then incubated with DSS and DMSO as described and electrophoresed on SDS-polyacrylamide gels. Affinity cross-linking was performed in the absence (T) or presence (NS) of 100 nM IL-1β to define the nonspecific binding. EL-4 6.1, AtT-20, and mouse pituitary all demonstrated specific covalent labeling of an identical protein with an apparent molecular weight (of the complex) of 100,000. Molecular weight standard markers were included on each individual gel in order to calculate the apparent molecular weights of the labeled species.

of the type I IL-1 receptor. The molecular weight observed following SDS-PAGE is consistent with the previously reported molecular weight of the type I receptor (~80,000), because the apparent molecular weight observed represents the sum of the molecular weight of the receptor-binding site (~80,000) and the ligand itself (^{125}I-IL-1α; 17,000). In mouse pituitary homogenates, identical labeling was observed, again identifying the type I receptor. In the absence of competing unlabeled ligand (T), ^{125}I-IL-1α was covalently incorporated into a protein with an apparent molecular weight of 100,000. In the presence of a saturating concentration (100 nM) of unlabeled IL-1β (NS) the covalent incorporation of ^{125}I-IL-1α could be completely inhibited. In addition, compounds that have been shown not to bind to the type I IL-1 receptor in membrane homogenates (TNF or CRF) did not affect the covalent attachment of IL-1α to the type I receptor in any of the tissues examined (data not shown), suggesting that the binding site labeled was specific for IL-1.

Autoradiographic Localization of ^{125}I-IL-1α and ^{125}I-IL-1ra Binding in Mouse Hippocampus, Pituitary, Spleen, Testis, and Kidney

A comparison of the autoradiographic distribution of ^{125}I-IL-1ra-labeled and ^{125}I-IL-1α-labeled IL-1 receptors is shown in Figs. 7 and 8. Overall, low densities of ^{125}I-IL-1α (Fig. 7A) and ^{125}I-IL-1ra (Fig. 7B)-binding sites were present throughout the brain. High densities and a discrete localization of IL-1 receptors were evident in the hippocampal formation and in the choroid plexus (Fig. 7). Within the hippocampus, IL-1 receptors were present in the molecular and granular layers of the dentate gyrus and were virtually absent in the CA1 to CA3 pyramidal region. As shown in Table IV, the pharmacological binding characteristics of ^{125}I-IL-1α were similar in the dentate gyrus and in the choroid plexus and, for the most part, comparable to the characteristics seen in homogenates of hippocampus. Interleukin 1α and IL-1β inhibited binding in both areas with comparable potencies [50% inhibitory concentration (IC$_{50}$) values of less than 100 pM]. The weak IL-1β analog, IL-1β$^+$, inhibited 80–85% of the specific binding at the high concentration of 50 nM, whereas comparable concentrations of TNF and CRF were essentially ineffective in inhibiting ^{125}I-IL-1α binding (Table IV). There was an absence of specific ^{125}I-IL-1ra or ^{125}I-IL-1α binding in the hypothalamus, cerebral cortex, and other brain areas.

In the peripheral tissues, the distribution of ^{125}I-IL-1ra-binding sites (Fig. 8B) was comparable to ^{125}I-IL-1α-labeled IL-1 receptors (Fig. 8A). There was a homogeneous distribution of ^{125}I-IL-1α (Fig. 8A) and ^{125}I-IL-1ra (Fig. 8B)-binding sites throughout the anterior pituitary, suggesting that IL-1 may

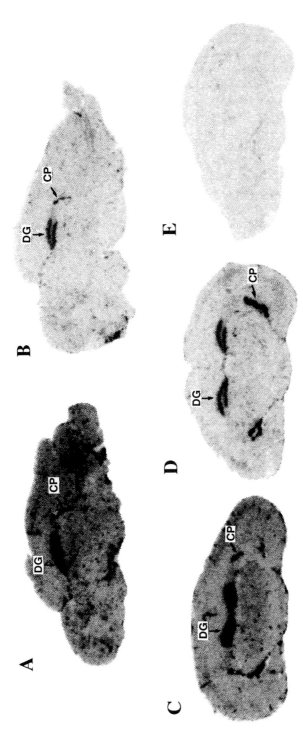

Fig. 7 (A–D) Autoradiographic localization of ^{125}I-IL-1α and ^{125}I-IL-1ra binding in mouse brain cut in sagittal (top) and coronal (bottom) planes. The tissues were incubated for 120 min with 40 pM ^{125}I-IL-1ra and 100 pM ^{125}I-IL-1α. The images were computer generated, using autoradiograms on Hyperfilm. The darker areas in the autoradiograms correspond to brain regions displaying higher densities of binding. (E) ^{125}I-IL-1ra binding is absent in this adjacent section coincubated with 100 nM IL-1α. DG, Dentate gyrus; CP, choroid plexus. [Reproduced with permission from Takao et al. (43).]

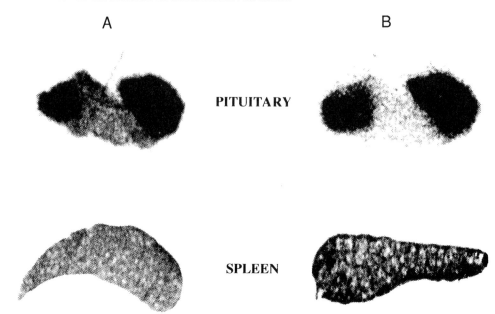

FIG. 8   Autoradiographic localization of (A) ^{125}I-IL-1α and (B) ^{125}I-IL-1ra binding in mouse pituitary and spleen. The tissues were incubated for 120 min with 40 pM ^{125}I-IL-1ra and 100 pM ^{125}I-IL-1α. The images were computer generated, using autoradiograms on Hyperfilm. The darker areas in the autoradiograms correspond to regions displaying higher densities of binding. [Reproduced with permission from Takao *et al.* (43).]

modify the release of multiple anterior pituitary hormones as well as ACTH. No specific ^{125}I-IL-1ra or ^{125}I-IL-1α binding was present in the intermediate and posterior lobe of the pituitary. High densities of IL-1-binding sites were found in the red pulp of spleen (Fig. 8), which consists of venous sinuses and splenic cord (58). Of note, there was low to negligible binding of ^{125}I-IL-1α and ^{125}I-IL-1ra in the white pulp regions of the spleen, which are enriched in lymphocytes. These data suggest that ^{125}I-IL-1ra and ^{125}I-IL-1α-binding sites are located primarily on resident macrophages. The highest densities of IL-1 receptors were found in the interstitial area of testis and lumenal borders of the epididymus (Fig. 9). The evidence that moderate to high densities of ^{125}I-IL-1α- and ^{125}I-IL-1ra-binding sites and type I IL-1 receptor mRNA (59) are present in the interstitial regions of testis supports that the endocrine effecs in the testis are mediated by specific IL-1 receptors. The autoradiographic distribution of ^{125}I-IL-1α-labeled receptors in kidney was also studied (50). Significantly higher densities of ^{125}I-IL-1α-binding sites were found in the medulla than in the cortex, which, in turn, had significantly

TABLE IV   Effects of IL-1-Related and -Unrelated Peptides on
Inhibition of ^{125}I-IL-1α Binding in Dentate Gyrus of
Hippocampus and in Choroid Plexus[a]

| Incubation condition | ^{125}I-IL-1α binding (fmol/mg tissue equivalent) | |
	Dentate gyrus	Choroid plexus
Total (50 pM ^{125}I-IL-1α)	132.3 ± 0.5 (100)	182.3 + 0.9 (100)
+ 100 pM IL-1α	54.0 ± 0.5 (34.1)	58.1 ± 0.4 (26.4)
+ 300 pM IL-1α	20.3 ± 0.4 (5.7)	24.3 ± 0.3 (6.4)
+ 1000 pM IL-1α	17.6 ± 0.3 (3.5)	20.3 ± 0.4 (4.0)
+ 50 nM IL-1α (blank)	13.5 ± 0.2 (0)	13.5 ± 0.3 (0)
+ 100 pM IL-1β	51.3 ± 0.5 (31.8)	78.3 ± 0.8 (38.4)
+ 300 pM IL-1β	27.0 ± 0.5 (11.4)	27.0 ± 0.3 (8.0)
+ 1000 pM IL-1β	24.3 ± 0.3 (9.1)	17.6 ± 0.3 (2.4)
+ 50 nM IL-1β (blank)	13.5 ± 0.2 (0)	13.5 + 0.1 (0)
+ 50 nM IL-1β^{+}	37.8 ± 0.3 (20.5)	37.8 ± 0.5 (14.4)
+ 50 nM CRF	139.1 ± 0.7 (105.7)	168.8 ± 1.0 (92.0)
+ 50 nM TNF	132.3 ± 0.5 (100)	155.3 ± 0.5 (84.0)

[a] Serial slide-mounted sagittal sections of mouse brain were incubated with ^{125}I-IL-1α with increasing concentrations of IL-1 related and -unrelated peptides to define the characteristics of ^{125}I-IL-1α binding in dentate gyrus and in choroid plexus. Autoradiograms of these brain sections and ^{125}I-labeled standards (Amersham) were generated with Ultrofilm. Interleukin 1-binding sites were labeled with 50 pM ^{125}I-IL-1α (total). Nonspecific binding (blank) was determined in the presence of 50 nM IL-1α or IL-1β and was comparable under both conditions. The relative densities of ^{125}I-IL-1α-binding sites in the absence (total) or presence of varying concentrations of IL-1α or IL-1β, 50 nM IL-1β^{+} (a weak analog of IL-1β), human tumor necrosis factor (TNF), and rat/human corticotropin-releasing factor (CRF) are shown. The values in parentheses represent the percentage specific binding of ^{125}I-IL-1α under the various experimental conditions. [Reproduced from Ref. 49 (T. Takao, D. E. Tracey, W.M. Mitchell, and E. B. De Souza, Interleukin-1 receptors in mouse brain: Characterization and neuronal localization, *Endocrinology*, 1990, **127**, 3070–3078) with permission. © The Endocrine Society.]

higher densities than in the interzone between cortex and medulla. There was a heterogeneous distribution pattern of ^{125}I-IL-1α binding within the renal cortex, suggesting that IL-1 receptors may be preferentially localized to a particular substructure (glomeruli or proximal tubules) within the kidney cortex.

Quinolinic Acid Lesions of Hippocampus

Quinolinic acid lesions of the hippocampus were utilized to determine if the ^{125}I-IL-1α-binding sites were localized to specific neuronal systems. In the hippocampus, intrinsic neurons were destroyed by local injection of quinolinic acid. This treatment abolished ^{125}I-IL-1α-binding sites in both the granu-

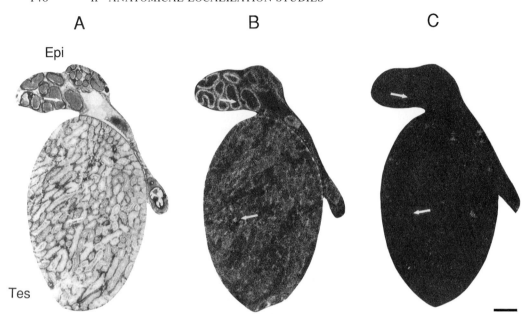

FIG. 9   Autoradiographic localization of ^{125}I-IL-1α-binding sites in intact mouse testis. (A) Bright-field photomicrograph showing the histology of a Cresyl Violet-stained section of mouse testis. (B) Dark-field photomicrograph (using Ultrofilm as a negative) showing the total distribution of ^{125}I-IL-1α-binding sites in mouse testis and epididymis. In dark-field illumination, the highest densities of binding sites show up as the lighter areas and the tissue is not visible. Note the high densities of IL-1-binding sites in the epididymis (most notably in the head region; arrow) and in the interstitial areas of the testis. Note the lower density of ^{125}I-IL-1α binding in the lumen of the seminiferous tubules (arrow). In (C), note the absence of specific ^{125}I-IL-1α binding in an adjacent section coincubated with 100 nM IL-1β. Tes, Testis; Epi, epididymis. Bar: 1 mm [Reproduced from Ref. 42 (T. Takao, W.M. Mitchell, D. E. Tracey, and E. B. De Souza, Identification of interleukin-1 receptors in mouse testis, *Endocrinology*, 1990, **127**, 251–258) with permission. © The Endocrine Society.]

lar and molecular layers of the dentate gyrus (49) (Fig. 10). Another study demonstrated type I IL-1 receptor mRNA over the granule cell layer of the dentate gyrus (60), indicating that IL-1 receptors were localized to intrinsic neurons.

In Vivo Modulation of IL-1 Receptors in Mouse

Effects of Hypophysectomy

In view of the effects of IL-1 on both the hypothalamic–pituitary–adrenocortical (16–18) and the hypothalamic–pituitary–gonadal (19) axes, we examined

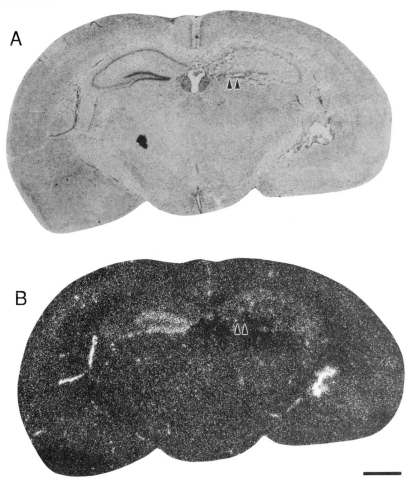

FIG. 10   Effect of quinolinic acid lesions of the hippocampus on ^{125}I-IL-1α binding. (A) Bright-field photomicrograph of a Nissl-stained coronal section of mouse brain at the level of the hippocampus. Note the absence of the molecular and granular cells in the area of the brain lesion (arrowheads). (B) Dark-field photomicrograph showing the distribution of ^{125}I-IL-1α-binding sites in (A). Note the presence of high densities of IL-1-binding sites in the unlesioned saline-injected dentate gyrus (left side) and the absence of binding in areas injected with 300 nM quinolinic acid (arrowheads; right side). The effects of the quinolinic acid lesions were confirmed in five mice. Bar: 2 mm. [Reproduced from Ref. 49 (T. Takao, D. E. Tracey, W.M. Mitchell, and E. B. De Souza, Interleukin-1 receptors in mouse brain: Characterization and neuronal localization, *Endocrinology*, 1990, **127**, 3070–3078) with permission. © The Endocrine Society.]

the effects of hypophysectomy on the relative density of IL-1 receptors in the hippocampus and testis to define the involvement of trophic pituitary hormones on regulation of IL-1 receptors (42, 49). Two to 3 weeks after hypophysectomy, the hippocampus weighed less in hypophysectomized than in sham-operated animals. Hippocampus weights in hypophysectomized and sham-operated mice were 23.1 ± 1.92 mg ($n = 9$) and 30.6 ± 1.32 mg ($n = 7$), respectively ($p < 0.005$). A saturating concentration of ^{125}I-IL-1α (120 pM) was utilized in this study to detect primarily changes in receptor density rather than receptor affinity. There was no significant change in the relative density of receptors between sham-operated (1.15 ± 0.50 fmol/mg protein; $n = 7$) and hypophysectomized (1.04 ± 0.40 fmol/mg protein; $n = 9$) mice. Because of the multiple effects of hypophysectomy, these data do not rule out possible effects of glucocorticoids and/or sex steroids on hippocampal IL-1 receptors. On the other hand, 2 to 3 weeks after hypophysectomy, the testes were significantly atrophied relative to those of sham-operated animals. Testis weights in hypophysectomized and sham operated mice were 57.2 ± 7.2 mg ($n = 10$) and 136.1 ± 12.5 mg ($n = 8$), respectively ($p < 0.0001$). Although the total number of ^{125}I-IL-1α-binding sites per testis was significantly decreased in hypophysectomized mice (sham-operated versus hypophysectomized: 8.04 ± 0.93 fmol/testis versus 3.08 ± 0.31 fmol/testis, respectively; $p < 0.001$) in proportion to the reduction in testicular mass, there was no significant change in the relative density of receptors. These data suggest that IL-1 receptors are present on testicular cells that are, in part, dependent on maintenance by trophic pituitary hormones. However, the observation that the relative density of IL-1-binding sites in some other regions of the testis remains the same following hypophysectomy also suggests that some receptors are also localized to cells within the testis that are not under pituitary control.

Effects of Lipopolysaccharide Treatment

In an attempt to define the involvement of endogenous IL-1 in the regulation of IL-1 receptors in mouse tissues, we examined ^{125}I-IL-1α binding in the kidney after ip injection of lipopolysaccharide (LPS) (50). Twenty-four hours after ip LPS injections, kidney weights were not statistically different between LPS-treated mice [142.2 ± 4.7 mg ($n = 6$)] and saline-injected control [136.5 ± 4.7 mg ($n = 6$)]. In homogenate-binding studies using a single concentration (100 pM) of radioligand, ^{125}I-IL-1α binding was significantly decreased in LPS-treated mice (LPS group, 0.130 ± 0.027 fmol/mg protein, vs control group, 0.385 ± 0.017, $n = 6$, $p < 0.001$). The autoradiographic studies (also carried out with a single radioligand concentration of 80 pM) confirmed the differential density of ^{125}I-IL-1α binding in kidney in control mice (cortex, 34.7 ± 6.2 fmol/mg tissue equivalent; medulla, 52.7 ± 8.1; $p < 0.05$) and demonstrated that the LPS-induced reductions in binding in kidney were evident in both the renal cortex (11.3 ± 0.3; $p < 0.05$) and medulla (26.0 ± 1.0; $p < 0.05$); the relative decrease in cortex (~67%) was somewhat larger than that seen in the medulla (~50%). Subsequently, saturation experiments were carried out in whole-kidney homogenates to determine whether the LPS-induced decreases in ^{125}I-IL-1α binding were due primarily to alterations in the affinity (i.e., K_D) and/or density of the receptor (i.e., B_{max}). Lipopolysaccharide treatment resulted in a significant decrease in K_D value (control, 79.1 ± 4.7 pM; LPS, 30.9 ± 6.1 pM; $n = 4$, $p < 0.001$) and a substantial reduction in B_{max} value (control, 0.91 ± 0.08 fmol/mg protein; LPS, 0.19 ± 0.02 fmol/mg protein; $n = 4$, $p < 0.005$). The data of the present study provide indirect evidence in support of the contention that LPS treatment increases endogenous IL-1 production. We observed a down regulation of IL-1 receptors following LPS treatment, an effect that is characteristically evident following hypersection of the homologous ligand, that is, IL-1. These effects of LPS are evident throughout the kidney (i.e., cortex and medulla), suggesting a generalized effect of the endotoxin to increase IL-1 production in the kidney. Alternatively, LPS treatment may have resulted in elevated circulating levels of IL-1, which in turn could act in kidney to down regulate the receptors. Similar effects of LPS treatment to down regulate IL-1 receptors were also observed in other tissues such as the hippocampus and spleen. The dramatic compensatory homologous down-regulation of IL-1 receptors in the kidney and other tissues further underscores the importance of the cytokine in regulating brain-endocrine-immune function.

In Vitro Modulation of IL-1 Receptors in Mouse AtT-20 Pituitary Tumor Cells

To further characterize the mechanisms regulating the interactions of IL-1 and CRF, we examined ^{125}I-IL-1α and ^{125}I-Tyr^0-ovine CRF (^{125}I-oCRF) binding at 24 hr following treatment of AtT-20 cell cultures with rat/human CRF (61). The treatment of AtT-20 cells for 24 hr with CRF produced a dose-dependent increase in ^{125}I-IL-1α binding and a dose-dependent decrease in ^{125}I-oCRF binding. The CRF-induced increase in ^{125}I-IL-1α binding in AtT-20 cells appears to be mediated through specific membrane receptors for CRF because the CRF receptor antagonist, α-helical ovine CRF(9–41), blocked the CRF-induced increase in IL-1 receptors without producing any change in ^{125}I-IL-1α binding by itself (Fig. 11). ^{125}I-Labeled IL-1α saturation assays were performed in CRF-treated and control cell cultures to determine whether the increase in ^{125}I-IL-1α binding following CRF treatment was related to changes in the affinity and/or concentration of IL-1 receptors on

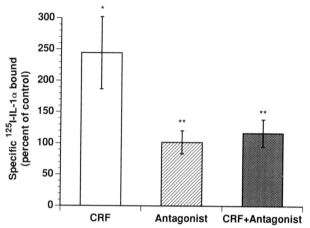

Fig. 11   Effect of CRF antagonist, α-helical oCRF (9–41), on the CRF-induced increase of ^{125}I-IL-1α binding to AtT-20 cell membrane homogenates. AtT-20 cells were incubated with vehicle, 10 nM rat/human CRF, 1 mM CRF antagonist, or 10 nM rat/human CRF + 1 mM CRF antagonist for 24 hr. Data are expressed as a percentage of vehicle-treated controls and represent the mean ± SEM of four independent experiments. Control values were 1.2 ± 0.1 fmol/mg protein for ^{125}I-IL-1α binding. *, $p < 0.01$ vs control; **, $p < 0.01$ vs 10 nM rat/human CRF as determined by one-way ANOVA and Duncan's multiple range test. [Reproduced from Ref. 61 (E. L. Webster, D. E. Tracey, and E. B. De Souza, Upregulation of interleukin-1 receptors in AtT-20 pituitary tumor cells following treatment with corticotropin-releasing factor, *Endocrinology*, 1991, **129**, 2796–2798) with permission. © The Endocrine Society.]

AtT-20 cells. Scatchard analysis of the saturation data indicated that the K_D values in the control and CRF-treated cells were similar, 18.8 ± 2.3 pM and 15.3 ± 2.6 pM, respectively, whereas the density of receptors in the CRF-treated cultures (B_{max} = 6.8 ± 0.8 fmol/mg protein) was significantly ($p < 0.05$, Student's t-test) higher than in the control-treated cells (B_{max} of 3.5 ± 1.8 fmol/mg protein). The increased density of IL-1 receptors following CRF treatment may involve a variety of mechanisms, including increased synthesis of IL-1 receptors, unmasking of cryptic receptors, and/or a decrease in internalization of IL-1 receptors. If increased CRF concentrations produce an up regulation of IL-1 receptors in the anterior pituitary similar to that observed in AtT-20 cells, then one might speculate that IL-1 (which increases in stressful situations) may act as the pituitary level to maintain the elevated plasma ACTH seen following stress.

Summary and Conclusions

Interleukin 1 receptors were identified, characterized, and localized in mouse brain, endocrine, and immune tissues with ^{125}I-IL-1α and ^{125}I-IL-1ra as radioligands. ^{125}I-Labeled IL-1 binding in mouse brain, endocrine, and immune tissues was linear with membrane protein concentration, saturable, reversible, and of high affinity. The binding sites for ^{125}I-IL-1 exhibited a pharmacological specificity for IL-1 and its analogs in keeping with relative biological potencies of the compounds in the thymocyte proliferation assay. The pharmacological specificity of the IL-1-binding site in brain, endocrine, and immune tissues was further strengthened by the lack of inhibitory activity of peptides such as CRF and TNF. The kinetic and pharmacological characteristics and molecular weight of ^{125}I-IL-1 binding in brain, endocrine, and immune tissues and AtT-20 cells were similar to those previously observed in EL-4 6.1 mouse thymoma cells membranes (62, 63), T lymphocytes (64), and fibroblasts (65) and appear to correspond to type I receptors. Autoradiographic localization studies revealed comparable distribution patterns of ^{125}I-IL-1α- and ^{125}I-IL-1ra-binding sites in the brain and peripheral tissues. The demonstration of the presence of high-affinity binding sites that are discretely localized in the mouse tissues and corticotropes provides further support for the proposed role of IL-1 in modulating the function in each tissue. Interleukin 1 receptors may play an important role in communication in the brain–endocrine–immune axis.

Acknowledgments

The data presented in this chapter involved collaborative studies with Steven G. Culp, Robert C. Newton, Daniel E. Tracy, W. Mark Mitchell, and Elizabeth L. Webster. We thank them for their contributions.

References

1. J. J. Oppenheim, E. J. Kovacs, K. Matsushima, and S. K. Durum, *Immunol. Today* **7**, 45 (1986).
2. S. B. Mizel, *FASEB J.* **3**, 2379 (1989).
3. C. A. Dinarello, *FASEB J.* **2**, 108 (1988).
4. A. Fontana, F. Kristensen, R. Dubs, D. Gemsa, and E. Weber, *J. Immunol.* **129**, 2413 (1982).
5. D. Giulian, T. J. Baker, L. N. Shih, and L. B. Lachman, *J. Exp. Med.* **164**, 594 (1986).
6. D. Giulian, D. G. Young, J. Woodward, D. C. Brown, and L. B. Lachman, *J. Neurosci.* **8**, 709 (1988).
7. D. Giulian and L. B. Lachman, *Science* **228**, 497 (1985).
8. V. H. Perry, M. C. Brown, and S. Gordon, *J. Exp. Med.* **165**, 1218 (1987).
9. A. Fontana, E. Weber, and J. M. Dayer, *J. Immunol.* **133**, 1696 (1984).

10. F. A. Lue, M. Bail, R. Gorczynski, and H. Moldofsky, *Sleep Res.* **16**, 51 (1987).
11. M. M. Mustafa, M. H. Lebel, O. Ramio, K. D. Olsen, J. S. Reisch, B. Beutler, and G. H. McCracken, Jr., *J. Pediatr.* **115**, 208 (1989).
12. W. L. Farrar, J. M. Hill, A. Harel-Bellan, and M. Vinocour, *Immunol. Rev.* **100**, 361 (1987).
13. E. Heier, J. Ayala, P. Denefle, A. Bousseau, P. Rouget, M. Mallat, and A. Prchiantz, *J. Neurosci. Res.* **21**, 39 (1988).
14. C. D. Breder, C. A. Dinarello, and C. B. Saper, *Science* **240**, 321 (1988).
15. C. D. Breder and C. B. Saper, *Soc. Neurosci. Abstr.* **15**, 715 (1989).
16. R. Sapolsky, C. Rivier, G. Yamamoto, P. Plotsky, and W. Vale, *Science* **238**, 522 (1987).
17. A. Uehara, P. E. Gottschall, R. R. Dahl, and A. Arimura, *Endocrinology* (*Baltimore*) **121**, 1580 (1987).
18. F. Berkenbosch, J. Van Oers, A. Del Rey, F. Tilders, and H. Besedovsky, *Science* **238**, 524 (1987).
19. C. Rivier and W. Vale, *Endocrinology* (*Baltimore*) **124**, 2105 (1989).
20. K. Bomsztyk, J. E. Sims, T. H. Stanton, J. Slack, C. J. McMahan, M. A. Valentine, and S. K. Dower, *Proc. Natl. Acad. Sci. U. S. A.* **86**, 8034 (1989).
21. R. Chizzonite, T. Truitt, P. L. Kilian, S. A. S., P. Nunes, K. P. Parker, K. L. Kaffka, A. O. Chua, D. K. Lugg, and U. Gubler, *Proc. Natl. Acad. Sci. U.S.A.* **86**, 8029 (1989).
22. C. A. Dinarello, *Blood* **77**, 1627 (1991).
23. R. Horuk, J. J. Huang, M. Covington, and R. C. Newton, *J. Biol. Chem.* **262**, 16275 (1987).
24. R. Horuk and J. A. McCubrey, *Biochem. J.* **260**, 657 (1989).
25. D. B. Carter, M. R. Deibel, C. J. Dunn, C.-S. C. Tomich, A. L. Laborde, J. L. Slightom, A. E. Berger, M. J. Bienkowski, F.F. Sun, R. N. McEwan, P. K. W. Harris, A. W. Yem, G. A. Waszak, J. G. Chosay, L. C. Sieu, M. M. Hardee, H. A. Zurcher-Neely, I. M. Reardon, R. L. Heinrikson, S. E. Truesdell, J. A. Shelly, T. E. Eessalu, B. M. Taylor, and D. E. Tracey, *Nature* (*London*) **344**, 633 (1990).
26. S. P. Eisenberg, R. J. Evans, W. P. Arend, E. Verderber, M. T. Brewer, C. H. Hannum, and R. C. Thompson, *Nature* (*London*) **343**, 341 (1990).
27. D. J. Dripps, E. Verderber, K. N. Ray, R. C. Thompson, and S. P. Eisenberg, *J. Biol. Chem.* **266**, 20311 (1991).
28. E. V. Granowitz, B. D. Clark, J. Mancilla, and C. A. Dinarello, *J. Biol. Chem.* **266**, 14147 (1991).
29. E. B. De Souza, *J. Neurosci.* **7**, 88 (1987).
30. O. H. Lowry, N. J. Rosenbrough, A. L. Farr, and R. J. Randall, *J. Biol. Chem.* **193**, 265 (1951).
31. D. B. Carter, K. A. Curry, C.-S. Tomich, A. W. Yem, M. R. Diebel, D. E. Tracey, J. W. Paslay, J. B. Carter, N. Y. Thériault, P. K. W. Harris, I. M. Reardon, H. A. Zurcher-Neely, R. L. Heinrickson, L. L. Clancy, S. W. Muchmore, K. D. Watenpaugh, and H. M. Einspahr, *Proteins* **3**, 121 (1988).
32. U. K. Laemmli, *Nature* (*London*) **227**, 680 (1970).
33. P. J. Munson and D. Rodbard, *Anal. Biochem.* **297**, 220 (1980).

34. E. B. De Souza, T. R. Insel, M. H. Perrin, J. Rivier, and W. W. Vale, *J. Neurosci.* **5**, 3189 (1986).

35. B. M. Slotnic and C. M. Leonard, "A Stereotaxic Atlas of the Albino Mouse Forebrain." U.S. Gov. Printing Office, Washington, DC, 1975.

36. C. H. Hannum, C. J. Wilcox, W. P. Arend, F. G. Joslin, D. J. Dripps. P. L. Heimdal, L. G. Armes, A. Sommer, S. P. Eisenberg, and R. C. Thompson, *Nature* (*London*) **343**, 336 (1990).

37. W. P. Arend, *J. Clin. Invest.* **88**, 1445 (1991).

38. C. A. Dinarello and R. C. Thompson, *Immunol. Today* **12**, 404 (1991).

39. S. K. Dower, S. R. Kronheim, T. P. Hopp, M. Cantrell, M. Deeley, S. Gillis, C. S. Henney, and D. L. Urdal, *Nature* (*London*) **324**, 266 (1986).

40. N. J. Busbridge, M. J. Dascombe, F. J. H. Tilders, J. W. A. M. Van Oers, E.A. Linton, and N. J. Rothwell, *Biochem. Biophys. Res. Commun.* **162**, 591 (1989).

41. A. Uehara, P. E. Gottschall, R. R. Dahl, and A. Arimura, *Biochem. Biophys. Res. Commun.* **146**, 1286 (1987).

42. T. Takao, W. M. Mitchell, D. E. Tracey, and E. B. De Souza, *Endocrinology* (*Baltimore*) **127**, 251 (1990).

43. T. Takao, S. G. Culp, R. C. Newton, and E. B. De Souza, *J. Neuroimmunol.* **41**, 51 (1992).

44. M. R. Opp, F. Obal, Jr., and J. M. Krueger, *Am. J. Physiol.* **260**, R52 (1991).

45. M. K. Hellerstein, S. N. Meydani, M. Meydani, K. Wu, and C. A. Dinarello, *J. Clin. Invest.* **84**, 228 (1989).

46. G. Katsuura, A. Arimura, K. Koves, and P. E. Gottschall, *Am. J. Physiol.* **258**, E163 (1990).

47. C. Rivier and W. Vale, *Endocrinology* (*Baltimore*) **129**, 384 (1991).

48. J. Honegger, A. Spagnoli, R. D'urso, P. Navarra, S. Tsagarakis, G. M. Besser, and A. B. Grossman, *Endocrinology* (*Baltimore*) **129**, 1275 (1991).

49. T. Takao, D. E. Tracey, W. M. Mitchell, and E. B. De Souza, *Endocrinology* (*Baltimore*) **127**, 3070 (1990).

50. T. Takao, W. M. Mitchell, and E. B. De Souza, *Endocrinology* (*Baltimore*) **128**, 2618 (1991).

51. I. Gery, R. K. Gershon, and B. H. Waksman, *J. Exp. Med.* **136**, 128 (1972).

52. C. A. Caamano, H. N. Fernandez, and A. C. Paladini, *Biochem. Biophys. Res. Commun.* **115**, 29 (1983).

53. L. Petruzzelli, R. Herrera, R. Garcia-Arenas, and O. M. Rosen, *J. Biol. Chem.* **260**, 16072 (1985).

54. C. L. Wood and M. S. O'Dorisio, *J. Biol. Chem.* **260**, 1243 (1985).

55. R. L. Vandlen, K. E. Arcuri, and M. A. Napier, *J. Biol. Chem.* **260**, 10889 (1985).

56. D. E. Grigoriadis and E. B. De Souza, *J. Biol. Chem.* **263**, 10927 (1988).

57. D. E. Grigoriadis and E. B. De Souza, *Peptides* (*N. Y.*) **10**, 179 (1989).

58. T. Fujita, M. Kashimura, and K. Adachi, *Experientia* **41**, 167 (1985).

59. E. T. Cunningham, Jr., E. Wada, D. B. Carter, D. E. Tracey, J. F. Battey, and E. B. De Souza, *Neuroendocrinology* **56**, 94 (1992).

60. E. T. Cunningham, Jr., E. Wada, D. B. Carter, D. E. Tracey, J. F. Battery, and E. B. De Souza, *J. Neurosci.* **12**, 1101 (1992).

61. E. L. Webster, D. E. Tracey, and E. B. De Souza, *Endocrinology* (*Baltimore*) **129**, 2796 (1991).
62. D. E. Tracey and E. B. De Souza, *Soc. Neurosci. Abstr.* **14**, 1052 (1988).
63. E. B. De Souza, E. L. Webster, D. E. Grigoriadis, and D. E. Tracey, *Psychopharmacol. Bull.* **25**, 299 (1989).
64. J. W. Lowenthal and H. R. MacDonald, *J. Exp. Med.* **164**, 1060 (1986).
65. S. K. Dower, S. M. Call, S. Gillis, and D. L. Urdal, *Proc. Natl. Acad. Sci. U.S.A.* **83**, 1060 (1986).

[9] c-*fos*-Based Functional Mapping of Central Pathways Subserving Effects of Interleukin 1 on the Hypothalamo–Pituitary–Adrenal Axis

Anders Ericsson and Paul E. Sawchenko

Introduction

Systemic administration of interleukin 1 (IL-1) has been shown to result in a rapid increase in adrenocorticotropic hormone (ACTH) and corticosterone secretion in rats (1–6). These endocrine events have been suggested as reflecting a negative feedback inhibition on the activity of the immune system, including the synthesis of cytokines, during the course of inflammatory and infectious processes (1, 7, 8). The mechanisms by which circulating IL-1 comes to modify pituitary–adrenal output are still poorly understood, although most data now tend to favor the hypothesis that the effects of IL-1 are ultimately exerted at the level of the hypothalamus to increase corticotropin-releasing factor (CRF) secretion into the hypophysial portal circulation (2–4, 9), and hence the central drive on the pituitary–adrenal system.

The existence of a blood–brain barrier (BBB) to macromolecules raises a formidable question as to how circulating IL-1 gains access to the brain parenchyma to exert its effects, directly or indirectly, on hypothalamic neurosecretory neurons. A frequently advocated hypothesis is that signaling by IL-1 may be transduced by one or more of the circumventricular organs (CVOs) of the brain, which lack a functional BBB, and that are anatomically closely interconnected with the neuroendocrine hypothalamus (10, 11). Alternatively, it has been suggested that IL-1 may be subject to active transport across the BBB, thereby affording it direct and privileged access to as yet unspecified neuronal populations (12, 13). The possibilities also exist that IL-1 may interact with its own receptor on endothelial cells of postcapillary venules (14) to cause increased leakage of blood-borne substances into the brain parenchyma, or to stimulate the synthesis and secretion of secondary signaling molecules, such as prostaglandins (15, 16), which may ultimately trigger or otherwise modify local neuronal responses.

Neurons have been shown to respond to a variety of extracellular stimuli, including potassium- or neurotransmitter-induced depolarization and stimulation by growth factors or hormones, by manifesting rapid and transient

Methods in Neurosciences, Volume 16

synthesis of several so-called cellular immediate early genes (cIEGs), including the protooncogene encoding the transcription factor, Fos (17, 18). The gene products of the cIEGs have been suggested as mediating the translation of short-term intercellular signaling events to longer term changes in cellular phenotype, via targeted alterations in gene expression. Analyses of changes in expression of cIEGs have proved to be powerful tools for evaluating the circuitry and cell groups that are affected by various physiological and pharmacological stimuli (19, 20).

In this article we outline a strategy with which to analyze the central circuitry, cell groups, and molecules that may subserve the response(s) to elevated circulating levels of the β subtype of IL-1 (21). This includes an initial mapping of cells within the CNS that respond to intravenous injection of IL-1β with increased synthesis of Fos, which is taken to serve as an index of increased cellular activity. This technique provides a sensitive, inducible, and highly resolute marker for cells that are responsive to systemic IL-1β; in these aspects, it compares favorably with alternative methods for activity mapping, such as the 2-deoxyglucose method. These data are utilized as an entry point for a more detailed analysis of the biochemical phenotype of targeted neurons, and of their anatomical and functional relationship to neurosecretory structures in the hypothalamus. This involves the use of various combinations of immuno- and *in situ*-hybridization histochemistry, axonal transport experiments, and discrete surgical and pharmacological manipulation of circuits implicated in the central responses to elevated circulating levels of IL-1β.

Systemic Administration of IL-1 to Freely Moving Rats

Adult male Sprague-Dawley albino rats, weighing 280–320 g, are used. The rats are individually housed for at least 1 week prior to the experiment in a germ- and virus-free environment under standard lighting, temperature, and feeding conditions. To further acclimate the animals, and minimize the risk of unrelated stress effects, they are subjected to daily handling during the adaptation period.

To allow for effective remote administration of IL-1 into the systemic circulation, cannulas are implanted into the jugular vein 2 days prior to the experiment. An approximately 15-cm long PE-50 cannula containing a sterile saline–heparin (500,000 IU/liter; Sigma, St. Louis, MO) solution is connected to a 3.5-cm length of Silastic tubing (Dow Corning, Midland, MI). The Silastic end is inserted into the jugular vein to the site of the cannula–tubing junction, and secured to the vein with ligatures. The free end of the assembly is sealed and exteriorized at an intrascapular position. This procedure places the tip of the silastic tubing at the site of the junction of the jugular vein and the atrium and assures a prompt delivery of injected cytokines directly into the systemic circulation. The ligatures securing the cannula–silastic tubing in the vein must be placed in such a way as not to clamp the silastic tubing at a position where it is not supported internally by the more rigid PE-50 cannula. It is also critical to keep the saline–heparin solution sterile and free of bacterial contamination, which can itself effect a powerful induction of Fos immunoreactivity in both cytokine- and vehicle-injected animals. We routinely prepare the saline–heparin solution fresh for every experiment. Body weight, drinking, and feeding are monitored after the implantation of the cannula as an index of their postsurgical recovery. Typically, a 300-g rat will lose approximately 10 g of body weight during the first 24 hr postsurgery but regains this weight during the remaining time before injection.

Interleukin 1 is administered intravenously in the home cages of the animals, via a long PE-20 cannula that is counterbalanced and allows for unrestricted movement of the animals. A sterile-filtered 40 mM sodium phosphate buffer (pH 7.4 at 25°C), containing 0.1% (w/v) ascorbic acid is prepared fresh on the day of IL-1 administration; this serves as the vehicle for IL-1 administration. Vehicle-filled 40-cm lengths of PE-20 are connected to the PE-50 cannula of each animal via a short piece of Silastic tubing and attached to the balanced device outside the cage. In our experience, the most commonly encountered pitfalls in this delivery system derive from nonsterile solutions in the cannulas, clamping of the silastic tubing when securing the tubing to the jugular vein, and destruction of cannulas by animals before or after connection.

We utilize a mature, 152-amino acid form of the recombinant human interleukin 1β peptide (kindly provided by Immunex Research and Development Corporation, Seattle, WA). This peptide, which has a specific activity of 1×10^8 U/mg [A375 assay (22); 1 A375 U $\simeq$ 2.7 LAF U (23); 17 ng of endotoxin/mg protein], is initially diluted 1:1 in sterile-filtered 200 mM Tris-HCl buffer (pH 7.4 at 25°C), containing 0.2% (w/v) bovine serum albumin (BSA), aliquoted into 1.5-μg batches and refrozen at −70°C. The BSA protects the protein during refreezing and stabilizes its biological activity once thawed. The BSA itself has not been found to promote Fos induction in any CNS region in independent control experiments. Thawed peptide may be stored at 4°C for up to 1 week with only a slight loss in activity (less than 50%). The biological activity of the protein, however, was found to be unpredictable if the peptide was stored at 4°C in a non-BSA-containing buffer.

Interleukin 1β peptide is administered in doses ranging between 0.21 and 3.58 μg/kg body weight in a total volume of 300 μl delivered over 3 min 1–4 hr prior to perfusion fixation. The final concentration of BSA and Tris buffer in the injectate is kept constant at 0.01% and 70 mM, respectively. Control animals receive injections of the same buffers with no IL-1 added.

Injected rats are anesthetized between 1:00 and 2:00 pm, weighed, and perfused via the ascending aorta with 500 ml of ice-cold 4% (w/v) paraformaldehyde in sodium borate buffer, pH 9.5, for 25 min. The brain is subsequently dissected out and postfixed in paraformaldehyde with 10% sucrose (w/v) for 3 hr. The brains are cryoprotected overnight in 10% sucrose/0.05 M potassium phosphate-buffered saline (KPBS) at pH 7.4. The following day the brains are frozen in dry ice and sectioned at 30 μm on a sliding microtome; evenly spaced series of sections are saved in a cryoprotectant solution (24) consisting of 150 g of sucrose and 300 ml of ethylene glycol diluted to a final volume of 1 liter by addition of 0.05 M sodium phosphate buffer. This allows long-term (months to years) storage at $-20°C$ of sections with minimal loss in antigenicity or hybridizability, and permits tissue from similarly treated groups of animals to be processed in tandem, facilitating direct comparisons of numbers of cells displaying Fos immunoreactivity and quantitative analysis of the strength of c-*fos* mRNA signal in positively hybridized neurons. The relatively short postfixation time enhances the sensitivity of immunolocalization. However, sections that are processed for *in situ* hybridization histochemistry are postfixed in neutral buffered 4% paraformaldehyde overnight to enable them to better withstand the rigors of protease digestion, which is needed to optimize sensitivity with this localization technique. Finally, the tissues are then processed for immunohistochemical or *in situ* hybridization analysis or various combined staining applications.

Time Course

Our initial study was aimed at determining whether the transcription factor Fos could serve as a useful marker for identifying cell groups that are activated following intravenous (iv) administration of IL-1β to rats. It was important to determine first that hypothalamic CRF neurons do themselves manifest Fos induction in response to IL-1 at doses known to result in increased hypothalamo–pituitary–adrenal (HPA) axis output. Then, by comparing the dose response and time course of Fos induction in hypothalamus and other central loci, a list of afferent cell groups that might be involved in conveying IL-1-related signals to the endocrine hypothalamus could be generated. Expression of both c-*fos* mRNA and Fos protein were monitored. The use of two independent indices of c-*fos* expression allows confirmation of localization patterns. Moreover, each individual method has distinct advantages when used singly (18) or in various combined applications. In general, isotopic hybridization methods are generally more sensitive in detecting c-*fos* expression, and are more amenable to quantitative analysis, whereas immunolocalization methods offer greater resolution and ease of combination with other anatomical tracing and staining techniques.

Hybridization histochemical localization of c-*fos* mRNA was accomplished with an ^{35}S-labeled antisense cRNA probe generated from a full-length 2.1-kb rat c-*fos* cDNA (25), subcloned into an *Eco*RI site of the Bluescript SK$^+$ plasmid vector (Stratagene, La Jolla, CA). Protocols for probe synthesis and hybridization are virtually identical to those described elsewhere in this volume (see Chapter 7) (26), and will not be reiterated here. The most important control involves application of labeled sense strand probes to sections adjoining those used for analysis; this procedure has consistently failed to yield any suggestion of a positive signal under any of the conditions described here.

For immunohistochemical localization, we employ a conventional avidin–biotin–immunoperoxidase technique. Sections are first pretreated for 10 min with 0.3% hydrogen peroxide in KPBS (to quench endogenous peroxidase activity), rinsed twice (5 min each) in KPBS, and then in 1.0% (w/v) sodium borohydride in KPBS (to reduce free aldehydes, and repeated (up to 10) 10-min rinses in KPBS, until the solution is free of bubbles. Neither of these pretreatment steps is essential, but each helps to minimize background. Sections are then incubated for 48 hr at 4°C in a polyclonal antiserum (Oncogene Sciences, Inc., Uniondale, NY) raised against the N-terminal portion (residues 4 to 17) of the Fos protein, which shows little homology with known Fos-related antigens (18). The serum is diluted at 1:7500 in KPBS with 2% normal goat serum and 0.3% Triton X-100. Following incubation in primary antiserum, an avidin–biotin–immunoperoxidase localization system, available in kit form (Vector Laboratories), is applied, with reaction product developed by nickel-enhanced glucose oxidase methods (27). This involves rinsing twice (10 min each) in 0.1 M acetate buffer (pH 6.0), and then exposing the sections to a freshly prepared reaction mixture consisting of 0.5 g of nickel ammonium sulfate, 40 mg of β-(D)-glucose, 8 mg of ammonium chloride, 0.6 mg of glucose oxidase, and 10 mg of diaminobenzidine in 20 ml of ice-cold 0.1 M acetate buffer. The reaction is terminated after 20–60 min by transferring the sections to acetate buffer. After three final rinses (10 min each) in KPBS, sections are mounted onto gelatin-coated slides, dehydrated, and coverslipped.

Using these procedures, the temporal expression of c-*fos* mRNA and protein in rat brain were examined following iv administration of interleukin 1β (1.87 μg/kg). This dose corresponds to an approximate dose of 0.5 μg of IL-1β/300-g rat, and has been shown to result in a significant increase in circulating ACTH and corticosterone (3, 6). *In situ* hybridization histochemistry revealed a positive hybridization signal over cells concentrated in the parvocellular division of the paraventricular nucleus of the hypothalamus (PVH), whose topography closely mirrored that of hypophysiotropic CRF-expressing neurons (Fig. 1). Labeling was maximal at 1 hr, and returned to near-background levels at 3 hr, after iv administration of IL-1β (Fig. 1).

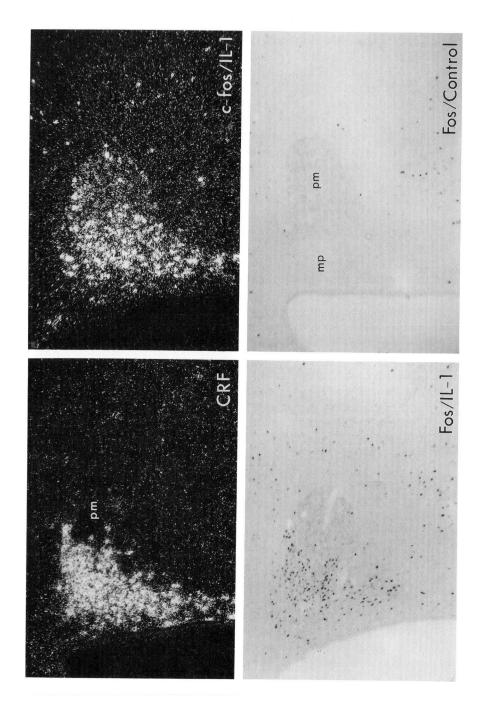

Immunostaining of neighboring sections for Fos protein revealed a pattern of nuclear staining whose distribution closely approximated that seen in the hybridization material. Predictably, the time course of Fos protein expression was distinct, and whereas a few immunostained cells were detected at 1 hr after IL-1β injection, maximal numbers were detected at 3 hr postinjection. Preadsorption of the Fos antisera resulted in a complete blockade of labeling in the PVH, and rats receiving vehicle alone did not display Fos immunoreactivity in the PVH. These findings indicate increased synthesis of c-*fos* mRNA and Fos protein in the parvocellular neurons of the PVH that are known to secrete CRF into pituitary portal plasma and that are known to play an obligate role in the regulation of the HPA axis.

Interleukin 1β-stimulated Fos induction was not limited to the PVH. Positive labeling for c-*fos* mRNA and Fos immunoreactivity were also observed in the caudal part of the nucleus of the solitary tract (NTS) and the ventrolateral medulla, areas that are known to serve as relays for the distribution of interoceptive information to the PVH (28). Other areas in the CNS that consistently displayed Fos induction in response to systemic IL-1β included circumscribed portions of the supraoptic nucleus, the parabrachial nucleus, the central nucleus of the amygdala, and the bed nucleus of the stria terminalis.

Interestingly, at the dose of IL-1β utilized, no consistent labeling for Fos mRNA or protein was observed in any of the circumventricular organs. These structures have been suggested as areas where blood-borne macromolecules, including IL-1β, may gain access to neurons within the CNS (11). In addition, we did not detect evidence of Fos synthesis in major sites of IL-1 receptor expression and/or ligand binding (11, 14, 29–31), including the dentate gyrus, the choroid plexus, the cerebral vasculature, and the brainstem raphesystem.

It is worthy of mention that several structures within the CNS displayed Fos immunoreactivity in both IL-1β- and vehicle-injected controls. These

---

Fig. 1 IL-1β-induced c-*fos* expression in the parvocellular division of the PVH. *Top:* Dark-field photomicrographs of coronal sections through the PVH to show the distribution of neurons positively hybridized for CRF (for reference) and those hybridized for c-*fos* mRNA 1 hr following iv injection of IL-1β. Both markers show a similar staining pattern, with positively labeled cells concentrated in the parvocellular division of the nucleus (mp), with scant or no specific signal in the magnocellular division (pm). *Bottom:* Bright-field photomicrographs of avidin–biotin–immunoperoxidase staining for Fos protein in animals sacrificed 3 hr after injection with IL-1β (left) or vehicle (right). Stimulated rats show a pattern of nuclear staining that is fully compatible with the hybridization patterns, whereas no specific staining is apparent in the PVH of control animals.

areas include the cingulate cortex, several midline thalamic nuclei, and scattered neurons in the lateral hypothalamic area. Labeling for c-*fos* mRNA and Fos immunoreactivity was also observed under all conditions in the suprachiasmatic nucleus, an area that has been shown to display a circadian pattern of Fos expression. Because we consistently harvested our animals between 1:00 and 2:00 pm we did not observe any significant variation of Fos expression in this nucleus, or in the PVH, where levels of CRF mRNA expression, at least, show distinctive diurnal variation (32).

Dose–Response Relationships

We next reasoned that comparison of the dose relatedness of IL-1β-stimulated Fos induction in the PVH and other CNS regions could provide an *a priori* basis for including or excluding specific extrahypothalamic cell groups as potential sites through which IL-1β signaling to the PVH might be mediated. We carried out an analysis of the pattern of labeling for Fos immunoreactivity in the CNS at 3 hr following iv injection of IL-1β at doses ranging from 0.21 to 3.58 μg/kg body weight. The results are summarized in Fig. 2, and reveal coarsely comparable thresholds for Fos induction in all IL-1β-responsive regions except the circumventricular organs, where reliable localization required roughly 5- to 10-fold higher dose levels than did the parvocellular division of the PVH.

Taken together, these initial data indicate that several groups of neurons that are known to be functionally interconnected and related to the regulation of the HPA axis are capable of manifesting a rapid and transient induction of Fos synthesis in response to intravenous injection of IL-1β. Our findings of significant levels of c-*fos* mRNA and Fos protein in, for example, the PVH and the caudal NTS as early as 1 hr postinjection suggest that these neurons are responding to systemic IL-1β within a time frame that is generally compatible with previous findings of elevated levels of ACTH and corticosterone in the blood following administration of IL-1 (3, 5–7). Moreover, our findings of a half-maximal induction of Fos immunoreactivity in the PVH and the NTS at a dose on the order of 0.87 μg of IL-1β/kg, with a weak but clearly detectable induction at 0.21–0.47 μg of IL-1β/kg, are in agreement with previous studies documenting significantly elevated plasma levels of ACTH and corticosterone after iv injection of IL-1β at doses on the order of 0.04–0.4 μg/kg (3, 6, 7). Thus our data suggest that Fos may serve as a useful marker for identifying neurons that are candidate mediators of an integrated neurosecretory response to circulating IL-1β.

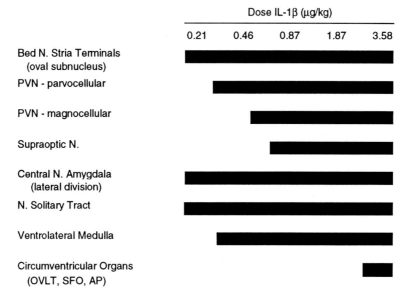

FIG. 2 Minimum iv doses of IL-1β required for consistent Fos protein induction in rat brain cell groups.

Characterization of IL-1 Responsive Neurons

Because of the extreme biochemical and connectional heterogeneity of the neural systems under consideration, and because of the fact that exogenous cytokines are capable of provoking responses from neuroendocrine axes apart from the HPA, it is important to establish directly that stimulated Fos induction is indeed targeting the systems of interest before investing time and effort in attempting to experimentally pursue suggestions gleaned from patterns of c-*fos* mRNA or protein expression alone. This may be achieved by employing the above-mentioned techniques for localization of c-*fos* mRNA and Fos protein in the contexts of multiple immunolabeling, combined immuno- and hybridization histochemistry, and combined immunolabeling and axonal transport techniques.

A protocol for combined immuno- and hybridization histochemical labeling has been published (33) and this provides a powerful means with which to phenotype Fos immunoreactive neurons. This further offers the potential for carrying out quantitative analyses of an mRNA species of interest in neurons identified, by virtue of displaying nuclear Fos immunoreactivity, as being responsive to a particular stimulus. In this combined application, immunostaining is carried out first, and the individual methods are modified as follows to allow concurrent dual staining: (1) pretreatments in hydrogen peroxide and sodium borohydride are omitted; (2) nonimmune (blocking) sera, potential sources of RNase, are replaced with 2% BSA and 2% heparin sulfate; and (3) nickel enhancement steps are eliminated from the immunostaining protocol, as the nickel–diaminobenzidine (DAB) reaction product does not withstand the hybridization protocol. Figure 3 provides an example of combined immunohistochemical labeling for Fos immunoreactivity and hybridization histochemical labeling for CRF mRNA from an IL-1β-stimulated animal. The use of this approach provided confirmation that systemic cytokine did indeed provoke Fos induction in CRF-expressing neurons. Interestingly, Suda et al. (34) have demonstrated with Northern blot analysis that elevated levels of CRF mRNA can be detected in the rat hypothalamus 3 and 5 hr after intraperitoneal injection of relatively high doses of IL-1β. These findings suggest that the CRF-secreting neurons rapidly increase transcriptional activity in response to IL-1β in the blood, although this awaits confirmation with the more satisfying anatomical resolution provided by in situ hybridization.

In addition to establishing the chemical phenotype of the ultimate target

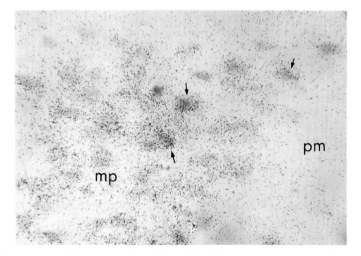

FIG. 3   IL-1β-induced Fos expression in identified CRF neurons. Bright-field photomicrograph of a combined immuno- and hybridization histochemical preparation from an animal sacrificed 3 hr following iv IL-1β showing Fos immunoreactive nuclei amid a field of reduced silver grains representing positive hybridization signal for CRF mRNA in the medial parvocellular subdivision (mp) of the PVH. Examples of neurons expressing both labels are shown (arrows). Note the paucity of both labels in the magnocellular division of the nucleus (pm) at this level.

neurons, it is also of interest to carry out similar characterization of cell groups implicated by the Fos mapping component as providing potentially relevant afferents, and, moreover, to determine that cells displaying Fos induction do in fact project to the neuroendocrine target neurons of interest. Based on the topography of cells displaying Fos induction in response to lower doses of Il-1β, those in the NTS and ventrolateral medulla, in particular, have been identified as prominent sources of predominantly catecholaminergic afferent projections to the PVH. We therefore performed a concurrent double-immunohistochemical analysis for Fos- and dopamine-β-hydroxylase (DBH; a marker for adrenergic and noradrenergic neurons) in brainstem sections from rats that had received a stereotaxic deposit of the retrograde tracer, true blue, in the PVH 30 days prior to iv cannulation and subsequent injection with 1.87 μg of IL-1β/kg 3 hr prior to perfusion. For this application, conventional indirect immunofluorescence detection of Fos-immunoreactive nuclei was employed, using the same polyclonal antiserum, raised in rabbit, and localized with affinity-purified, fluorescein-conjugated goat anti-rabbit IgG (Tago, Burlingame, CA). The DBH was localized with a mouse-derived monoclonal antibody (Pel-Freez, Rogers, AK), which was detected with affinity-purified, rhodamine-conjugated goat anti-mouse IgG (American Qualex, La Mirada, CA). Thus the distinct emission spectra of fluorescein, rhodamine, and true blue allowed all three markers to be detected concurrently. The most important controls for this kind of analysis include provisions to ensure that fluorochrome-labeled secondary antisera do not cross-react with the inappropriate primary antiserum, or with each other. In addition, controls to ensure that the presence of the retrograde tracer did not itself compose a stimulus for Fos induction are obligatory, and were negative in our experiments.

The results confirmed that some Fos-expressing neurons in the NTS, and a substantial majority of those in the ventrolateral medulla, were in fact catecholaminergic, and that these included neurons that project to the region of the PVH (Fig. 4). Thus our data suggest that catecholaminergic cells in the caudal brainstem that are activated following iv injection of IL-1β, as indicated by increased nuclear staining for Fos immunoreactivity, are also anatomically related to the neurosecretory hypothalamus.

Experimental Manipulation

The results summarized above are consistent with the hypothesis that the effects of IL-1β on the HPA axis may be mediated via aminergic afferents to CRF-expressing neurons in the PVH. This prompted us to examine whether the increased functional activity of neurons in the PVH following

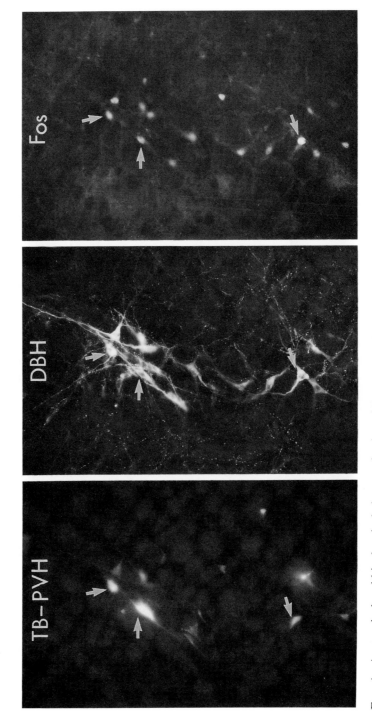

FIG. 4 Anatomical and biochemical characterization of IL-1β-responsive neurons. Fluorescence photomicrographs of a field in the C1 region of the ventrolateral medulla from an IL-1β-injected animal stained concurrently for Fos immunoreactivity, dopamine-β-hydroxylase (DBH, a marker for adrenergic and noradrenergic neurons), and the retrograde tracer true blue (TB), which was previously injected into the PVH. A substantial majority of all Fos-immunoreactive neurons stain positively for DBH, and at least some of these neurons also project to the region of the PVH.

iv injection of IL-1β, as monitored by increased nuclear staining for Fos immunoreactivity, is dependent on intact ascending pathways from aminergic neurons in the caudal medulla. We used a retracting wire knife (35) to administer discrete transections intended to unilaterally interrupt ascending catecholaminergic fibers near their origins in the medulla. After a 2-week survival period (to allow for degeneration of relevant afferents) these animals, along with sham-operated controls, were cannulated for iv administration of IL-1β or vehicle, using the 1.87-μg/kg dose, and a 3-hr postinjection survival. The effectiveness of the cuts were evaluated by staining for DBH at the lesion site and in the PVH; responsiveness of cells in the parvocellular division of the PVH was followed by immunoperoxidase staining for Fos. Well-placed transections markedly decreased the density of DBH-immunoreactive varicosities in the PVH on the side ipsilateral to the lesion. In addition, these transections resulted in an 80–90% reduction in the number of Fos-immunoreactive nuclei in the PVH on the ipsilateral side (Fig. 5). Control cuts, placed in the forebrain at sites designed to interrupt inputs from circumventricular cell groups associated with the lamina terminalis, did not result in any apparent modification of IL-1β-stimulated Fos induction in the PVH. These findings suggest that increased activity of neurons in the PVH in response to systemically administered IL-1β is dependent on intact catecholaminergic afferents from the medulla oblongata. Whether this effect is also manifest in altered CRF mRNA levels and/or altered HPA axis output remains to be determined.

Discussion

The approach outlined here provides a means with which to identify and characterize the central circuitry that may be involved in mediating responses of the HPA axis, or other neuroendocrine systems, to an acute exogenous cytokine challenge. The sensitivity and resolution afforded by c-*fos* and other cIEG mapping methods provides a powerful *entrée* with which to begin to define possibilities as to the central pathways that may mediate adaptive responses to increased circulating cytokines. It is to be emphasized that the appearance of Fos in a particular cell type is not, from a systems-level perspective, a meaningful end point. Fos induction cannot be taken as either a necessary or sufficient condition for inferring that a gene of interest is transcriptionally activated. In fact, direct effects of Fos on CRF gene expression seem unlikely, as no binding site for the transcriptionally active Fos/Jun complex (AP-1) have been described in the CRF promoter sequence, suggesting that other transcription factors, distinct from Fos, are induced in these neurons in response to elevated levels of IL-1β in the blood, and

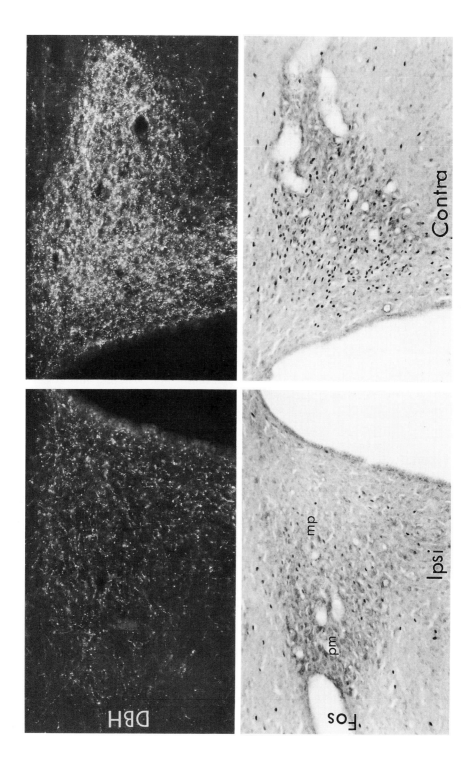

may interact with regulatory elements in the CRF gene promoter to effect increased CRF gene transcription. To determine whether other cIEGs may be directly involved in the regulation of the CRF gene expression under these conditions we performed a hybridization histochemical analysis of the temporal pattern of expression for NGFI-B (36), a member of the steroid hormone receptor superfamily, in the PVH of rats that had received intravenous injection of 1.87 μg of IL-1β/kg. The promoter regions of the CRF gene contain a sequence that resembles a binding site for NGFI-B (37), and may therefore be potential targets for NGFI-B-mediated gene regulation. Interestingly, a significant induction of NGFI-B mRNA was detected in cells in the PVH and other CNS regions following iv administration of IL-1β, with spatial and temporal patterns of expression that closely overlapped those of c-*fos* under the same conditions (38). Such convergent functional mapping data, using distinct, and ostensibly unrelated, cIEGs, also lends confidence to the negative aspects of the results obtained in monitoring c-*fos* expression, as it is by no means clear that all cells have the capacity to manifest induction of c-*fos*, or any other cIEG, with roughly equivalent sensitivities.

One important issue that remains to be addressed for the type of analysis outlined here is whether the amounts of IL-1β peptide administered exogenously in any way mimic plasma levels that may be encountered during the course of infectious or inflammatory processes. Reimers *et al.* (39) showed that IL-1β injected intravenously has a short half-life of approximately 2.9 min in the rat circulation, and that most IL-1β protein is rapidly taken up in the liver and the kidney. Based on their findings, an iv dose of 0.47 μg of IL-1β/kg, which resulted in a significant induction of Fos immunoreactivity in the PVH and NTS, would yield an initial plasma concentration of IL-1β on the order of 0.35 nM, which decreases to roughly 26 pM within 15 min. In humans, sepsis may result in plasma levels of IL-1β up to 16 pM (40), which is lower than the lowest levels of IL-1β that give rise to a detectable Fos induction in the PVH in our experiments. On the other hand, septic

---

FIG. 5 Effects of catecholamine-depleting knife cuts on IL-1β-stimulated Fos expression in the PVH. *Top:* Dopamine-β-hydroxylase (DBH) stained fibers and varicosities in the PVH on the side ipsilateral (ipsi; left) and contralateral (contra; right) to a discrete medullary knife cut designed to interrupt ascending DBH-containing projections. A marked diminution on the ipsilateral side is evident. *Bottom:* Neighboring sections from the same animal, which received iv IL-1β 3 hr prior to sacrifice. An 80–90% reduction in the number of Fos-immunoreactive nuclei in the parvocellular division of the PVH (mp) is apparent. The magnocellular division of the nucleus is labeled (pm) for reference.

patients are exposed to chronically elevated levels of IL-1β, which are commonly accompanied by increased titers of other cytokines. Cytokines are well known to act synergistically within the immune system, and tumor necrosis factor α and interleukin 6, among others, are able to stimulate the HPA axis when injected alone (41, 42). It will therefore be of importance to investigate whether intravenous injection of IL-1β does in fact stimulate the release of other cytokines, and to determine if IL-1β may be effective at even lower doses when coinjected with other cytokines or when administered chronically.

The fundamental question of how elevated levels of IL-1β are transduced to exert effects within the brain parenchyma remains unanswered. Several groups of neurons that are located within the BBB respond with increased activity, that is, Fos induction, to iv injection of IL-1β. However, these neurons are not known to be capable of binding IL-1, and appear not to express at least the type 1 IL-1 receptor (11, 14, 29–31), suggesting that they are not direct targets for circulating cytokine. Furthermore, the absence of IL-1 receptors in the circumventricular organs, as well as the fact that we do not detect Fos induction in these regions in response to doses of IL-1β that are high enough to stimulate the HPA axis, indicate that IL-1 may exert a stimulatory effect on the CNS via an alternative route of entry. Our findings indicate, instead, that intact projections from neurons in the caudal brainstem to the PVH are required for neuronal activation in the hypothalamus. Although this does not establish a causal relationship (permissive effects need to be considered), these results do raise the possibility that fluctuations in circulating IL-1 may be recorded by the peripheral nervous system and subsequently transmitted via the vagus or glossopharyngeal nerves to the NTS for distribution to the endocrine hypothalamus, among other CNS regions. Although alternative mechanisms cannot be ruled out, this hypothesis is testable, and its generation represents an example of how cIEGs may be used as starting points with which to sort the grain from the chaff in deciphering complex CNS–immune system interactions.

Acknowledgments

The work summarized here was supported by NIH Grant NS-21182, and was conducted in part by the Foundation for Medical Research. P.E.S. is an Investigator of the Foundation for Medical Research. A.E. has been supported by a Fogarty International Research Fellowship (TW-04658), the Foundation Blanceflor Boncompagni-Ludovisi, née Bildt, The Royal Swedish Academy of Sciences, The Swedish Medical Research Council, and Svenska Läkaresällskapet. We are grateful to the

Immunex Research and Development Corporation for generously supplying recombinant human IL-1β and to Mr. Kris Trulock for expert photographic assistance.

References

1. H. Besedovsky, A. Del Rey, E. Sorkin, and C. A. Dinarello, *Science* **233,** 652 (1986).
2. F. Berkenbosch, J. van Oers, A. Del Rey, F. Tilders, and H. Besedovsky, *Science* **238,** 524 (1987).
3. R. Sapolsky, C. Rivier, G. Yamamoto, P. Plotsky, and W. Vale, *Science* **238,** 522 (1987).
4. A. Uehara, P. E. Gottschall, R. R. Dahl, and A. Arimura, *Endocrinology (Baltimore)* **121,** 1580 (1987).
5. A. J. Dunn, *Life Sci.* **43,** 429 (1988).
6. C. Rivier, W. Vale, and M. Brown, *Endocrinology (Baltimore)* **125,** 3096 (1989).
7. E. M. Sternberg, J. M. Hill, G. P. Chrousos, T. Kamilaris, S. J. Listwak, P. W. Gold, and R. L. Wilder, *Proc. Natl. Acad. Sci. U.S.A.* **86,** 2374 (1989).
8. E. M. Sternberg, W. S. Young, III, R. Bernardini, A. E. Calogero, G. P. Chrousos, P. W. Gold, and R. L. Wilder, *Proc. Natl. Acad. Sci. U.S.A.* **86,** 4771 (1989).
9. S. Tsagarakis, G. Gillies, L. H. Rees, M. Besser, and A. Grossman, *Neuroendocrinology* **49,** 98 (1989).
10. C. M. Blatteis, *Int. J. Neurosci.* **38,** 223 (1988).
11. J. T. Stitt, *Yale J. Biol. Med.* **63,** 121 (1990).
12. W. A. Banks, A. J. Kastin, and D. A. Durham, *Brain Res. Bull.* **23,** 433 (1989).
13. W. A. Banks and A. J. Kastin, *Life Sci.* **48,** 117 (1991).
14. E. T. Cunningham, Jr., E. Wada, D. B. Carter, D. E. Tracey, J. F. Battey, and E. B. De Souza, *J. Neurosci.* **12,** 1101 (1992).
15. T. Watanabe, A. Morimoto, Y. Sakata, and N. Murakami, *Experientia* **46,** 481 (1990).
16. P. Navarra, S. Tsagarikis, M. Faria, L. H. Rees, M. Besser, and A. B. Grossman, *Endocrinology (Baltimore)* **128,** 37 (1991).
17. M. Sheng and M. E. Greenberg, *Neuron* **4,** 477 (1990).
18. J. I. Morgan and T. Curran, *Annu. Rev. Neurosci.* **14,** 421 (1991).
19. M. Hamamura, D. J. R. Nunez, G. Leng, P. C. Emson, and H. Kiyama, *Brain Res.* **572,** 42 (1992).
20. R. K. W. Chan and P. E. Sawchenko, *Soc. Neurosci. Abstr.* **17,** 614 (1991).
21. A. Ericsson, K. Kovacs, and P. E. Sawchenko, *Proc. 74th Annu. Meet. Endocr. Soc.,* p. 441 (1992).
22. S. Nakai, K. Mizuno, M. Kaneta, and Y. Hirai, *Biochem. Biophys. Res. Commun.* **154,** 1189 (1988).
23. K. Nakano, K. Okugawa, H. Hayashi, S. Abe, Y. Sohmura, and T. Tsuboi, *Dev. Biol. Stand.* **69,** 93 (1988).

24. R. E. Watson, Jr., S. J. Wiegand, R. W. Clough, and G. E. Hoffman, *Peptides* (*N.Y.*) **7,** 155 (1986).

25. T. Curran, M. B. Gordon, K. L. Rubino, and L. C. Sambucetti, *Oncogene* **2,** 79 (1987).

26. E. T. Cunningham, Jr. and E. B. DeSouza, *Methods Neurosci.* **16,** 112 (1993).

27. S. Shu, G. Ju, and L. Fan, *Neurosci. Lett.* **89,** 169 (1988).

28. P. E. Sawchenko and L. W. Swanson, *Brain Res. Rev.* **4,** 275 (1982).

29. G. Katsuura, P. E. Gottschall, and A. Arimura, *Biochem. Biophys. Res. Commun.* **156,** 61 (1988).

30. T. Takao, D. E. Tracey, W. M. Mitchell, and E. B. De Souza, *Endocrinology* (*Baltimore*) **127,** 3070 (1990).

31. E. Ban, G. Milon, N. Prudhomme, and F. Haour, *Neuroscience* **43,** 21 (1991).

32. A. G. Watts and L. W. Swanson, *Endocrinology* (*Baltimore*) **125,** 1734 (1989).

33. A. G. Watts and L. W. Swanson, *in* "Methods in Neurosciences" (P. M. Conn, ed.), Vol. 1, p. 127. Academic Press, San Diego, 1989.

34. T. Suda, F. Tozawa, T. Ushiyama, T. Sumitomo, M. Yamada, and H. Demura, *Endocrinology* (*Baltimore*) **126,** 1223 (1990).

35. R. M. Gold, G. Kapatos, and R. J. Carey, *Physiol. Behav.* **10,** 813 (1973).

36. J. L. Milbrandt, *Neuron* **1,** 183 (1988).

37. T. E. Watson, T. J. Fahrner, M. Johnston, and J. Milbrandt, *Science* **252,** 1296 (1991).

38. A. Ericsson and P. E. Sawchenko, *Soc. Neurosci. Abstr.* **18,** 1013 (1992).

39. J. Reimers, L. D. Wogensen, B. Welinder, K. R. Hejnæs, S. S. Poulsen, P. Nilsson, and J. Nerup, *Scand. J. Immunol.* **34,** 597 (1991).

40. J. G. Cannon, R. G. Tompkins, J. A. Gelfand, H. R. Michie, G. G. Stanford, J. W. M. van der Meer, S. Endres, G. Lonnemann, J. Corsetti, B. Chernow, D. W. Wilmore, S. M. Wolff, J. F. Burke, and C. A. Dinarello, *J. Infect. Dis.* **161,** 79 (1990).

41. Y. Naitu, J. Fukata, T. Tominaga, Y. Nakai, S. Tamai, K. Mori, and H. Imura, *Biochem. Biophys. Res. Commun.* **155,** 1459 (1988).

42. R. Bernardini, T. C. Kamilaris, A. E. Calogero, E. O. Johnson, M. T. Gomez, P. W. Gold, and G. P. Chrousos, *Endocrinology* (*Baltimore*) **126,** 2876 (1990).

[10] Anatomical and Functional Approaches to Study of Interleukin 2 and Its Receptors in Brain

David Seto, Uwe Hanisch, Françoise Villemain,
Alain Beaudet, and Rémi Quirion

Introduction

Interleukin 2 (IL-2), a 133-amino acid 15.42 kDa, protein is a cytokine secreted by T lymphocytes, known to act on receptors present on a subset of these cells (1). Receptors for IL-2 (IL-2R) are membrane-associated proteins that exist either as single units or as heterodimers. The low-affinity unit (p55, IL-2Rα, Tac) binds IL-2 with an affinity in the range of 10–20 nM, whereas an intermediate-affinity unit (p70, IL-2Rβ) has a K_d of 0.5–1.0 nM. The combination of these two units in a heterodimer demonstrates high affinity for IL-2 [K_d = 10–50 pM (2)].

Biochemical and immunohistochemical evidence has revealed the presence of IL-2-like immunoreactivity in mammalian brain (3–6). Moreover, IL-2 was found to induce various biological effects in the CNS following either direct injection into the brain or peripheral administration. For example, intracerebroventricular administration of IL-2 produces sedation, sleep, and synchronization of electrocorticogram spectra (7). Interleukin 2 is also able to suppress the induction and expression of long-term potentiation (LTP) in the rat hippocampus, and to modulate K^+-evoked acetylcholine release in rat brain slices (3, 9, 10). These effects appear to be exerted through specific membrane receptors of the type found on the surface of T cells (3, 5).

Here we briefly describe some of the methods and approaches that have been used thus far to investigate the presence and distribution of IL-2-like immunoreactivity and IL-2 receptors in the central nervous system (CNS), as well as the possible modulatory role of this cytokine on neurotransmitter release.

Immunohistochemical Detection of Brain IL-2-like Materials

The topographic distribution of IL-2-like immunoreactivity has been reported for the rat and mouse brain (4, 5). The major advantage of mouse studies rests with the availability of homologous antibodies against IL-2 and IL-2 receptors of this species. For the rat, studies had to rely on heterologous antibodies against recombinant human IL-2 in the absence of commercially available homologous probes. However, the anti-human serum demonstrated good cross-reactivity toward rat IL-2, as expected from the structural homologies between human and rat IL-2 and the high potency of human IL-2-like molecules in rat brain (3, 6, 7–10).

Immunoautoradiography

For regional localization of IL-2 immunoreactivity, adult male Sprague-Dawley rats (200–250 g) or adult CD-1 mice (4–5 weeks old) are deeply anesthetized with chloral hydrate [3.5 mg/kg, intraperitoneal (ip)] and perfused transaortically with a mixture of 4% paraformaldehyde and 0.2% saturated picric acid in 0.1 M phosphate buffer (pH 7.4). Brains are then removed from the skull, postfixed in the same solution for 1 hr at 20–21°C, and immersed overnight in a 30% sucrose phosphate-buffered solution. Next, tissues are snap frozen by immersion in 2-methylbutane at −40°C, after which they are kept frozen at −80°C until use. Coronal sections (30 μm thick) are cut on an American Optical (Buffalo, NY) freezing microtome and collected in 0.1 M sodium-potassium phosphate buffer. Sections are then preincubated for 30 min at room temperature in Tris-HCl (100 mM, pH 7.4) containing 0.2% bovine serum albumin (Sigma Chemicals, St. Louis, MO) and 1.8% lysine (Sigma Chemicals) and sequentially incubated in normal donkey serum (rats; Sigma Chemicals; dilution 1 : 30) or normal rabbit serum [mice; ICN Immunobiologicals (Costa Mesa, CA) dilution 1 : 30] for 30 min at room temperature. Sections from rat brain are then incubated with a rabbit antiserum directed against recombinant human IL-2 (3) (dilution 1 : 8000; Amersham, Arlington Heights, IL) for 18–20 hr at room temperature. This antiserum is documented to cross-react only marginally with other interleukins, such as human IL-1β (<0.19%), IL-1α (0.39%), IL-3 (<0.30%), IL-4 (<0.04%), and to exhibit <0.01% cross-reactivity with human tumor necrosis factor and interferon γ. Control sections are incubated under the same conditions, either by omitting the primary antiserum or by preabsorbing it with human recombinant IL-2 [Sigma Chemicals or UBI (Lake Placid, NY); 30.1 μM solution of IL-2 in Tris-NaCl buffer overnight at 4°C]. Sections from mouse brain are incubated in the same fashion, using a rat antimouse IL-2 monoclonal antibody (5 μg/ml) derived from the S4B6 hybridoma cell line (11). Rat brain sections are then incubated with donkey anti-rabbit and mouse brain sections with rabbit anti-rat ^{125}I-labeled immunoglobulins (0.2 mg/ml; Amersham) for 30 min at room temperature. All sections are next rinsed thoroughly in Tris-HCl, followed by a rinse in distilled water. Sections are mounted onto gelatinized glass slides, dehydrated in graded ethanols, cleared in xylene, and rehydrated. They are finally air dried in a dust-free atmosphere and juxtaposed against tritium-sensitive Hyperfilm (Amersham).

Prototypical examples of results obtained in the rat by using this protocol are illustrated in Fig. 1. Comparable selective, albeit widespread, immuno-staining patterns are evident in sections from mouse brain (F. Villemain and A. Beaudet, unpublished). Low to moderate labeling densities are apparent in cerebral cortex, neostriatum, lateral septum, thalamus, and the cerebellar cortex. High immunostaining densities are confined in both species to the pyramidal cell layer of the hippocampus, the granule cell layer of the dentate gyrus, and a number of hypo- and epithalamic nuclei including the arcuate nucleus–median eminence complex, the zona incerta, and the habenula (4, 5).

Peroxidase–Anti-peroxidase Immunohistochemistry

For cellular localization of IL-2-like immunoreactivity, sections from selected mouse brain regions are prepared and immunolabeled as above, using the S4B6 anti-IL-2 monoclonal antibody. After overnight incubation in S4B6, sections are washed three times (10 min each) in Tris-saline containing 0.2% bovine serum albumin (BSA) and 1% normal rabbit serum (NRS) and sequentially incubated at room temperature with (1) a 1/50 dilution of rabbit anti-rat IgGs (Jackson Immunoresearch Laboratories, Bar Harbor, ME) for 1 hr and (2) a 1/100 dilution of polyclonal rat peroxidase–anti-peroxidase (PAP) complex (Sternberger-Meyer Immunocytochemicals, Baltimore, MD) for 1 hr. These two steps are then each repeated once for 30 min. After two rinses in Tris-NaCl, the sections are reacted for 6 min with 0.5% 3,3'-diaminobenzidine (DAB) in 0.1 M Tris-HCl buffer containing 0.01% H_2O_2. Sections are then briefly rinsed in distilled water, mounted onto gelatin-coated slides, dehydrated in graded ethanols, defatted in xylene, coverslipped, and examined with a Leitz Aristoplan (Wetzlar, Germany) microscope.

At low magnification, the regional distribution of IL-2-like immunoreactivity conforms to that observed by immunoautoradiography. At high magnification, reaction product is seen to be accumulated over both neuronal perikarya and intervening neuropil. Perikaryal labeling was most evident in areas of high labeling density, such as the arcuate nucleus (Fig. 2a) and the hippocampus (Fig. 2b). Electron microscopic examination of the arcuate

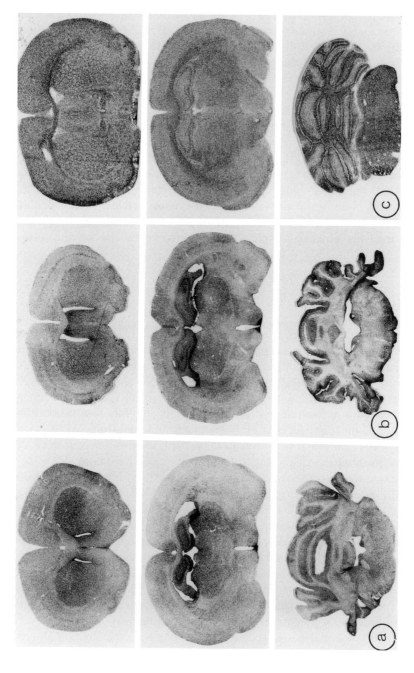

Fig. 1 Comparative distribution of IL-2-like immunoreactivity (a), Tac antigen-like immunoreactivity (b), and ^{125}I-labeled IL-2-binding sites (c) in rat brain sections. Film autoradiograms prepared after tagging anti-IL-2 (a) and anti-Tac (b) primary antibodies with iodinated IgGs, or after incubation of fresh frozen sections with ^{125}I-labeled human recombinant IL-2 (c). Note the similarity between the distributions of IL-2 and Tac antigen immunoreactivity. By contrast, ^{125}I-labeled IL-2-binding distribution shows both points of similarity (e.g., in the hippocampus) and divergence (e.g., in the hypothalamus) with that of Tac immunolabeling.

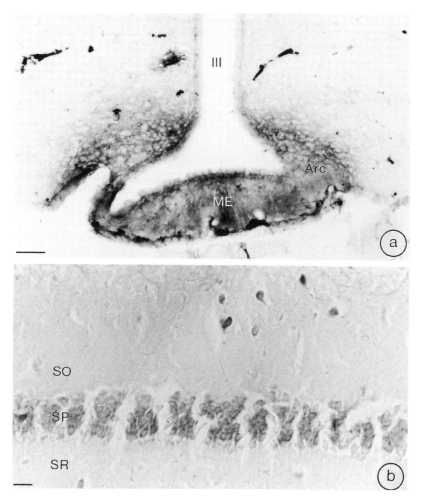

FIG. 2   Light microscopic localization of IL-2-like immunoreactivity as revealed by the PAP technique in the arcuate nucleus–median eminence complex of the hypothalamus (a) and in the hippocampus (b). (a) In the arcuate nucleus (Arc), IL-2-like immunoreactivity is intense and distributed over both perikarya and neuropil. (b) In the hippocampus, the immunoreactivity is mainly confined to the perikarya of pyramidal cells (SP, stratum pyramidale). Note that the reaction product pervades the cytoplasm of the cells but spares the nucleus. III, Third ventricle; ME, median eminence; SO, stratum oriens; SR, stratum radiatum. Scale bars: 50 μm.

nucleus confirmed the association of IL-2 immunolabeling with neuronal perikarya and indicated that dendritic processes accounted for the bulk of neuropil labeling (5).

Immunohistochemistry of Brain IL-2 Receptors (Tac Antigen-like Immunoreactivity)

One possible means to study the presence and distribution of putative IL-2 receptors in the CNS is to use immunohistochemical approaches to reveal the presence of the Tac (p55) receptor subunit in this tissue (4).

For this purpose, rat brains are fixed and sectioned as described above for IL-2 immunostaining. Following a preincubation in Tris-NaCl buffer containing BSA and lysine, sections are incubated for 30 min in normal sheep serum followed by a monoclonal antibody directed against the Tac antigen of the human IL-2 receptor (dilution, 1 : 500) for 18–20 hr at room temperature. The anti-human Tac monoclonal antibody has been shown to detect IL-2 receptors in primary cultures of rat cerebral cortex neurons (12, 13) and on rat sympathetic neurons (14). Preabsorption of the anti-human Tac monoclonal antibody with recombinant human IL-2 (0.1 μM solution of IL-2 in Tris-NaCl buffer overnight at 4°C) did not reduce the intensity of Tac immunostaining. However, immunolabeling was reduced somewhat if IL-2 (0.1 μM) was added to the antibody during the overnight incubation period, suggesting that the latter recognizes an epitope onto or close to the IL-2-binding site. Control sections are incubated under the same conditions, either in the presence of a mouse anti-human monoclonal antibody (Sigma Chemicals) or in the absence of the anti-Tac monoclonal 1gG antibody. All sections are then incubated with sheep anti-mouse ^{125}I-labeled immunoglobulin (0.2 mg/ml; Amersham) for 30 min at room temperature. Following this last incubation, sections are autoradiographically processed, using tritium-sensitive film as described above.

As shown in Fig. 1b, human Tac immunoreactivity is present and selectively distributed in the rat brain. As for IL-2 immunoreactivity (compare Fig. 1a and b), the highest densities of labeling are detected in the hippocampal formation (stratum pyramidale of Ammon's horn and granule cell layer of the dentate gyrus), the arcuate nucleus of the hypothalamus, the median eminence, and the molecular layer of the cerebellar cortex. Preliminary results in the mouse obtained with a monospecific anti-mouse IL-2Rα chain antibody reveal a distribution comparable to that seen in the rat (F. Villemain and A. Beaudet unpublished), thereby strengthening the validity of the results observed in the rat.

Quantitative IL-2 Receptor Autoradiography

In vitro receptor autoradiography has also been used to study the discrete distribution of IL-2 receptor-binding sites in rat brain (4). However, because of the low abundance of receptors in the normal rat brain (poor signal-to-noise ratio), only highly sensitive probes and optimal assay conditions allow the detection of specific labeling by this approach. Slides must be cleaned and gelatinized, and sections prepared as described (15). Additionally, radio-iodinated IL-2 must be used as fresh as possible and even repurified before its use in the binding assay. Otherwise, the level of specific labeling is too low for meaningful analysis.

Rats are sacrificed by decapitation and their brains rapidly removed from the skull, frozen in 2-methylbutane at $-40°C$, and stored at $-80°C$. Sections (20-μm thick) are cut with a cryostat at $-17°C$, mounted on pre-cleaned gelatin-coated slides, air dried, and stored at $-80°C$ until use. For labeling of ^{125}I-labeled IL-2-binding sites, sections are preincubated for 30 min at 22°C in a buffer of the following composition: 20 mM N-2-hydroxyethylpiperazine-N'-2-ethanesulfonic acid (HEPES), 120 mM NaCl, 5 mM KCl, 2 mM CaCl$_2$, and 1 mM MgCl$_2$ (pH 7.4), also containing bovine serum albumin (1 mg/ml). The sections are then incubated (2 hr, 22°C) in the same buffer containing 50 pM ^{125}I-labeled human IL-2 (700–1100 Ci/mmol; Amersham). Specific binding is determined in the presence of an excess (0.1 μM) of unlabeled IL-2 (Sigma Chemicals). At the end of the incubation, slides are rinsed in five washes (1.5 min each) of cold Tris-HCl (50 mM, pH 7.4, 4°C) buffer. Slides are then dipped in cold distilled water to remove salts and air dried before exposing against Hyperfilms with ^{125}I-labeled microscale standards (Amersham) for up to 3 months, depending on the brain regions studied. Films are then developed as described earlier (4, 15) and autoradiograms are quantitated by computerized image analysis.

Under these assay conditions, ^{125}I-labeled IL-2-binding sites are distributed in a manner similar, but not identical, to that described above for Tac immunoreactivity (Fig. 1c). For example, both signals are highly enriched in the hippocampal formation, whereas the arcuate hypothalamic nucleus is better stained with the Tac antiserum than with ^{125}I-labeled IL-2 (compare Fig. 1b and c). This may relate to the existence, in certain brain regions, of only one subunit of the IL-2 receptor (i.e., Tac/p55) with too low an affinity for

IL-2 for autoradiographic detection using picomolar concentrations of radio-ligand.

Modulatory Role of IL-2 on Acetylcholine Release

The presence of IL-2-like immunoreactivity and receptor-binding sites in the CNS strongly argues for biological roles for this cytokine in the brain. As a means to address its possible role as neuromodulator, we investigated the action of IL-2 on the release of acetylcholine (ACh) in slices of rat hippocampus, in view of the concomitant enrichment in ACh terminals, IL-2 immunoreactivity, and IL-2 receptor-binding sites in this structure. A superfusion method was preferred here to static incubations (3) as it allows the tissue slices to be continuously exposed to fresh, oxygenated incubation medium, and permits a better evaluation of time onset and duration of drug effects.

The protocol described here was established for adult (300–350 g) rat brain but is applicable to other species as well as to other tissues, the critical variable being the use of a sufficient amount of tissue to ensure reliable measurements of ACh levels.

Various brain regions (hippocampus, striatum, cortex) are removed on ice and sliced with a McIlwain tissue chopper (Mickle Laboratory Engineering, Gomshall, Surrey, England) at 0.4 mm. An entire sliced hemispheric region is transferred to a superfusing chamber (Brandel Instruments, Gaithersburg, MD) and perfused with Krebs buffer (composition: 120 mM NaCl, 4.6 mM KCl, 2.4 mM CaCl$_2$, 1.2 mM KH$_2$PO$_4$, 1.2 mM MgSO$_4$, 9.9 mM glucose, 25 mM NaHCO$_3$) at pH 7.4, 37°C, using a flow rate of 0.5 ml/min for 30–45 min to equilibrate the tissue and establish a stable basal efflux of ACh. The buffer also contains physostigmine (30 μM; Sigma Chemicals), an esterase blocker, and choline chloride (10 μM; Sigma Chemicals) to ensure the stability of the released ACh and to support a constant supply of its precursor. Collection of the superfusate is initiated at various intervals depending on the time resolution required in a given experiment. The tissue is then stimulated with either a high-K$^+$ (26.2 mM) Krebs buffer (with a concomitant reduction of NaCl to conserve isotonicity) or electrical stimulation, in the presence or absence of various concentrations of human IL-2 (Sigma Chemicals or UBI). After variable periods of stimulation and exposure to IL-2, tissues are returned to superfusion with normal Krebs buffer.

The collected superfusates are next spun (13,000 rpm; 4 min; 25°C; Biofuge, Baxter Co., Montréal, Quebec, Canada) to remove extraneous protein and an aliquot is either frozen at −70°C or subjected immediately to ACh analysis. The superfused tissues are removed at the end of the experiment and kept for protein determination according to Lowry et al. (16).

Samples for ACh analysis are subjected to extraction according to Fonnum (17) as modified by Goldberg and McCaman (18), and to a radioenzymatic reaction for its quantification. The protocol used is as follows.

1. Acetylcholine is extracted from a volume (400 μl) of superfusate by the addition of an equal volume of tetraphenylboron in butyronitrile (Aldrich Chemicals, Milwaukee, WI) (10 g/liter), mixed, and spun (13,000 rpm, 25°C) for 4 min each.

2. Each volume (300 μl) of the organic phase is removed and placed in clean plastic tubes and a half volume of AgNO$_3$ (20 g/liter; 150 μl) is added, mixed, and spun (13,000 rpm, 25°C) for 4 min each to recover the ACh from the organic phase.

3. Each volume (110 μl) of aqueous phase is removed and placed in another set of clean plastic tubes and excess silver is precipitated by adding 10 μl of MgCl$_2$ (1 M) per 110 μl of sample, mixed, and spun (13,000 rpm, 25°C) for 4 min each.

4. A final volume (100 μl) is then removed for evaporation under vacuum, and either stored at -20°C or subjected immediately to the radioenzymatic reaction.

5. For this reaction each sample is redissolved in 32 μl of a mixture containing ATP (0.8 mM; Boehringer Mannheim, Indianapolis, IN), dithiothreitol (5 mM; Boehringer Mannheim), MgCl$_2$ (12.5 mM), glycylglycine at pH 8.0 (25 mM; Sigma), and choline kinase (0.005 unit; Sigma) and incubated at 30°C for 25 min to phosphorylate the choline but not the ACh contained in the samples.

6. Ten microliters of a solution containing acetylcholinesterase (2 units; Sigma) and [^{32}P]ATP (0.45 μCi; New England Nuclear, Boston, MA) is added to each sample, which are then incubated at 30°C for 20 min. During this second incubation period, ACh is hydrolyzed and the choline formed phosphorylated to [^{32}P]phosphorylcholine.

7. The reaction is then stopped by the addition of 100 μl of NaOH (50 mM) and radioactive phosphorylcholine is separated from radiolabeled ATP by ion-exchange chromatography on a 5 $\times$ 20 mm column of Amberlite CG-400 (converted to formate form; Sigma) that had previously been equilibriated with 50 mM NaOH (Fisher, Pittsburgh, PA). Phosphorylcholine is eluted by adding 3 ml of NaOH (50 mM).

8. Radioactivity is determined by liquid scintillation counting, using Eco($+$)lite (ICN, Costa Mesa, CA) as the solvent system.

For each set of extractions, internal ACh standards dissolved in the Krebs' buffer used for experimental samples are extracted and analyzed along with these samples to determine recovery and generate standard curves.

A prototypical example of the effects of IL-2 on hippocampal ACh release is shown in Fig. 3. Interleukin is an extremely potent modulator of ACh

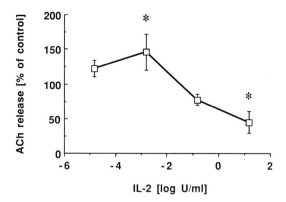

FIG. 3 Modulatory effects of human IL-2 on acetylcholine release in superfused rat hippocampal slices *in vitro*. Low concentrations of IL-2 potentiate K^+-stimulated acetylcholine release whereas higher concentrations significantly inhibit the release of the transmitter. Means $\pm$ SEM of at least six to eight determinations. *$p < 0.05$.

release, acting as a stimulatory agent at low concentrations (femto- to picomolar range) but inhibiting release at higher concentrations (nanomolar). These results reveal that IL-2 immunoreactivity and IL-2-binding sites present in the rat hippocampal formation are biologically relevant and involved in the regulation of neurotransmitter release. It remains to be established if the inhibitory and stimulatory effects of IL-2 on ACh release are mediated by similar or different transduction mechanisms.

Conclusions

It is now clear that IL-2, by acting on specific receptor sites, can induce a variety of biological effects in the CNS, including neuromodulation of transmitter release. However, major questions are still pending, among which are those concerned with the nature of the IL-2-like immunoreactivity present in the CNS. For example, is the primary sequence of brain IL-2 identical to that of IL-2 produced by T lymphocytes? Already, some evidence suggests that in the mouse, T lymphocyte IL-2 mRNA is present in the brain (19) but it remains to be established if it is fully translated and if the posttranscriptional maturation is identical in the CNS and immune cells. Attempts have been made to extract and purify IL-2-like materials directly from brain tissues (6, 11), but it has until now proved difficult to exclude possible contamination from blood-borne IL-2.

The present results clearly identify neuronal cells as the primary source of IL-2-like materials in regions such as the arcuate nucleus and the hippocampus. However, these findings do not exclude the possibility that in other brain regions some of the immunoreactive IL-2 might be produced by glial cells, particularly by resident microglial cells, which bear resemblance to immune cells. Further studies will also be needed to determine the cellular localization of brain IL-2 receptors, of which virtually nothing is currently known (4, 13, 14). Moreover, it remains to be established if the functional organization of brain IL-2 receptors is identical to that of its peripheral counterparts. For example, are the respective roles of the two IL-2 receptor subunits (p55 and p70) the same in the CNS as in the immune system? Are these subunits identical molecular moieties in brain and periphery? Is their association necessary to ensure high affinities for IL-2 in the CNS? Is an identical structural organization required to ensure functional activities in all brain regions? Are brain IL-2 receptors coupled to transduction mechanisms similar to those of T lymphocyte IL-2 receptors? It is also of interest that the p55/Tac antigen is widely expressed under normal resting conditions in the brain. This is in contrast to the immune cells, in which expression is seen only on challenge. It may suggest unexpected functions for this protein in the CNS as well as differential mechanisms of expression for the Tac antigen in brain vs immune cells. Information regarding most of these questions should be available soon, as research activities in this field have markedly expanded. It should then be easier to establish the genuine functional relevance of IL-2 in normal brain organization and function.

Acknowledgments

Supported by grants from the Medical Research Council of Canada to A. Beaudet and R. Quirion. D. Seto and R. Quirion are holders of studentship and "Chercheur-Boursier" awards from the "Fonds de la Recherche en Santé du Québec," respectively. F. Villemain and U. Hanisch are fellows of the Human Frontiers Science Program. The expert secretarial assistance of Mrs. J. Currie is acknowledged.

References

1. J. G. Sinkovics, *Rev. Immunol.* **8,** 217 (1988).
2. W. A. Kuziel and W. C. Greene, *J. Invest. Dermatol.* **94,** 27S (1990).
3. D. M. Araujo, P. A. Lapchak, B. Collier, and R. Quirion, *Brain Res.* **498,** 257 (1989).
4. P. A. Lapchak, D. M. Araujo, R. Quirion, and A. Beaudet, *Neuroscience* **44,** 173 (1991).
5. F. Villemain, J. M. Girard, T. Owens, and A. Beaudet, *Soc. Neurosci. Abstr.* **16,** 1213 (1990).

6. J. E. Merrill, *Ann. N.Y. Acad. Sci.* **594,** 188 (1990).
7. B. De Sarro, Y. Masuda, C. Asciotti, M. G. Audino, and G. Nistico, *Neuropharmacology* **29,** 167 (1990).
8. V. Tancredi, C. Zona, F. Velotti, F. Eusebi, and A. Santoni, *Brain Res.* **525,** 149 (1990).
9. D. Seto, U. K. Hanisch, J.-G. Chabot, and R. Quirion, *Soc. Neurosci. Abstr.* **17,** 782 (1991).
10. U. Hanisch, D. Seto, and R. Quirion, *J. Neurosci.* (in press).
11. T. R. Mosmann, H. Cherwinski, M. W. Bond, M. A. Giedlin, and R. L. Coffman, *J. Immunol.* **136,** 2348 (1986).
12. R. P. Saneto, A. Altman, R. L. Knobler, H. M. Johnson, and J. de Vellis, *Proc. Natl. Acad. Sci. U.S.A.* **83,** 9221 (1986).
13. R. P. Saneto, F. Chiappelli, and J. de Vellis, *J. Neurosci. Res.* **18,** 147 (1987).
14. P. Keely Haugen and P. C. Letourneau, *J. Neurosci. Res.* **25,** 443 (1990).
15. R. Quirion and T. V. Dam, *in* "Methods in Neurosciences" (P. M. Conn, ed.), Vol. 12, p. 223. Academic Press, San Diego (1992).
16. O. H. Lowry, N. J. Rosebrough, A. L. Farr, and R. J. Randall, *J. Biol. Chem.* **193,** 165 (1951).
17. F. Fonnum, *Biochem. J.* **113,** 291 (1969).
18. A. M. Goldberg and R. E. McCaman, *J. Neurochem.* **20,** 1 (1973).
19. F. Villemain, T. Owens, T. Renno, and A. Beaudet, *Soc. Neurosci. Abstr.* **17,** 1199 (1991).

Section III

Neuroendocrine Actions

[11] Endocrine Aspects of Neuroimmunomodulation: Methods and Overview

Samuel M. McCann, Ljiljana Milenkovic,
M. Carmen Gonzalez, Krzysztof Lyson,
Sharada Karanth, and Valeria Rettori

This article presents methods used to evaluate the actions of cytokines at the hypothalamic and pituitary level and then summarizes the current status of our knowledge of their actions on the hypothalamic–pituitary unit. This field has developed explosively in the last few years, following the discovery of the structure of these small proteins produced by the immune system.

Methods of Study

In Vivo Studies

In our *in vivo* studies we have used conscious, freely moving animals because results obtained in anesthetized animals are relevant only to that particular anesthetic and the depth of anesthesia. Frequently, results with various brain transmitters can be opposite in unanesthetized animals from those obtained in conscious animals (1). In such studies it is essential that the method of administration of the cytokine not cause pain or discomfort to the animal. Consequently, we inject substances to be studied either intravenously (iv) in animals bearing indwelling intrajugular catheters (2, 3) or into the third ventricle (3V) in animals with implanted third ventricular cannulae (4, 5).

Intravenous and Third Ventricular Injection

Substances injected intravenously are distributed throughout the body and, therefore, it is difficult to assign a locus of action following this route of injection. If an effect can be obtained following third ventricular (3V) injection with a lower dose than that effective by intravenous injection, one can reasonably assign a site of action to central structures. The action would be mediated on sites adjacent to the third ventricle following the uptake of the compound in question from the ventricle.

Methods in Neurosciences, Volume 16

Many previous studies have shown that practically all molecules can be taken up by the brain by the 3V route. These range in size from low molecular weight transmitters, such as dopamine, norepinephrine, and γ-aminobutyric acid (GABA) (5, 6), to γ-globulins, as revealed by effective immunoneutralization of brain peptides following intraventricular administration of antisera directed against them (7, 8). Studies with intraventricular injection of labeled dopamine revealed that it was primarily distributed to structures adjacent to the 3V, but it is distributed in much smaller amounts to the median eminence, so that 3V-injected substances can enter hypophysial portal capillaries and reach the pituitary gland via the hypophysial portal veins (E. Vijayan and S. M. McCann, unpublished; Ref. 9). Measurements indicate that only about one-hundredth of a dose of atrial natriuretic peptide injected into the 3V reached the gland (J. Antunes-Rodrigues, J. Gutkowska, and S. M. McCann, unpublished).

Therefore, although 3V injections point to an action of the substance in question on sites adjacent to the 3V, it is still possible that the action is mediated on more distant structures in the CNS or in fact even on the pituitary gland. High doses of an intraventricularly injected substance could even reach the peripheral circulation via the pituitary route and have an action in peripheral organs. However, if the dose required to produce an effect intravenously is much greater than that given intraventricularly, then this possibility is rendered unlikely.

An action at the pituitary level following 3V injections can be determined by evaluating the sensitivity of the pituitary gland to the releasing or inhibiting hormone in question. If the action is mediated at the pituitary directly, a modification of the response to the releasing or inhibiting hormone of interest should be evident. If, on the other hand, the action is mediated by an action on the release of hypothalamic hormones that control pituitary function, then the action of the hypothalamic hormone on the pituitary would not be modified, except as could be predicted from the action of the substance at the hypothalamic level (10).

An advantage of the 3V injection technique is that it appears to do little damage to neural tissue. For example, reproducible drinking responses can be obtained to repeated injections of hypertonic saline solution into the 3V (11), whereas when it is microinjected into hypothalamic tissue, drinking can be induced only two or three times, probably because of damage produced by the hypertonic solution (12).

Microinjection into Brain or Pituitary

To further localize the site of action of the compound, it is desirable to microinject it into specific loci in the hypothalamus or other brain structures.

This has the drawback mentioned before of possible damage to tissue, causing loss of responsiveness. However, in general, we and others have found this an effective approach. One potential problem is that unless cannulae are placed bilaterally, the compound will be acting largely unilaterally to produce its effect. Usually this will be sufficient; however, there could be a compensatory opposite action mediated on the contralateral side that could diminish the effect unless the microinjection is made bilaterally. Therefore, if one does not obtain an effect, one should do bilateral injections. Even this approach does not eliminate the possibility of diffusion away from the injection site with an action on an adjacent site. By injecting at sites around the presumed site and finding lesser or no activity, one can localize the site. In the case of substances that are not water soluble, it may be necessary to implant them at the tip of the needle either in the ventricle or in the brain tissue (13).

To establish a pituitary site of action *in vivo,* it is possible to microinject or implant the substance into the pituitary gland itself (14, 15); however, this approach has been largely neglected and replaced by *in vitro* studies, except for evaluating pituitary responsiveness by intravenous injection of releasing or inhibiting hormones following 3V injection of the substance to evaluate a direct pituitary action (10).

Other classic approaches to determine the localization of the action concern electrolytic or radio-frequency lesions (16, 17) and cuts made with the Halasz knife or modifications thereof (18). These approaches have been little used in the case of cytokines, and not by us, and will not be further discussed here.

Push–Pull Cannulae in Brain or Pituitary

To determine the effect of administration of cytokines on the output of brain transmitters, one implants a push–pull cannula in the relevant area and measures the output of various transmitters or releasing hormones from the cannula placed either in the brain (19) or in the pituitary gland (20). There are advantages and disadvantages to this technique; however, we have found it useful and have been able to measure the output of growth hormone-releasing hormone (GRH) and somatostatin into the pituitary push–pull cannula (21). We found that the output of both of these peptides was pulsatile and that the release of both peptides was increased following application of ether anesthesia, with the increase in growth hormone releasing-inhibiting hormone (SRIH, somatostatin) release outlasting that of GRH. Ether stress suppresses growth hormone release in the rat and this was measured by peripheral blood samples. It could also have been measured in samples from the push–pull cannula. The fact that GRH was also released by ether and yet plasma growth hormone decreased may be explained by the ability of the released somatostatin to counteract the stimulatory effect of GRH at the pituitary level.

Hypophysial Portal Blood Collection

The method of hypophysial portal blood collection was pioneered by Porter, who collected portal blood by placing a catheter over the cut end of the pituitary stalk following removal of the lower jaw and aspiration of the pituitary gland in animals under urethane anesthesia (22). This method was valuable in showing that substances secreted into the hypophysial portal vessels were present in much higher concentration than those in peripheral circulation, proving secretion of the substances into portal blood. An alternative method developed by Worthington (23), in which the stalk is simply cut, leaving the pituitary gland intact, suffers from the problem of possible retrograde flow of blood from the pituitary gland and contamination of the sample with substances of pituitary origin. These techniques have been used to show the secretion of many releasing hormones, other peptides, and dopamine into portal blood (24, 25). With respect to interleukin 1 (IL-1), the secretion of corticotropin-releasing hormone (CRH) and to a lesser extent of vasopressin into portal blood following the lateral ventricular injection of the monokine was demonstrated (26). Portal blood collections have also been used to follow the release of epinephrine, vasopressin, and CRH under various stress conditions (26).

The technique demonstrates that a substance is secreted into the portal blood; however, it cannot determine the amounts of any substance secreted in unanesthetized animals, because urethane is an irreversible deep anesthetic. This problem has been circumvented to a degree by the use of a steroidal anesthetic, althesin, which allows the determination of increased levels of luteinizing hormone-releasing hormone (LHRH) in portal blood at the time of the proestrous surge of gonadotropins (27). Even this is not sufficient to eliminate the possible effects of anesthetics.

Another problem is the stress of the extensive surgery needed to place the catheter in position. In the technique of Porter, the pituitary gland itself is removed, which could cause loss of short-loop feedback mechanisms emanating from the pituitary. Therefore this technique is not satisfactory for estimating the basal secretion of substances to the pituitary gland from the median eminence. It also fails to determine the amounts of substances that reach the anterior lobe via the short portal vessels that transmit information from the neural lobe to the anterior lobe and constitute approximately one-third of the blood flow of the anterior pituitary gland (28).

The portal blood collection technique has been improved by a modification introduced by Clarke in sheep, which consists of opening a passage via the nose to the pituitary stalk (29). Subsequently, the stalk is scarified in conscious sheep so as to cause dripping of portal blood into the sinus below, which then can be aspirated. This procedure does not give a quantitative collection of portal blood and there is also the possibility of back flow from the anterior pituitary; however, it goes a long way toward removing most of the problems encountered with the original classic technique. This technique has been used to show pulsatile release of LHRH (29). It would certainly be of interest to do studies in sheep with intraventricular injection or peripheral injection of cytokines to determine the effects on the release of releasing and inhibitory hormones into the portal vessels under these conditions.

In Vitro Studies

Hypothalamic

Many different methods have employed incubation of various-sized pieces of the hypothalamus. We have found that incubation of stalk–median eminence fragments gives good results, either in a static (30, 31) or perifusion system (32). We explored the responsivity of different-sized pieces to prostaglandin E_2 and norepinephrine in early studies and found that the median eminence–stalk explant gave the best results (30, 31). Larger fragments have been used; for example, to study IL-1 effects on CRH release, we and others (34) have employed medial hypothalamic pieces that include the paraventricular nucleus, the major site of origin of the CRH neurons, and extend basally to the median eminence. We have studied the actions of various cytokines with such explants. Interleukin 2 has even had effects on the entire medial hypothalamus incubated *in vitro* in our experiments (35).

In the case of a number of transmitters acting on the hypothalamus, it appears that the action of the transmitter in the medial basal hypothalamus may be opposite in sign near the terminals of the releasing hormone neurons in the median eminence to that at the cell bodies, usually located more rostrally, such as in the paraventricular region, the preoptic region, or the median preoptic nucleus (36–38). Consequently, it is important to do incubations of various-sized pieces to determine whether the action of a given cytokine is the same with each of these types of fragments.

We have employed a dorsomedial hypothalamic cube of tissue that includes only the periventricular nucleus. Using this piece, we found that insulin-like growth factor I and growth hormone will stimulate release of somatostatin and increase the messenger RNA for somatostatin (39). In this case most of the effects may be mediated either directly on the perikarya of the somatostatinergic neurons or via adjacent interneurons that synapse on these perikarya.

None of these procedures is physiological because they all involve cutting of many nerve fibers, frequently of the neuron in question as well. However, if one combines results from these techniques and compares them to the results from the *in vivo* studies, it is usually possible to draw a reasonably coherent picture concerning the action of a given cytokine at the hypothalamic level.

Furthermore, with these *in vitro* incubation systems, it is easy to determine the mechanism of action of a cytokine in altering release of the releasing hormones. The mechanism of action can also be approached *in vivo*, but it is much more difficult to draw meaningful conclusions.

One can also evaluate whether or not there are interneurons interposed between the action of the cytokine and its action on the releasing or inhibiting hormone neuron. This can be studied either *in vivo* (40, 41) or *in vitro* (42, 43) by use of transmitters that stimulate the release of the particular releasing hormone and receptor blockers that block their action. Thus one can determine the effects and role of interneurons in resting and stimulated releasing hormone release. Following the incubations, the release of peptides and releasing hormones into the incubation medium can be quantitated by radioimmunoassay.

Pituitary

Several different types of static incubation systems have been devised, the earliest one (and the one used almost exclusively in the early days of neuroendocrine research) being the hemipituitary system. It is critical to employ a preincubation period to lower the basal release of the hormones. The high initial release may be due to cutting of tissue, but this high background confounds the observation of the effects of putative stimulators or inhibitors of pituitary hormone secretion.

One can obtain good results with single hemipituitaries provided that, after the initial preincubation, one uses still another preincubation to obtain the basal release of hormone and then adds to the same medium the stimulant in question and incubates again. One can then determine the change in hormone release induced by the putative agent (44). Then the shortest time of incubation with the putative agent to obtain a clear response is the best to use, because of possible negative feedback of released hormones to suppress additional release. Also, metabolism of the added compound can cause the obliteration of transient effects when one incubates tissue for a period of time longer than the duration of action of the stimulant. In that case, continued basal release can mask the short stimulatory phase of the compound. This problem does not arise in the case of perifusion systems.

Portanova et al. (45) introduced short-term culture of dispersed pituitary cells. The dispersion was carried out by trypsin. This preparation was almost immediately responsive to CRH with the release of adrenocorticotropic hormone (ACTH). Dispersed cell incubation has the advantage that diffusion barriers would be eliminated. Also, one has a large population of cells, so that variance in response of individual cells is practically eliminated, giving uniform responses to various secretogues in different samples from the same gland. In many instances trypsinization with immediate use of the tissue causes loss of responsiveness, perhaps related to loss of the receptors during the trypsinization and/or other unknown factors. If dispersion is produced by collagenase we found that one had immediate responsiveness to LHRH, whereas there was no response to LHRH of trypsinized cells (46); however, trypsinized cells overnight cultured gave satisfactory responses to most agents (47).

Presumably, differences from batch to batch and relatively low sensitivity led Brazeau et al. (48) to develop the 4-day monolayer cultured cell system, which is excruciatingly sensitive to LHRH and somatostatin and has become the standard in this field. If this is responsive to the putative agent, then it is an ideal system; however, it is more cumbersome than the short-term incubation or overnight culture systems, because of the time required and the necessity to use sterile technique.

Sometimes 4-day cultured cells are unresponsive. A good example is incubation with IL-1, which showed no immediate release of ACTH in the 4-day monolayer culture system (49). Some workers have, however, incubated samples for much longer periods of time and shown responsiveness (50). Why does this preparation not respond immediately? The reasons have not been determined, but it could be due to a loss of receptors during the initial dispersion or to a down regulation of the receptors for IL-1, during culture in vitro in the absence of the endogenous ligand.

Therefore, before concluding that pituitaries are unresponsive to a given agent, it is necessary to try the hemipituitary system. This has the disadvantage that one is looking at the responsiveness of individual hemipituitaries, so that variability increases. Also, possible diffusion barriers may exist and there may be cell death near the center of the pituitary. However, hemipituitaries seem to be responsive to anything that acts on the anterior pituitary, in contrast to the cultured cell systems, in which responsiveness is often lost.

Why is this so? One possibility is the down regulation of receptors referred to above. Another possibility is that important paracrine or autocrine actions may occur when the normal architecture is maintained in hemipituitaries. In the dispersed pituitary cell cultures, in which the cells are separated from each other, even autocrine effects may not be apparent; certainly paracrine effects are not. Indeed, paracrine effects have been demonstrated by Vankelekom *et al.* (51) in the case of prolactin and luteinizing hormone (LH) cells in a series of experiments using aggregates of pituitary cells in culture.

The aggregate pituitary cell culture technique has been developed by Vankelekom *et al.* (51), as indicated above. It is this author's view that although it has led to some interesting findings, it has no particular advantage over hemipituitaries. Some investigators have even used quartered glands, and so on. The disadvantage of this technique is the increased tissue damage caused by such slicing procedures.

Using these pituitary incubation systems, it is possible to monitor the effect of a given agent on the output of the various pituitary hormones, and it has been found that the pituitary secretes not only pituitary hormones but also IL-6 *in vitro* (52). Vankelekom *et al.* (51) have pointed to its probable production in the folliculostellate cells of the gland. It may well be that most of the cytokines are actually produced in these cells, which appear to be modified macrophages, of the pituitary gland.

Again, incubation of the anterior pituitary can be carried out in either a static or perifusion system. For both hypothalamic and pituitary tissue, the static system has the advantage of ease of performance, but the disadvantage is that the concentrations of various hormones can increase in the medium and tissue and can generate ultra-short-loop negative feedback effects that can result in a flattening or even inversion of the dose–response curve (53–56). The perifusion systems have the advantage that these effects do not occur; however, the disadvantage is that many more samples need to be assayed. Our feeling has been that if one obtains the same result with both of these systems, it is much easier, at least in initial studies, to use a static system. The perifusion system allows easier determination of the time course of response of the tissue to a given cytokine. It is also necessary to determine possible pulsatile release.

Immunocytochemistry, in Situ Hybridization, and Receptor Autoradiography

Immunochemistry is the method *par excellence* to demonstrate the presence of these cytokines in the hypothalamus, pituitary, or other CNS regions and, when coupled with measurements of release *in vitro* or into push–pull cannulae, can determine whether or not the cytokine is actually made and released in the tissue and its site of origin.

In this connection, IL-1α (57) and IL-1β (58) neuronal systems have been described in the hypothalamus on the basis of immunocytochemical studies. This should be coupled with attempts to demonstrate the messenger RNA for the cytokine, reported for IL-1β in the hypothalamus (59), and its localization by *in situ* hybridization.

Receptors for the cytokine should also be localized in brain and pituitary. These latter aspects are the subjects of other chapters in this volume and will not be further discussed here.

These are the major methods that have been used so far in studying the possible roles of the various mono- and cytokines on the hypothalamic–pituitary axis.

Overview of Actions of Mono- and Cytokines on Hypothalamic–Pituitary Axis

A new field, known as neuroimmunomodulation, has developed, in which it is apparent that CNS activity modulates the immune system by the autonomic nervous system and by alterations in the output of anterior pituitary hormones. In turn, the immune system, which releases several monokines, feeds back to modulate the activity of the hypothalamic–pituitary unit (60, 61).

It has been known as far back as 1936 from the pioneering work of Selye (62) that noxious stimuli of one type or another, called stresses, activate the release of ACTH, which in turn releases adrenal cortical steroids. These then bring about a series of reactions in the body that consist of thymic involution, decrease in size of lymph nodes, lymphopenia, and eosinopenia. The role of the nervous system in these phenomena was not established at that time; however, we now know that the nervous system plays a profoundly important role in control of the release of pituitary hormones by means of a series of releasing and inhibiting hormones that are released in the median eminence of the tuber cinereum and pass down the hypophysial portal vessels to the hypophysial sinusoids, where they act to stimulate or inhibit the release of particular pituitary hormones.

Following infection, the introduction of bacterial endotoxins, or most immunization procedures, a stresslike response of the hypothalamic–pituitary unit occurs (63). The response to stress extends beyond the activation of ACTH secretion to the activation of prolactin (PRL) and growth hormone (GH) release in humans. Prolactin and GH release is augmented by nearly all stresses in lower forms; however, the rat is an exception in that stress, instead of stimulating, inhibits GH release. In addition, stress results in inhibition of the release of the glycoprotein hormones [thyroid-stimulating hormone (TSH), LH, and to a lesser extent follicle-stimulating hormone (FSH)]. Therefore in the acute phase of infection one would have the stimulation of ACTH and adrenal corticoid release, which tends to suppress the immune response, which in turn would be counterbalanced by the stimulatory effects on the immune response of GH (except in the rat) and PRL released during stress (64).

Multiple pathways mediate the activation of the hypothalamic–pituitary unit that takes place during stress (65). This can occur via emotional stimuli, painful stimuli, damage to tissue which produces pain; products of the immune cells themselves may evoke the response. For example, bacterial pyrogens evoke the release of endogenous pyrogens from these cells, which circulate through the blood to the hypothalamus to evoke fever by affecting temperature-regulating centers and activate the pituitary–adrenal system (66, 67).

Hypothalamic Control of Pituitary Secretion

The hypothalamic control of pituitary hormone secretion is brought about by a series of peptidic transmitters. For ACTH, the most important transmitter (at least in humans and rats) is CRH, a 41-amino acid peptide (68). The first hypothalamic peptide shown to release ACTH was vasopressin, and it is now apparent that vasopressin plays a physiologically significant role in the release of ACTH (69); in sheep it has even been stated to be more important than CRH (70). Both of these are released into the hypophysial portal vessels and each augments the action of the other to bring about the stress-induced release of ACTH.

Prolactin release is particularly under the control of prolactin-inhibiting factors (PIFs), in particular dopamine; however, it appears that GABA, acetylcholine, and a peptide inhibitor, which may be the gonadotropin-releasing hormone-associated peptide (GAP), also play important roles. On the other hand, there are at least 10 stimulatory factors, which include oxytocin, vasoactive intestinal polypeptide (VIP), peptide histidine isoleucine (PHI), thyrotropin-releasing hormone (TRH), and oxytocin (71). The evidence for the physiological significance of oxytocin, VIP, PHI, and TRH is strengthened on the basis of studies with antiserum directed against each of these peptides. In particular, oxytocin is released by suckling and may be an important component of the suckling-induced prolactin release, as supported by studies with antisera directed against the peptide. Oxytocin may be involved in the stress-induced release of prolactin, because it is released into portal vessels during stress (72).

The control of growth hormone is complex because it is controlled by GRH on the one hand and by somatostatin on the other (73).

Hypothalamic control of TSH is mediated primarily by TRH but vasopressin also releases TSH; however, the physiological significance of this action is unknown (73, 74). The release of LH is under the control of LH-releasing hormone (LHRH) (73) and an FSH-releasing factor (FSHRF) has been postulated (75). The existence of the latter is supported by many examples of dissociation in the release of FSH and LH. FSHRF has not yet been isolated; however, GAP(1–13) has specific FSH-releasing activity, as does an analog of LHRH, leading to the view that this factor will ultimately be isolated (76).

Hypothalamic–Pituitary Response to Infection

In infection, or following injection of bacterial pyrogens, a fever occurs that is also accompanied by alterations in the release of pituitary hormones producing the pattern of pituitary hormonal release that occurs in infection. In earlier work (67) we injected a purified bacterial pyrogen intravenously into dogs and found that after a delay fever occurred. This fever was paralleled by an increase in plasma cortisol, indicating that a release of ACTH had occurred (67). Studies by others at that time led to the conclusion that the delay in the induction of fever following injection of bacterial pyrogens was accounted for by the time required for the release of an endogenous pyrogen that acted directly on the hypothalamic temperature-regulating centers. It was shown that the major source of the endogenous pyrogen in plasma was the circulating monocytes (77). We speculated that the elevation of plasma cortisol that we observed in these dogs injected with bacterial pyrogens was due to the action of endogenous pyrogen within the hypothalamus to induce not only fever but also activation of ACTH secretion. Finally, in the early 1980s the first endogenous pyrogen was isolated, its structure determined, and it was synthesized. It was named IL-1 (66).

Interleukin 1

Interleukin 1 has now become available for study and it is apparent that intraperitoneal administration of the peptide activates ACTH secretion (78). Similarly, intravenous administration of IL-1 increases plasma ACTH in the rat (79). The supposition that the peptide acts by release of CRH was supported by other experiments in which, following systemic administration of the peptide, there was an increase in CRH in portal blood and a borderline increase in vasopressin as well (79). Both of these peptides are capable of directly stimulating a release of ACTH from the pituitary gland and vasopressin potentiates the action of CRH to release ACTH (80). In other studies antisera directed against CRH have been shown to block the response to systemic administration of IL-1, again indicating that the response may be mediated by release of CRH (26).

A possible action of IL-1 to affect ACTH release directly is controversial. In AtT-20 tumor cells, which consist of abnormal corticotrophs, IL-1 stimulates ACTH release *in vitro* (81). In three studies it has been found to have no effect on the release of ACTH from normal pituitary cells *in vitro* (26, 78, 82) and furthermore it failed to alter the response to CRH (78); however, in one study, employing quartered anterior pituitaries, a dose-related release of ACTH was found (83). The reason for these discrepant results is not apparent, but it may be related to use of dispersed cells in the negative experiments. This could have resulted in loss of paracrine effects and possible decreases in receptors as discussed earlier. Indeed, in subsequent studies, effects in dispersed cells have been observed after prolonged incubation (50), perhaps related to up regulation of interleukin receptors on exposure to their natural ligand.

In our studies we obtained an increase in GH and PRL release and an inhibition of TSH release following the 3V administration of IL-1 at a dose of 5 ng (0.3 pmol) that produced a slight elevation of body temperature (84); however, the responses vanished at the higher dose of 25 ng (1.5 pmol), which produced a frank fever (84).

Incubation of IL-1 with rat hypothalamic fragments *in vitro* produced a release of prostaglandin E_2 (PGE_2) but not $PGF_{2\alpha}$ into the medium at a concentration of 10^{-14} M, whereas as in the *in vivo* studies with pituitary hormones, a higher dose at 10^{-11} M was without effect. Similar results were obtained with IL-2 (V. Rettori and M. Gimeno, unpublished). Perhaps the ACTH responses to IL-1 may be mediated by release of prostaglandins. The bell-shaped dose–response curve of hormonal responses observed *in vivo* with IL-1 may be caused by the decreased prostaglandin release at higher doses of the monokine.

We have expanded our studies on IL-1 to its effects on gonadotropin release in conscious castrate male rats. The 3V injection of 0.06 pmol of recombinant human IL-1α caused a suppression of pulsatile LH but not FSH release in the animals. There was no interference with the pulsatile release of both gonadotropins in diluent-injected controls and in these rats there was a significant number of instances in which the pulses of FSH and LH were asynchronous. Following administration of the monokine, LH pulses ceased completely with a varying delay, such that all LH release had stopped pulsing in animals by 1 hr and there were no pulses during the second hour after 3V injection. In sharp contrast, pulsatile release of FSH was barely altered, the only change being a borderline significant increase in the height of the FSH pulses. We postulated that IL-1 selectively blocked pulsatile release of LH and not FSH, supporting our previous findings indicating a separate hypothalamic control of LH and FSH, LH being controlled by LH-releasing hormone and FSH being controlled by FSH-releasing factor (85).

To determine the mechanism of blockade of pulsatile LH release, we incubated medial basal hypothalami *in vitro* and evaluated the effect of IL-1α (10^{-11} M) on LHRH release into the medium in a static incubation system. Interleukin 1α lowered slightly the basal release of LHRH and completely blocked the norepinephrine (5×10^{-5} M)-induced release of LHRH. It also completely blocked the release of PGE_2 induced by norepinephrine. We postulated that IL-1 reacted with its newly discovered receptors in the basal hypothalamus to block the norepinephrine-induced release of PGE_2, thereby blocking the release of LHRH (85).

Intraventricular injection of IL-1 has also been found capable of blocking the proestrous release of LH (86). This action may be mediated as described above by blocking the action of norepinephrine.

Cachectin (Tumor Necrosis Factor)

We have carried out extensive studies with tumor necrosis factor (TNF). Our results on the *in vitro* effects of this monokine on the release of pituitary hormones, using incubation of either hemipituitaries or dispersed pituitary cells cultured overnight (53), indicate that after at least 1 hr of incubation the monokine can stimulate the release of ACTH, GH, TSH, and minimally prolactin, in these *in vitro* systems. The effect on prolactin was not observed in every experiment.

Interestingly, the minimal effective dose (MED) for these actions of cachectin was 100-fold greater with dispersed cells than with hemipituitaries. We speculate that this may be due either to loss of receptors in the former preparation and/or to some paracrine actions of various pituitary cells to augment the effects in the hemipituitaries, as discussed earlier.

The data indicate a role for prostaglandins in these effects because indomethacin, an inhibitor of cyclooxygenase, completely or partially blocked the effects. Interestingly, cachectin produced a dose-related suppression of cyclic AMP levels in the pituitary and this effect was blocked by somatostatin, which brought out a remarkable stimulation of prolactin release by TNF. Possibly this was caused by the elevation of cyclic AMP, which occurred in the presence of both cachectin and somatostatin, because cyclic AMP is a known stimulator of prolactin release from the lactotrophs.

A bell-shaped dose–response curve was obtained and the MED of 10^{-12}

M for the hemipituitaries is within the levels that might be encountered *in vivo* in infection. Consequently, we concluded that cachectin may play an important role in altering pituitary hormone release by direct actions on the gland in infection.

We also studied the effects of injection of cachectin into the 3V of conscious male rats and found that it stimulated ACTH, PRL, and GH secretion and inhibited the secretion of TSH, the latter only after a delay of 2 hr (87). Cachectin had a lower MED to elevate body temperature than IL-2; however, at a dose of 0.06 pmol the effect was maximal with an elevation in rectal temperature of about 1–1.5°C, which remained constant even as the dose was increased 100-fold. This maximal elevation was much lower than that obtained with IL-1 (3–3.5°C). The effects on ACTH and GH secretion were obtained only with the highest dose evaluated (6 pmol), whereas in the prior experiments IL-1 stimulated PRL and GH release with a dose of 0.3 pmol and, as indicated earlier, the response vanished when the dose was increased to 1.5 pmol.

Thus the behavior with regard to cachectin was different from that previously found with IL-1. We evaluated the effects of 3V injection of the inhibitor of cyclooxygenase, indomethacin, to block prostaglandin synthesis. This completely blocked the fever induced by cachectin but had only a partial effect on the ACTH release induced.

The inhibitory action on TSH release *in vivo* was the opposite of that obtained with pituitaries *in vitro*. Thus the *in vivo* inhibition of TSH release must be mediated by structures near the 3V. Because of the delay in release of the other pituitary hormones from pituitary cells *in vitro*, it is unlikely that the other *in vivo* effects of 3V injection of cachectin were mediated at the pituitary gland; they were also probably mediated via a direct effect on the hypothalamus (87).

Interferon γ

We evaluated the effect of interferon γ (INF-γ) on hypothalamic–pituitary function (88, 89). This cytokine injected into the 3V at a low dose of 0.3 pmol produced a stimulation of ACTH release accompanied by a delayed inhibition of GH and TSH release, but produced no effect on prolactin. Not surprisingly, in view of the results with IL-1, a higher (1.5 pmol) dose was without effect. The lack of response to the higher dose of INF-γ is reminiscent of the results with IL-1; however, this monokine had little effect in elevating body temperature and consequently the argument used above, that this lack of response at high doses was due to further elevation of body temperature, is an unlikely explanation for this loss of effect of INF-γ at higher doses.

Incubation of INF-γ with hemipituitaries *in vitro* revealed no effect on the release of prolactin, TSH, and GH, but a stimulation of ACTH release occurred at the relatively high dose of 10^{-8} M. From these results it appears that INF-γ may play a role in inducing the hypothalamic–pituitary response to infection by actions primarily on the hypothalamus (88).

We have continued to analyze the actions of INF-γ by *in vitro* studies with medial basal hypothalami and hemipituitaries. In the case of the medial basal hypothalami incubated in a static incubation system, we found that the monokine would stimulate the release of somatostatin at concentrations of 10^{-8} and 10^{-9} M and that it would also lower GH release from pituitaries incubated *in vitro* at a concentration of 10^{-12} M. In the *in vitro* pituitary incubation at a high dose of 10^{-8} M, we found that it potentiated the response to GH-releasing factor; however, because this is a 10,000-fold increase in dose over that producing inhibition, we question whether this is of pathophysiological significance. Again, in the *in vitro* incubation of either hypothalami or pituitaries we noticed that the stimulatory action on somatostatin release and the inhibitory action on GH release vanished at higher doses, again giving this same strange, bell-shaped dose–response curve encountered before with the *in vivo* studies with IL-1 and INF-γ and the *in vitro* pituitary incubations with cachectin (53). It is obvious that this is a characteristic of the actions of at least some of these cytokines and it will be interesting to examine the mechanism further.

Interleukin 6

We have characterized the actions of IL-6 on the hypothalamic–pituitary axis. Following its injection into the 3V of conscious, castrate male rats, it elevated body temperature and this was accompanied by an elevation of plasma ACTH within 15 min, whereas TSH was significantly lowered. Prolactin and GH levels were not changed. Plasma gonadotropin levels were also unaltered by 3V injection of IL-6. The effects on rectal temperature and hormone release were directly related to the dose of the monokine injected, with an MED of 1.5 pmol. The pattern of hormonal responses was similar to that obtained with IL-1 and cachectin, except that there was no effect on PRL or GH levels.

When the monokine was incubated with pituitaries *in vitro*, it increased the release of ACTH and GH into the culture medium but only after a 2-hr period of incubation at the single concentration of 10^{-13} M. Concentrations of 10^{-14} or 10^{-12} M were ineffective. Again, we have a bell-shaped dose–response curve with abolition of the actions at higher doses. It appears that IL-6 has important actions at the hypothalamic and/or pituitary level to stimulate ACTH and GH secretion and to decrease TSH release (90).

We have also shown that IL-6 at a concentration of 10^{-13} M, increases

CRH release *in vitro* from a medial hypothalamic piece extending from the paraventricular to include the median eminence (34). The effect vanished at concentrations greater than 10^{-12} M. Therefore it is likely that the increased plasma ACTH observed following injection of IL-6 into the 3V was caused by CRH release, which in turn stimulated release of ACTH by the corticotrophs. Navarra *et al.* (33) have similarly found this stimulatory effect at concentrations of 10^{-13} M.

We have studied the mechanism by which IL-6 stimulates the release of CRH *in vitro*. We believe that it involves arachidonic acid metabolites. Dexamethasone, the synthetic glucocorticoid, may act after combination with the glucocorticoid receptors to inhibit ACTH release by blockade of phospholipase A_2, the enzyme that stimulates synthesis of arachidonic acid. Dexamethasone was capable of blocking the action of IL-6 to increase CRH release from medial basal hypothalamic fragments incubated *in vitro* at the low concentration of 10^{-11} M (91).

We then studied the effect of inhibitors of the three pathways of arachidonic acid metabolism and found that the most effective inhibitor was clotrimazole, which blocks the epoxygenase enzyme involved in synthesis of epoxides. This was effective at a dose of 10^{-9} M, whereas blockade of cyclooxygenase by indomethacin to inhibit prostaglandin synthesis or lipoxygenase to inhibit leukotriene synthesis by 5,8,11-eicosatriynoic acid was much less effective. Therefore the results suggest that IL-6 stimulates CRH release by activation of the arachidonic acid cascade and that the most effective compounds activating CRH release are the epoxides (91). Glucocorticoids inhibit IL-6-induced CRH release by blocking arachidonic acid synthesis.

α-MSH, which has important antipyretic (92) and antiinflammatory actions (93), blocks the release of CRH induced by IL-6 at a concentration of 10^{-13} M, an action shared by ACTH. Because the MED for the inhibitory effect of ACTH is 10–100 times less than that of α-MSH and α-MSH is ACTH(1–13), the action of α-MSH may result from its ability to combine with ACTH receptors.

These actions of ACTH and α-MSH might have therapeutic value by reducing the release of CRH, which has the ability to inhibit immune responses via its stimulation of ACTH release and consequent adrenal cortical steroid release. In this respect, because of the lack of action on the adrenal cortex, α-MSH could be more valuable in suppressing release of cytokines and blocking their peripheral action.

Interleukin 2

Interleukin 2, a lymphokine synthesized and secreted by T lymphocytes, has now been evaluated and appears from our results to be the most potent agent known to act directly on the pituitary to alter pituitary hormone release. At concentrations of 10^{-15} M it elevated prolactin and TSH release and inhibited release of FSH, LH, and GH. Adrenocorticotropic hormone release was stimulated at a higher concentration of 10^{-12} M. After reaching the minimal effective stimulatory or inhibitory dose, the dose–response curve was flat, but at much higher doses of 10^{-9} or 10^{-8} M responses tended to diminish to nonsignificant values, again a dose–response relationship reminiscent of that obtained with other cytokines (56).

We have also evaluated the action of IL-2 following its 3V injection into conscious rats and have determined that its actions *in vivo* are similar to those obtained with incubation of pituitaries *in vitro*, in that the interleukin-2 stimulated ACTH, prolactin, and TSH release, but inhibited FSH, LH, and growth hormone discharge (94). That these actions are at least in part due to direct effects on the hypothalamus is indicated by the fact that IL-2 can stimulate the release of CRH from medial basal hypothalamic fragments incubated *in vitro* (95), and at the same time inhibit the release of LHRH (96). Furthermore, it stimulated the release of somatostatin and blocked dopamine-induced GRF release, which can account for its ability to inhibit GH release (97). Thus this cytokine has actions at both the hypothalamic and pituitary levels, as in the case of the other monokines that we have evaluated.

Thymosin α_1

We have begun the evaluation of thymosin α_1 (Tα_1), the first thymic peptide to be synthesized. It produced a dose-related decrease of plasma TSH and ACTH following its injection into the 3V, together with a decrease of plasma prolactin, but there was no significant change in plasma GH concentrations (98). The decreases in ACTH and TSH were caused by decreased release of CRH and TRH, because *in vitro* incubation of medial basal hypothalami revealed that Tα_1 could suppress release of these neuropeptides.

In many previous instances we have found that a peptide will influence the release of another hypothalamic peptide but that in most instances these actions are mediated via interneurons. To test this hypothesis we incubated the hypothalami in the presence of metergoline, a blocker of serotonin receptors. Metergoline blocked the decrease of TRH release induced by serotonin and reversed the Tα_1-induced inhibition of TRH release, indicating that a serotoninergic receptor was probably involved in the pathway of inhibition of TRH by Tα_1 (99).

Incubated with hemipituitaries *in vitro*, Tα_1 evoked a dose-dependent release of TSH and ACTH whereas there was no effect on the release of prolactin and GH. The peptide evinced a remarkable ability to stimulate LH in a dose-related manner at doses as low as 10^{-12} M, whereas FSH release was unaltered (98). Because $T\alpha_1$ has been localized to both the hypothalamus and pituitary, it too may have physiological significance in neuroendocrine immunology. Thus both hypothalamic and pituitary sites of action may be of importance for the induction of changes in pituitary hormone with all cytokines.

Localization of Interleukin 1 and Its Receptors in Brain

Work on these important new small proteins has proceeded apace in other laboratories and receptors for IL-1 have been characterized in the hypothalamus (100). Interleukin 1 has been found in the hypothalamus in microglia (101), which are essentially brain macrophages, and it has also been reported to be present in astrocytes; the secretion from these cells is induced by bacterial pyrogens (102). Interleukin 1β has even been reported in humans in a neuronal system with cell bodies in the paraventricular nucleus and axons extending to the median eminence (58). In immunocytochemical studies in rats, we have found evidence for IL-1α in microglia and also in neurons in the lateral preoptic area and hypothalamus, but not in neuronal projections to the median eminence. The number of these neurons was dramatically increased by intravenous injection of lipopolysaccharide (LPS) at a dose that increased plasma ACTH (57).

Interleukin 6 is released by hypothalamic fragments incubated *in vitro* and its release is augmented by LPS (52). The current view is that the IL-6 from the hypothalamus is probably derived from glial elements; however, we cannot overrule the possibility that it may also be produced by neurons.

Receptors for IL 1 have been characterized in the hypothalamus by radioautography, and it appears that IL-1α and IL-1β utilize the same receptors (100). There have been reports of differences in potency of the two forms of IL-1 (49); whether these are real or related to the species and source of the monokine has not yet been clearly demonstrated.

Penetration of Cytokines into Brain

During bacterial or viral infection, cyto- and monokines are released from cells of the immune system and circulate through the blood stream. It appears that they penetrate into the brain through the circumventricular organs, particularly the organum vasculosum lamina terminalis (OVLT) (101–103). These are areas in which the blood–brain barrier is broken down and the concept has been advanced that the monokines interact with the modified glial cells in the OVLT to induce the production of prostaglandin E_2. These cells are visualized as having long processes, so that they can then interact with neurons within the temperature-regulating centers or releasing and inhibiting hormone neurons by releasing prostaglandin E_2 (104).

Thus in infection there are multiple pathways by which the mono- and cytokines can reach the brain, that is, via the circulating blood, via local production in glial elements, and also via production in neuronal elements (105).

Pituitary Production of Cytokines

In addition, these substances are probably made within the pituitary gland itself. Evidence is strong that IL-6 is made by folliculostellate cells in the anterior pituitary (51, 52). These were of unknown function but now appear to be modified macrophages, and they have been shown to produce IL-6 (52). It has been shown that IL-1 will induce IL-6 production by anterior pituitaries *in vitro* (106). Evidence suggests that IL-1β can also be synthesized in the gland (107). Thus, in the pituitary as well as in the brain, these cytokines reach the gland via the peripheral circulation or via local production within the tissue. Thus, the mono- and cytokines can act in the pituitary either by paracrine effects or via the concentrations in the blood reaching the gland.

The concentrations of the cytokines present in brain or pituitary gland are undoubtedly increased in cases of infection by the action of viral or bacterial endotoxins. The actual levels obtained are not known and this is the reason why the question of the pathophysiological significance of these various monokines must be evaluated by the use of antisera directed against them. Obviously, if the levels are of pathophysiological significance, antisera directed against the proteins should eliminate their action and thereby show the pathophysiological significance. An antagonist of the receptor of IL-1 has been found and this antagonist is available for study. In one report it was stated that the antagonist would block the response to LPS, which certainly suggests that IL-1 plays a role in this response (49).

Conclusions

It is apparent that the stress response is mimicked by infections and by most immunization procedures that lead to an altered pattern of pituitary hormone secretion. There is increased ACTH secretion, leading to immunosuppressive actions, and increased release of PRL and GH (except in the rat), which tends to augment immune responses. The effects of infection are brought about by a complex interplay of mono- and cytokines on hypothalamic neu-

TABLE I   Actions of Cytokines on the
Hypothalamic–Pituitary Unit

Cytokine	Fever	ACTH	PRL	LH	FSH	GH	TSH
IL-1	+ +	+ +	+	−	0	+	−
TNF[a]	+	+	+	?	?	+	−
INF-γ	+	+	0	?	?	−	−
IL-6	+	+	0	?	?	−	−
IL-2	?	+	+	−	−	−	+
Tα_1	+	−	−	+[b]	0	0	−

[a] TNF, Cachectin.
[b] *In vitro* on hemipituitaries.

rons, which results in altered release of hypothalamic peptides that in turn alter the release of the peptides into the hypophysial portal vessels to bring about the expected pituitary response.

It appears that all of these cytokines have actions at both the hypothalamic and pituitary levels, the rapid effects being produced by hypothalamic action to alter releasing hormone discharge and the pituitary actions being slower and probably more important in responses to prolonged release of monokines in infection. The pattern of modification of pituitary hormone release varies depending on the monokine studied and we are still not sure of their relative importance.

Thus it has become apparent that each of the monokines has its own particular pattern of response at the hypothalamic and pituitary levels. The mechanism of action involves combination with their receptors and is mediated at least in part by arachidonic acid metabolites. Table I summarizes the various actions of these powerful new compounds that we have observed. It is probable that the pattern of hormone response that is seen in infection depends on interactions at the hypothalamic and pituitary levels among these various agents.

Acknowledgment

This work was supported by NIH Grants DK40994, DK10073, and DK43900.

References

1. K. A. Pass and J. G. Ondo, *Endocrinology* (*Baltimore*) **100,** 1437 (1977).
2. P. G. Harms and S. R. Ojeda, *J. Appl. Physiol.* **36,** 391 (1974).

3. S. R. Ojeda, H. E. Jameson, and S. M. McCann, *Endocrinology (Baltimore)* **102,** 531 (1978).

4. J. Antunes-Rodrigues and S. M. McCann, *Proc. Soc. Exp. Biol. Med.* **133,** 1464 (1970).

5. E. Vijayan and S. M. McCann, *Neuroendocrinology* **25,** 150 (1978).

6. E. Vijayan and S. M. McCann, *Brain Res.* **155,** 35 (1978).

7. O. Khorram, J. Bedran de Castro, and S. M. McCann, *Proc. Natl. Acad. Sci. U.S.A.* **81,** 8004 (1984).

8. M. Arisawa, G. D. Snyder, W. H. Yu, L. R. De Palatis, R. H. Ho, and S. M. McCann, *Neuroendocrinology* **52,** 22 (1990).

9. L. Milenkovič, A. F. Parlow, and S. M. McCann, *Neuroendocrinology* **52,** 389 (1990).

10. W. H. Yu, S. M. McCann, and C. H. Li, *Proc. Natl. Acad. Sci. U.S.A.* **85,** 289 (1988).

11. B. Andersson, M. Jobin, and K. Olsson, *Acta Physiol. Scand.* **67,** 127 (1966).

12. B. Andersson and S. M. McCann, *Acta Physiol. Scand.* **33,** 333 (1955).

13. P. S. Kalra and S. M. McCann, *Neuroendocrinology* **19,** 289 (1975).

14. V. D. Ramirez, R. Abrams, and S. M. McCann, *Endocrinology (Baltimore)* **75,** 243 (1964).

15. V. D. Ramirez and S. M. McCann, *Endocrinology (Baltimore)* **75,** 206 (1964).

16. S. M. McCann, *Am. J. Physiol.* **175,** 13 (1953).

17. W. Bishop, C. P. Fawcett, L. Krulich, and S. M. McCann, *Endocrinology (Baltimore)* **91,** 643 (1972).

18. B. Halasz, *in* "Frontiers in Neuroendocrinology" (W. F. Ganong and L. Martini, eds.), p. 307. Oxford Univ. Press, London, 1969.

19. V. D. Ramirez, J. C. Cheng, E. Nudka, W. Lin, and A. D. Ramirez, *Ann. N.Y. Acad. Sci.* **473,** 434 (1986).

20. D. E. Dluzen and V. D. Ramirez, *Neuroendocrinology* **45,** 328 (1987).

21. M. C. Aguila, R. L. Pickle, W. H. Yu, and S. M. McCann, *Neuroendocrinology* **54,** 515 (1991).

22. J. C. Porter and K. R. Smith, *Endocrinology (Baltimore)* **81,** 1182 (1967).

23. W. C. Worthington, Jr., *Nature (London)* **210,** 710 (1966).

24. J. C. Porter, J. F. Sissom, J. Arita, and M. J. Reymond, *Vitam. Horm. (N.Y.)* **40,** 145 (1981).

25. O. M. Cramer, C. R. Parker, and J. C. Porter, *Endocrinology (Baltimore)* **104,** 419 (1979).

26. R. Sapolsky, C. Rivier, G. Yamamoto, P. Plotsky, and W. W. Vale, *Science* **238,** 522 (1987).

27. D. K. Sarkar and G. Fink, *Endocrinology (Baltimore)* **108,** 862 (1981).

28. J. C. Porter, R. S. Mical, N. Ben-Jonathan, and J. G. Ondo, *Recent Prog. Horm. Res.* **29,** 161 (1973).

29. I. J. Clarke and J. T. Cummins, *Endocrinology (Baltimore)* **111,** 1737 (1982).

30. S. R. Ojeda, A. Negro-Vilar, and S. M. McCann, *Endocrinology (Baltimore)* **104,** 617 (1979).

31. A. Negro-Vilar, S. R. Ojeda, and S. M. McCann, *Endocrinology (Baltimore)* **104,** 1749 (1979).

32. S. Kentroti, W. L. Dees, and S. M. McCann, *Proc. Natl. Acad. Sci. U.S.A.* **85,** 953 (1988).

33. P. Navarra, S. Tsagarakis, M. Faria, L. H. Rees, G. M. Besser, and A. B. Grossman, *Endocrinology (Baltimore)* **128,** 37 (1991).

34. K. Lyson, L. Milenkovič, and S. M. McCann, *Prog. NeuroEndocrinImmunol.* **4,** 161 (1991).

35. S. Karanth and S. M. McCann, in preparation (1992).

36. S. M. McCann, *Annu. Rev. Pharmacol. Toxicol.* **22,** 491 (1982).

37. V. Rettori, A. Karara, O. C. Narizzano, R. Ponzio, and S. M. McCann, *Neuroendocrinol. Lett.* **11,** 177 (1989).

38. S. M. McCann and E. Vijayan, *Int. Conf. Neurotensin, 2nd, 1991* (in press) (1992).

39. M. C. Aguila, V. Boggaram, and S. M. McCann, submitted for publication (1992).

40. O. Khorram, H. Mizunuma, and S. M. McCann, *Neuroendocrinology* **34,** 433 (1982).

41. K. S. Iyer and S. M. McCann, *Peptides (N.Y.)* **8,** 45 (1987).

42. L. Milenkovič, K. Lyson, M. C. Aguila, and S. M. McCann, *Neuroendocrinology* **56,** 674 (1992).

43. S. Karanth, M. C. Aguila, and S. M. McCann, *Neuroendocrinology* (in press) (1993).

44. V. Rettori, C. C. Pazos-Moura, E. G. Moura, J. Polak, and S. M. McCann, *Proc. Natl. Acad. Sci. U.S.A.* **89,** 3035 (1992).

45. R. Portanova, D. K. Smith, and G. Sayers, *Proc. Soc. Exp. Biol. Med.* **133,** 573 (1970).

46. H. Nakano, C. P. Fawcett, F. Kimura, and S. M. McCann, *Endocrinology (Baltimore)* **103,** 1527 (1978).

47. G. Snyder, Z. Naor, C. P. Fawcett, and S. M. McCann, *Endocrinology (Baltimore)* **107,** 1627 (1980).

48. P. Brazeau, W. W. Vale, R. Burgus, N. Ling, M. Butcher, J. Rivier, and R. Guillemin, *Science* **179,** 77 (1973).

49. C. Rivier, in "Circulating Regulatory Factors and Neuroendocrine Function" (J. C. Porter and D. Jezova, eds.), p. 295. Plenum, New York, 1990.

50. P. Kehrer, D. Turnhill, J. M. Dayer, and A. F. Muller, *Neuroendocrinology* **48,** 160 (1988).

51. H. Vankelecom, P. Carmeliet, J. Van Damme, A. Billiau, and C. Denef, *Neuroendocrinology* **49,** 102 (1989).

52. B. L. Spangalo, R. M. MacLeod, and P. C. Izakson, *Endocrinology (Baltimore)* **126,** 582 (1990).

53. L. Milenkovič, V. Rettori, G. D. Snyder, B. Beutler, and S. M. McCann, *Proc. Natl. Acad. Sci. U.S.A.* **86,** 2418 (1989).

54. K. Lyson and S. M. McCann, *Neuroendocrinology* **54,** 262 (1991).

55. M. C. Gonzalez, M. Riedel, V. Rettori, W. H. Yu, and S. M. McCann, *Prog. NeuroEndocrinImmunol.* **3,** 49 (1990).

56. S. Karanth and S. M. McCann, *Proc. Natl. Acad. Sci. U.S.A.* **88,** 2961 (1991).

57. V. Rettori, W. L. Dees, J. K. Hiney, L. Milenkovič, and S. M. McCann, *Proc. 74th Annu. Meet. Endocr. Soc.,* Abstr. No. 534, p. 185 (1992).

58. C. D. Breder, C. A. Dinarello, and C. B. Saper, *Science* **240,** 321 (1988).

59. G. A. Higgins and J. A. Olschowka, *Mol. Brain Res.* **9,** 143 (1991).

60. S. M. McCann, N. Ono, O. Khorram, S. Kentroti, and M. C. Aguila, *Ann. N.Y. Acac. Sci.* **496,** (1987).

61. S. M. McCann, V. Rettori, and L. Milenkovič, *in* "Interactions Among CNS, Neuroendocrine and Immune Systems" (J. W. Hadden, K. Masek, and G. Nistico, eds.), Chapter 8, p. 93. Pythagora Press, Rome-Milan, 1989.

62. H. Selye, *Nature* (*London*) **138,** 32 (1936).

63. H. O. Besedovsky, E. Sorkin, N. Keller, and J. Müller, *Proc. Soc. Exp. Biol. Med.* **150,** 466 (1975).

64. S. M. McCann, V. Rettori, L. Milenkovič, J. Jurcovicova, and M. C. Gonzalez, *in* "Circulating Regulatory Factors and Neuroendocrine Function" (J. C. Porter and D. Jezova, eds.), Vol. 274, p. 315. Plenum, New York, 1990.

65. F. E. Yates and J. W. Maran, *in* "Handbook of Physiology" (R. O. Greep and E. B. Aswood, eds.), Sect. 7, Vol. 4, Part 2. Am. Physiol. Soc., Washington, DC, 1974.

66. G. W. Duff and S. K. Durum, *Yale J. Biol. Med.* **55,** 437 (1982).

67. I. Chowers, H. T. Hammel, J. Eisenman, R. M. Abrams, and S. M. McCann, *Am. J. Physiol.* **210,** 606 (1966).

68. C. Rivier and W. W. Vale, *Fed. Proc., Fed. Am. Soc. Exp. Biol.* **44,** 189 (1985).

69. N. Ono, J. Bedran de Castro, O. Khorram, and S. M. McCann, *Life Sci.* **36,** 1779 (1985).

70. M. O. Familari, A. I. Smith, R. Smith, and J. W. Funder, *Neuroendocrinology* **50,** 152 (1989).

71. S. M. McCann, M. D. Lumpkin, H. Mizunuma, O. Khorram, A. Ottlecz, and W. K. Samson, *Trends Neurosci.* **7,** 127 (1984).

72. W. K. Samson, M. D. Lumpkin, and S. M. McCann, *Endocrinology* (*Baltimore*) **119,** 554 (1986).

73. S. M. McCann, *in* "Neuroendocrinology" (C. B. Nemeroff, ed.), Chapter 1, p. 1. CRC Press, Boca Raton, FL, 1992.

74. M. D. Lumpkin, W. K. Samson, and S. M. McCann, *Science* **235,** 1070 (1987).

75. M. D. Lumpkin, J. K. McDonald, W. K. Sambo, and S. M. McCann, *Neuroendocrinology* **50,** 229 (1989).

76. W. H. Yu, R. P. Millar, S. C. F. Milton, R. C. de L. Milton, and S. M. McCann, *Brain Res. Bull.* **25,** 867 (1990).

77. J. M. Lipton, ed., "Fever." Raven Press, New York, 1980.

78. F. Berkenbosch, J. Van Oers, A. Del Rey, F. Tilders, and H. Besadovsky, *Science* **238,** 524 (1987).

79. C. Rivier and W. W. Vale, *Endocrinology* (*Baltimore*) **124,** 2105 (1989).

80. S. M. McCann, M. D. Lumpkin, and W. K. Samson, *in* "Neuroendocrinology of Vasopressin, Corticoliberin and Opiomelanocortins" (A. J. Baertschi and J. J. Dreifuss, eds.), p. 319. Academic Press, London, 1982.

81. B. Woloski, E. M. Smith, W. J. Meyer, G. M. Fuller, and J. E. Blalock, *Science* **230,** 1035 (1985).

82. A. Uehara, S. Gillis, and A. Arimura, *Neuroendocrinology* **45,** 343 (1987).

83. E. W. Bernton, J. Beach, J. W. Holaday, R. C. Smallridge, and H. G. Fein, *Science* **238,** 519 (1987).
84. V. Rettori, J. Jurcovicova, and S. M. McCann, *J. Neurosci.* **18,** 179 (1987).
85. V. Rettori, M. F. Gimeno, A. Karara, M. C. Gonzalez, and S. M. McCann, *Proc. Natl. Acad. Sci. U.S.A.* **88,** 2763 (1991).
86. P. S. Kalra, A. Sahu, and S. P. Kalra, *Endocrinology (Baltimore)* **126,** 2145 (1990).
87. V. Rettori, L. Mikenkovič, B. A. Beutler, and S. M. McCann, *Brain Res. Bull.* **23,** 471 (1989).
88. M. C. Gonzalez, M. Riedel, V. Rettori, W. H. Yu, and S. M. McCann, *Prog. NeuroEndocrinImmunol.* **3,** 49 (1990).
89. M. C. Gonzalez, M. C. Aguila, and S. M. McCann, *Prog. NeuroEndocrinImmunol.* **4,** 222 (1991).
90. K. Lyson and S. M. McCann, *Neuroendocrinology* **54,** 262 (1991).
91. K. Lyson and S. M. McCann, *Neuroendocrinology* **55,** 708 (1992).
92. J. R. Glyn and J. M. Lipton, *Peptides (N.Y.)* **2,** 177 (1981).
93. J. M. Lipson, *Yale J. Biol Med.* **63,** 173 (1990).
94. S. Karanth and S. M. McCann, submitted for publication (1993).
95. S. Karanth and S. M. McCann, submitted for publication (1993).
96. S. Karanth and S. M. McCann, submitted for publication (1993).
97. S. Karanth and S. M. McCann, *77th Annu. Meet. Endocr. Soc.,* Abstr. No. 1383, p. 397 (1992).
98. L. Milenkovič and S. M. McCann, *Neuroendocrinology* **55,** 14 (1992).
99. L. Milenkovič, K. Lyson, M. C. Aguila, and S. M. McCann, *Neuroendocrinology* **56,** 674 (1992).
100. T. Takao, D. E. Tracey, W. M. Mitchell, and E. B. DeSouza, *Endocrinology (Baltimore)* **127,** 3070 (1990).
101. E. Hetier, J. Ayala, and P. Denefle, *J. Neurosci. Res.* **21,** 391 (1988).
102. A. Fontana, P. W. McAdam, and F. Kristensen, *Eur. J. Immunol.* **13,** 685 (1983).
103. J. T. Stitt, *Yale J. Biol. Med.* **59,** 137 (1986).
104. G. Katsura, P. E. Gottschall, R. R. Dahl, and A. Arimura, *Endocrinology (Baltimore)* **122,** 1773 (1988).
105. J. I. Koenig, *Prog. NeuroEndocrinImmunol.* **4,** 143 (1991).
106. B. L. Spangelo and R. M. MacLeod, *Proc. 73rd Annu. Meet. Endocr. Soc.* (1991).
107. J. I. Koenig, K. Snow, B. D. Clark, R. Toni, J. G. Cannon, A. R. Shaw, C. A. Dinarello, S. Reichlin, S. L. Lee, and R. M. Lechan, *Endocrinology (Baltimore)* **126,** 3053 (1990).

[12] Determining Role and Sources of Endogenous Interleukin 1 in Pituitary–Adrenal Activation in Response to Stressful and Inflammatory Stimuli

Frank Berkenbosch,† Nico Van Rooijen,
and Fred J. H. Tilders

Introduction

Interleukin 1 (IL-1) is one of the accessory signals necessary for antigen-induced T cell proliferation (1) Interleukin 1 activates T cells by inducing IL-2 production and expression of IL-2 receptors by these cells. In addition to its immunological activity, IL-1 is considered to play a signaling role in various other components of the so-called acute-phase response. This integrated response is defined as a set of local and systemic reactions following infection and/or injury. Prominent and long-term changes in pituitary–adrenal activity are now recognized as an important component of the acute-phase reaction (2). This pituitary–adrenal response can be considered as an important regulatory reaction to prevent excessive proliferation of antigen-committed immune cells and in addition to maintain a high level of tolerance to self-antigens, in this way preventing the initiation of autoimmune responses (3). Although not all criteria have been met (Table I), the available observations indicate that IL-1 may be one of the prime signals involved in the activation of the pituitary–adrenal response to infection/injury. In this article, we discuss the currently available methods that are used to study the cellular sources of IL-1 and the role of IL-1 (and other cytokines) in pituitary–adrenal activation to inflammatory stimuli. Moreover, some of the methods discussed, in particular those involving passive immunization as well as methods to determine the secretory activity peptidergic neurons, can also be used to address other scientific questions in the area of neuroscience.

Determination of Circulating IL-1 Concentrations

Introduction

To date, a variety of different bioassays have been employed to measure IL-1 concentrations in biological fluids such as plasma or cerebrospinal fluid

† His colleagues and students will remember his spirit and contributions to the field. We all sorely miss Frank.

TABLE I   Criteria for Interleukins as Mediators
for Pituitary–Adrenal Responses
to Immune Challenges

Criterion 1
   The putative interleukin released should have some quantitative and temporal relationship to the magnitude and time
   course of the pituitary–adrenal response, respectively
Criterion 2
   Injection of the putative interleukin must result in pituitary–adrenal activation
Criterion 3
   Substances that block the production and/or action of the
   putative interleukin should prevent the pituitary–adrenal response

(4). Bioassays have the disadvantage of being laborious and difficult to stan-
dardize and in addition the specificity of these assays is a major point of
concern. For instance, several IL-1 inhibitors have been characterized and
purified from plasma (5) and one of these is an endogenous IL-1 receptor
antagonist that has been cloned (6) and that is cosecreted with IL-1. Therefore, it can be anticipated that bioassays do not provide an accurate determination of IL-1 responses in the circulation, but rather reflect the net effect
of IL-1 and its endogenous inhibitors. To avoid such problems related to the
use of bioassays, we have developed radioimmunoassays (RIAs) that allow
more accurate examination of conditions during which rat or human IL-1
may be present in plasma (7, 8) and tissues. Details of the development,
validation, and application of these RIAs will be described below.

Storage of Recombinant IL-1 Proteins

To obtain reliable assays, stability of recombinant IL-1 preparations must
be ascertained over long time intervals. Sterile Tris-HCl buffer (10 mM Tris-
HCl, pH 7.3) is suitable for long-term and stable storage of human or rat
recombinant IL-1β or IL-1α preparations. At 4°C, biological activity (*in vitro*
and *in vivo*) of these IL-1 preparations is maintained up to 3 months after
storage. Long-term stability (at least up to 3–4 years) with minimal loss of
bioactivity can be obtained by storage of the cytokines in the same buffer
at −70°C. Aliquots of IL-1 preparations (in concentrations as low as 100
ng/ml) should contain high-grade bovine serum albumin (BSA) (e.g., Boseral;
Organon, Oss, The Netherlands) to reduce nonspecific adsorption to storage tubes.

Radioiodination of IL-1β

We compared various methods to radioionidate rat recombinant IL-1β (gift from Dr. E. Kawashima, Glaxo, Geneva, Switzerland). Strong oxidizing methods such as the use of chloramine-T favor the formation of aggregates, which are evident in elution profiles of Sephadex G-75 gel filtrations. Less aggregation can be obtained by using milder techniques such as Iodogen (9), which indicates that the strength of the oxidating agent relates to the extent of polymeric aggregation. Nonoxidizing radioiodination, such as by the Bolton and Hunter technique (10), is also useful to label rat and also human recombinant IL-1β preparations with minimal protein aggregation. However, in our studies with the rat protein, specific activity was lower and more variable (~6 μCi/μg) than was obtained after Iodogen labeling (~23 μCi/μg). Therefore we recommend the use of Iodogen as the most reliable technique to label rat recombinant IL-1β. Briefly, Iodogen (1,3,4,6-tetrachloro-3α,6α-diphenylglycouril; Pierce Chemicals, Rockford, IL)-coated polyethylene conical tubes (e.g., Greiner, the Netherlands) containing 2.5–5 μg of rat recombinant IL-1β dissolved in 10 μl of 0.1 M Tris-HCl buffer (pH 7.3) are incubated for 15 min at room temperature with 1 mM NaI (10 μl of an NaOH solution, pH 7–11; Amersham, England). To separate the labeled IL-1β protein from free iodine, the labeling mixture is loaded on a Sephadex G-25 medium column (15 × 1.5 cm; volume, 13 ml; flow rate, 24 ml/hr; fraction volume, 0.4 ml) and eluted with a buffer consisting of 0.1 M Tris-HCl (pH 7.3) containing 0.1% gelatin or 0.02% high-grade BSA to prevent adherence of labeled IL-1β to the column. In view of interference of aggregates in the IL-1 assay, the activity collected in the void volume is further purified by gel filtration, using Sephadex G-50 gel filtration (65 × 1.5 cm; volume, 120 ml; flow rate, 12 ml/hr; fraction volume, 2 ml) with 0.1 M Tris-HCl (pH 7.3) containing 0.02% high-grade BSA as elution buffer. In this way, the labeled monomers can be separated from aggregates. Successful purification of monomeric labeled IL-1β can also be achieved by passing the Sephadex G-25 fractions over a Microsep microconcentrator (Filtron Technology Co., Northborough, MA) containing a low-protein polyethersulfone (PES) membrane with a molecular weight cut-off of 30,000. Figure 1 illustrates antibodybinding curves for Sephadex G-50 and Microsep filter-purified radiolabeled recombinant rat IL-1β. The advantage of the Microsep separation procedure lies in its higher recovery (90% vs 60%, using Sephadex G-50 gel filtration) and rapidity (4 vs 24 hr) but is more costly. Although we did not systematically compare radioionidation procedures for human recombinant IL-1β,the Iodogen procedure as described here for rat recombinant protein also results in human recombinant IL-1β preparations with high specific

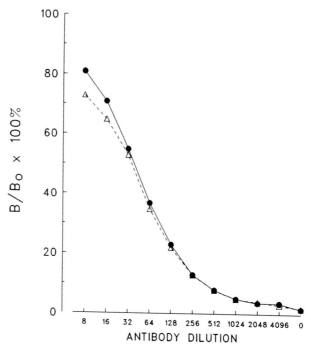

FIG. 1   Antibody dilution curves of Iodogen-labeled rat recombinant IL-1β purified by Sephadex G-50 gel filtration (△) or by Microsep microconcentrator (●) containing a low-protein polyethersulfone (PES) membrane with a molecular weight cut-off of 30,000. The antiserum used was raised to human recombinant IL-1β. This antiserum cross-reacts with rat recombinant IL-1β.

activity (approximately 100 μCi/μg) and minimal formation of aggregates.

Extraction

Although our developed RIAs did not suffer from plasma interference (Figs. 2 and 3), reliable protein detection utilizing RIAs usually requires extraction of plasma samples. Although the generally used extraction methods have not systematically been studied for IL-1 extraction, several reports indicate that chloroform extraction or polyethelene glycol precipitation results in high recovery and concentration of IL-1 proteins and in the additional removal of endogenous inhibitors in plasma (11, 12). Methods to extract IL-1 proteins from plasma by the use of glass particles such as activated Vycor (13), which

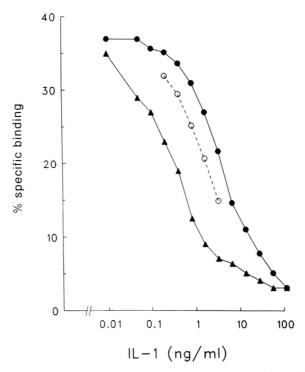

FIG. 2   Displacement of antiserum binding to labeled rat recombinant IL-1β by serial dilutions of recombinant preparations of IL-1β from different species (▲, human IL-1β; ●, rat IL-1β) or by serial dilutions of plasma (○) obtained from rats injected with endotoxin. The antiserum used was raised to human recombinant IL-1β.

has been used successfully for detection of a vast array of plasma proteins (14) that, like IL-1, show a high tendency to adhere to glass, have not been examined.

Standard Curves

Interleukin 1 standard displacement curves are generated by overnight incubation at 4°C with an IL-1 antiserum in an appropriate dilution (30–50% binding of the tracer) with serially diluted standard (recombinant IL-1β preparation) in assay buffer (PBS containing 0.1% Tween and 0.1% BSA or gelatin as carrier) or in heparinized rat plasma followed by another 24 hr of incubation after addition of tracer (10,000 cpm/tube). Separation of antibody-bound and free IL-1 can be achieved by a second antibody precipitation (Saccel; Well-

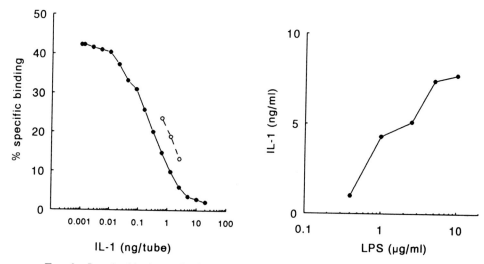

FIG. 3   Interleukin 1 standard curve (left) and dose-dependent IL-1 response curve of endotoxin (lipopolysaccharide, LPS) in whole human blood (right). The IL-1 standard curve (●) was constructed by determination of the extent of displacement of antiserum binding to radioiodinated human recombinant IL-1β by serial dilutions of unlabeled human recombinant IL-1β used as standard. Note that serial dilutions of plasma obtained from endotoxin-stimulated human blood (○) are parallel to that of IL-1β used as standard.

come Reagents, Beckenham, England) or by adding polyethylene glycol (20% solution in water). Figure 2 illustrates a typical standard displacement curve of our present rat IL-1β RIA.

Plasma Samples

Currently available IL-1 assays are too insensitive to detect circulating IL-1 in healthy animals or humans. In humans and animals, IL-1 plasma concentrations are below the 50-pg/ml level. Our findings that IL-1 can be detected after intravenous administration of rat recombinant IL-1β demonstrates the usefulness of the described assay to detect IL-1β in unextracted rat plasma (14a). The half-life of injected rat recombinant IL-1β was 5 min and the fictive distribution volume was 25 ml, indicating that the injected rat IL-1β distributes primarily over the blood and extracellular fluid compartments. Moreover, IL-1 is also induced in measurable quantities after injection of pyrogenic doses of endotoxin, also called bacterial lipopolysaccharide (LPS), in rats. From the displacement curves of serial dilution of plasma of endotoxin-treated rats (Fig. 2), it can be concluded that high levels of circulating concentrations of IL-1 can be detected by our assay as early as 90 min after endotoxin administration (Westphal 055.B5 preparation; Difco, Detroit, MI). Similar doses of endotoxin injected intraperitoneally are less effective to induce IL-1 in the circulation. It is worth noting that the preparations of endotoxin used should be defined in as detailed a manner as possible, because marked potency differences, using *Limulus,* exist between different LPS preparations. Furthermore, the potency *in vitro* appears to be a poor predictor for the adrenocorticotropic hormone (ACTH)-releasing activity *in vivo*. Endotoxin administration also leads to increases in circulation of IL-1 in humans (11), although responses are small due to restriction of the dosage of LPS. Because of the risks to induce shock by endotoxin administration to humans, it has been customary to analyze cytokine secretion from white blood cells *in vitro*. These cells are collected from human blood by the use of Ficoll or Percoll gradients, and the subsequent analysis of the cytokine responses is determined by incubating the isolated cells in microtiter plates for several hours after addition of endotoxin. As an alternative, we developed a whole-blood assay that avoids the unknown influences of Ficoll or Percoll and of culture media. Currently, we are studying this method for its usefulness as a diagnostic test for autoimmune disorders. Blood samples of 4.5 ml are drawn into ethylenediaminetetraacetic acid (EDTA)-coated glass vacutainer tubes (Becton-Dickinson, England). Under sterile conditions, 100 μl of a 2500-U solution of trasylol (aprotinin; Bayer, Leverkussen, Germany) diluted in PBS and increasing concentrations of endotoxin [Westphal 055.B5 (Difco); range, 0–50 μg/100 μl sterile PBS] are added. After a 24-hr incubation at 37°C, the vacutainer tubes are centrifuged (10 min, 1000 g). The supernatants are recentrifuged (5 min, 17,000 g) to eliminate cellular debris and blood cells. The supernatant is aliquoted and stored at -20°C until assayed for cytokines. Figure 3 (left) shows a typical standard displacement curve and serial dilution curve of human plasma obtained from blood treated with endotoxin; Fig. 3 (right) also shows a typical dose-dependent IL-1 response curve to endotoxin. The interassay and intraassay variation of the IL-1 responses is less than 8%.

Liposome-Mediated Macrophage Suicide Technique to Examine Role of Macrophages in Endotoxin-Induced Responses

Introduction

We examined the mediating role of macrophages in the pituitary–adrenal (8) and thermogenic response (14b) to endotoxin treatment in rats, using the liposome-mediated macrophage suicide technique. Moreover, the use of this technique led us to conclude that circulating IL-1 concentrations in rats

A

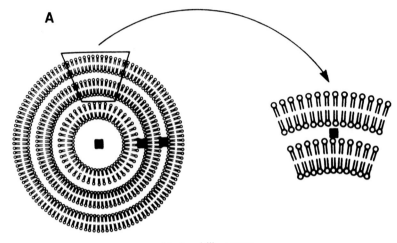

�␣ = Hydrophilic group
ᐈ = Hydrophobic fatty acid chains

$$\blacksquare \; = \quad \begin{array}{ccc} OH & Cl & OH \\ | & | & | \\ O=P\!-\!\!\!\!&C\!-\!\!\!\!&P=O \\ | & | & | \\ OH & Cl & OH \end{array}$$

B

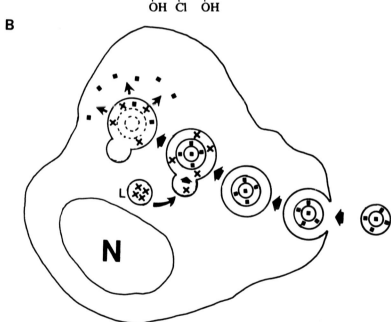

originate largely from cells of macrophage lineage (8). This liposome-mediated macrophage suicide technique involves specific liposome-mediated delivery of dichloromethylene diphosphonate (Cl_2MDP) to phagocytic cells (15). Cl_2MDP belongs to a new class of drugs developed for treatment of diseases of bone and calcium metabolism (16); it has a short half-life *in vivo* and will not be ingested by phagocytic cells per se. However, taking advantage of the natural fate of liposomes (i.e., their phagocytosis in particular by cells of the macrophage lineage), liposome-encapsulated Cl_2MDP targets Cl_2MDP to the interior of such cells (Fig. 4). Once ingested, the liposomes fuse with primary lysosomes, in which the phospholipid bilayers are disrupted by phospholipases, leading to release of the toxic Cl_2DMP in the cell. By administration of liposome-encapsulated Cl_2MDP via the appropriate routes, elimination of macrophages can be obtained in spleen, liver, lung, and lymph nodes. Repopulation of lymphoid organs by new macrophages originating from stem cells in the bone marrow occurs from day 7 after liposome-Cl_2MDP treatment. The efficacy of the elimination can be assessed by histochemical and immunocytochemical or ultrastructural techniques or by functional assays such as the capacity of macrophages to ingest carbon or latex particles. The selectivity of the technique has been demonstrated by observations showing that T and B cells as well as neutrophils and mast cells are not affected after injection of Cl_2MDP (8, 17).

Preparation of Cl_2MDP Liposomes

To prepare liposomes, 86 mg of phosphatidylcholine and 8 mg of cholesterol (molar ratio 6 : 1, Sigma Chemical Co., St. Louis, MO) are dissolved in 20 ml of methanol-chloroform (1 : 1) in a round-bottom flask. The thin film that forms on the interior of the flask after low-vacuum rotary evaporation at 27°C in 10 ml of phosphate-buffered saline (PBS) (10 mM; pH 7.4) containing 2.7 g of Cl_2MDP (a kind gift of Boehringer, Mannheim, Germany) is dispersed by gentle rotation for 10 min. The free Cl_2MDP is removed by rinsing with PBS, followed by centrifugation for 30 min at 100,000 g at 16°C. Subse-

---

FIG. 4   (A) Liposomes consist of concentric layers of phospholipids separated by aqueous compartments. The aqueous solution together with hydrophilic molecules such as Cl_2MDP (black squares) will be encapsulated during the formation of liposomes. (B) Liposomes with entrapped Cl_2MDP (squares) are ingested by macrophages. The ingested liposomes fuse with lysosomes (L) containing phospholipases (crosses). The drug Cl_2MDP is released in the cell after disruption of the bilayers of the liposomes by phospholipases.

quently, the liposomes are resuspended in 4 ml of PBS and can be stored at 4°C for up to 1 week.

Administration of Cl₂MDP

Table II shows a summary of the presence of macrophages in different organs after administration of liposome-encapsulated Cl_2MDP along various routes. For intravenous use, effective injection volumes of the liposome-encapsulated Cl_2MDP are approximately 2 ml for rats and 0.2 ml for mice. The optimum time intervals after Cl_2MDP-liposome treatment are discussed in detail elsewhere (18).

Cytochemical Identification of Macrophages

Histochemical identification of macrophages can be performed on paraformaldehyde- or acetone-fixed sections of tissues such as liver, spleen, and lymph nodes, or on cytospin preparations of peritoneal lavage by the use of acid phosphatase histochemistry (19). In addition, macrophages can be identified immunocytochemically by using monoclonal antibodies to rat surface antigens of macrophages as described in detail elsewhere (8, 19).

Methods to Assess Role and Sources of IL-1

Introduction

As indicated in the general introduction, the second criterion to be fullfilled to ascertain a physiological role of IL-1 in the pituitary–adrenal response is that injection of purified or recombinant IL-1 must result in pituitary–adrenal activation (Table I). Indeed, there is consensus that pituitary–adrenal activation is induced by peripheral or central administration of recombinant IL-1 preparations (2). However, it is conceivable that the physiological role of IL-1 (as with every other peptide or protein) is only demonstrated by studying the effects of blockade of the endogenously produced IL-1 in response to an inflammatory stimulus (criterion 3, Table I). In contrast to the relative ease by which the biological effect of IL-1 can be studied in the pituitary–adrenal system, studies to block the action of endogenously produced IL-1 during the pituitary–adrenal response to an inflammatory stimulus (e.g., endotoxin) are complicated or hampered by the lack of appropriate tools. An IL-1 receptor antagonist (IL-1RA) has been purified, characterized, and cloned

TABLE II Presence of Macrophage Populations in Different Organs after Administration of Liposome-Encapsulated Cl$_2$MDP along Various Routes[a]

Administration route of liposomes	Presence of macrophage populations[b]						
	Splenic macrophages	Kupffer cells in liver	Lymph node macrophages[c]	Alveolar macrophages in lung	Testis macrophages	Synovial macrophages[d]	Peritoneal macrophages
Intravenous	−	−	+	+	+	+	+
Intraperitoneal	−	−	+	+	+	+	−
Subcutaneous	+	+	−	+	+	+	+
Intratracheal	+	+	+	−	+	+	+
Local in testis	+	+	+	+	−	+	+
Intraarticular[d]	+	+	+	+	+	−	+

[a] See relevant references for optimum time intervals after treatment.
[b] +, Macrophages present in normal numbers; −, macrophages completely depleted or present in strongly reduced numbers.
[c] Popliteal lymph nodes.
[d] In knee joint.
[e] In footpad.

(6). The IL-1RA, which is coproduced with IL-1 in cells of the macrophage lineage, binds to both type I and type II IL-1 receptors and exerts no known physiological actions other than blocking receptor activation by IL-1α or IL-1β. This antagonist may represent a major tool for physiological studies and should therefore become easily accessible to researchers. In a limited number of studies, the IL-1RA has been used to establish the role of IL-1 in a variety of acute-phase responses, including changes in pituitary–adrenal activity in response to inflammatory stimuli. The data show that most of the effects of IL-1 can be blocked by the IL-1RA but the biological potency *in vivo* of the IL-1RA is at least 500–1000 times less than that for IL-1, limiting its use on a larger scale.

Another approach to study the physiological role of IL-1 (and other cytokines) is the use of passive immunization paradigms with antibodies that interfere with signal transfer of IL-1 either by binding to IL-1 or by occupying the receptors for IL-1. Immunoneutralization is widely used to study the physiological role of a variety of different proteins in biological functions. Concerning *in vivo* immunoneutralization studies, major conclusions are drawn from positive or negative findings of these studies, while surprisingly little is known about the mechanisms of action of biological active antibodies and their required physicochemical characteristics. Some years ago, we developed monoclonal antibodies to corticotropin-releasing factor (CRF) (20–22), and currently we are raising antibodies to rat IL-1β. The methods involved and the specific requirements for the antibodies to allow conclusions in passive immunization studies will be discussed.

Requirements and Methods in Passive Immunoneutralization Studies

In passive immunization or immunoneutralization experiments, antibodies are considered to bind to a specific biologically active compound and thereby prevent its action on target tissue. However, it is general experience that not all antibodies that bind to a given protein/peptide do in fact block its biological activity. In fact, the binding epitope, even for small peptides, appears to be an important factor determining the biological activity of a given antibody, as we have discussed earlier (22). Thus, before using a particular antiserum to study an unknown role of a peptide, the antiserum should be demonstrated to be biologically active with respect to an established effect. Obviously, data on the intrinsic biological activity of antibody–antigen complex derived from appropriate bioassay systems are of the utmost importance for the interpretation of the results obtained with passive immunization (Fig. 5). If we assume that the liquid-phase interaction with the antibody and the peptide is crucial for the observed biological effects of antibodies *in vivo,* it seems logical to study antibody-binding characteristics under conditions closely mimicking the situation *in vivo.* Another factor relevant to the biological activity of an immunoglobulin is its association constant (K_a). A first approximation of the necessary local antibody concentration to bind a given percentage of the peptide can be described as $K_d = AB/C$, where A is the molar concentration of free antigen, B is the molar concentration of the free antibody, C is the molar concentration of the complex, and K_d (reciprocal of K_a or association constant) is the dissociation constant of the antibody (molar concentrations). Under conditions in which the antibody concentration is considerably higher than the antigen concentration, which represents the situation in most passive immunization studies, the ratio of free (A) over bound (C) antigen, will be primarily dependent on the antibody concentration (B) and the K_d. Thus, by increasing the antibody concentration, the ratio of free/bound antigen declines proportionally. For instance, if we aim to bind 99% of the antigen, such experiments require antibody concentrations in the compartment involved in signal transfer that are approximately 100 times higher than the K_d. Under the assumption that radioiodination of the peptide does not interfere with the characteristics of antibody binding, several methods can be used to determine the K_d value of an antibody. These include Scatchard analysis of the RIA data (20, 23, 24). In addition, analysis of antiserum dilution curves can be used (25, 26), in which half-maximal antigen binding is obtained at antibody concentrations that equal the K_d. For both analyses, the concentrations of the specific antibodies are required. Analysis of antibody saturation curves (27) or Scatchard analysis of RIA data (20, 23) gives the concentrations of binding sites of an antibody preparation. Assuming that under saturation conditions most of the complexes have the A_2B configuration, the antibody concentration equals half the concentration of the binding sites. Alternatively, the concentration of specific antibodies can be determined by means of a specific sandwich enzyme-linked immunosorbent assay (ELISA) (Schotanus *et al.,* in preparation) or by antibody purification and protein determination (21).

Another relevant parameter for the biological activity of an antiserum is its binding kinetics. It is worth noting that equilibrium conditions are usually not relevant, because binding should occur within a limited time interval between secretion and receptor interaction of the ligand. For instance, the time that a neuropeptide such as CRF needs to reach receptors in the pituitary gland after its secretion can be approximately 3–5 sec (20). Thus it seems not sufficient that an antibody can bind a relevant proportion of the peptide, but it should do this within an extremely short interval. The association constant is a parameter that reflects the ratio between the on-rate constant and the off-rate constant of the binding. The higher the on-rate constant, the lower the antibody concentration required to bind a certain percentage of

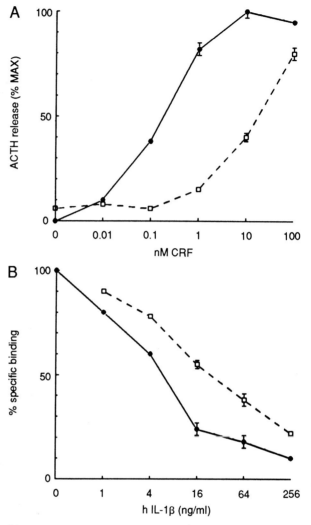

FIG. 5 Two bioassays to test the intrinsic biological activity of antibody–antigen complexes. (A) Effect of the CRF monoclonal antibody PFU 83 (1 μM) on ACTH release from cultured rat anterior pituitary cells in response to rat/human CRF. ACTH release is expressed as a percentage of maximal ACTH release (% MAX). To study the capacity of PFU 83 to block the bioactivity of CRF, culture supernatant was incubated with various concentrations of CRF for 1 hr before addition to the pituitary cells. The primary anterior pituitary cells were cultured as described else-where (21). ●, CRF; □, CRF after incubation with PFU 83. (B) Effect of rat IL-1β monoclonal antibody (SILK 3) on the binding of radioiodinated rat recombinant IL-1β to IL-1 receptors on EL4 cells. To study the capacity of SILK 3 to block

the peptide in a given time, as we have illustrated with the CRF monoclonal PFU 83 (20). We developed a method to determine the on-rate constant of antibody binding (20). Briefly, antiserum or control IgG (diluted in rat plasma; final volume, 75 μl) is added to the relevant radioiodinated peptide (50,000 cpm in 50 μl of rat plasma), mixed, and incubated at 37°C. After various time intervals (5–60 sec), 1.5 ml of cold (-20°C) methanol (96%) is added, mixed, and centrifuged for 15 sec at 10,000 g, and the supernatants are aspirated immediately. Nonspecific binding is measured by the addition of methanol followed by antibody to test tubes containing radioiodinated peptide. Nonspecific binding is less than 7% and tracer binding to control IgG is less than 6%.

Methods to Determine Mechanism of Action of IL-1 and Other Stressful Stimuli

Introduction

One of the important arguments indicating that IL-1 increases pituitary–adrenal activity via CRF release from the hypothalamus is based on the observation that IL-1 increases the turnover of CRF in the median eminence (28), the site from which CRF is released into the hypothalamic portal vessels. In general, current methods to determine the activity and secretory activity of neuropeptidergic neurons are based on measurements of indirect parameters such as the level of mRNA encoding neuropeptides or the level of expression of the oncogene c-*fos* in neuropeptidergic neurons or the levels of neuropeptides in the cerebrospinal fluid. The widely used technique to study the secretory activity of hypohysiotrophic neurons, that is, neuropeptide concentration measurements in portal blood draining from the median eminence to pituitary gland, suffers from the limitation of major surgery and the use of anesthetics (29). Over the last few years we have developed a novel and useful approach that utilizes the rate of peptide decline after axonal transport

---

binding of rat IL-1β to EL4 cells, different dilutions of ammonium sulfate-precipitated hybridoma culture supernatant were added together with labeled IL-1β (30,000 cpm) to the EL4 cells (1 million cells/tube) and incubated for 4 hr at 4°C. After centrifugation (1000 g, 10 min) cells were washed with PBS containing 0.01% Triton X-100. Tubes were recentrifuged and pellets were counted. ●, Diplacement of binding with dilutions of unlabeled rat recombinant IL-1β; □, dispacement of binding with dilutions of the IL-1β monoclonal antibody SILK 3.

blockade to assess turnover rates of neuropeptides in the brain. Several studies have been published demonstrating the value of this approach to quantify the secretory activity of CRF and vassopressin (AVP) neurons in the hypothalamus (28, 30–32). Although the peptide content can easily be determined by neurochemical techniques, the use of quantitative immunocytochemistry has greatly facilitated the resolution of this approach, potentially allowing the determination of changes in secretory activity of peptidergic neurons at the cellular level.

Peptide Turnover

The approach to determine peptide turnover is reminiscent of that developed many years ago to determine turnover of monoamines in monoaminergic neurons. The latter involved measurements of the decline of monoamine stores after pharmacological blockade of monoamine synthesis. In contrast to monoaminergic neurons, in which synthesis occurs in nerve terminals, the terminals of peptidergic neurons have stores of neuropeptides that reflect a dynamic equilibrium between release of neuropeptide and supply of newly synthesized neuropeptide from the cell body. This last process involves mRNA translation mechanisms, enzymatic cleavage, and fast axonal transport (33). Accordingly, we have demonstrated that the rate of decline of CRF and AVP in the median eminence after axonal transport blockade by a minimal nontoxic dose of colchicine that still blocks axonal transport (34) is a reflection of the secretory activity of these neurons (28, 30–32). To block axonal transport, rats receive an intracisternal injection of 5 μg of colchicine dissolved in 10 μl of saline into the cisterna magna under light ether anesthesia. Control rats receive only intracisternal injection of saline. For intracisternal injections, rats are fixed by the use of ear bars in a horizontal position, with the trunk in a vertical position. After a small incision in the skin at the level of the foramen magnum, intracisternal injections are made with a bladded needle (free length, 6 mm). At this non-toxic dose, no colchicine-induced change in pituitary or adrenal activity and no time-dependent change in CRF or AVP concentration in the median eminence are observed for up to 6 hr (31). Accordingly, the depletion rate of CRF or AVP from the median eminence will reflect secretion rates, if blockade of axonal transport does not interefere with the neural activity. To determine the stimulus-induced secretion rate of neuropeptides, groups of colchicine-treated rats are exposed to a stimulus (e.g., injection of IL-1 or insulin, or hemorrhage) and decapitated at various time intervals thereafter. Although processing of the tissue for quantitative immunocytochemistry is most appropriate for studying the depletion rate of CRF and AVP in the median eminence, immunoassays can be used to determine changes in concentrations of the neuropeptides in other brain regions. Changes in the peptide content in colchicine-treated rats can be expressed as the depletion rate (turnover) over different time domains, describing the time dependency of changes in secretory activity of neuropeptidergic neurons under study (Fig. 6).

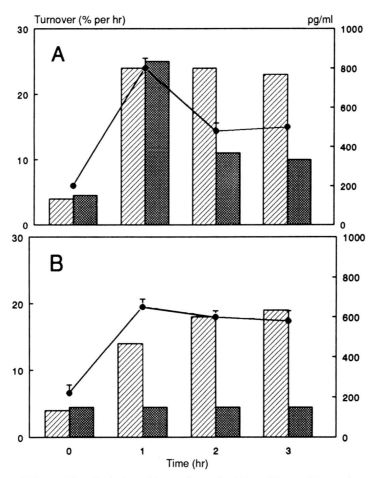

FIG. 6   Effect of insulin-induced hypoglycemia (A) or IL-1β (B) on the turnover (depletion rate) of CRF (striped bars) and AVP (black bars) in the external zone of the median eminence of rats. Bars represent average turnover as computed from the differences in peptide content of groups of colchicine-treated rats sacrificed 1, 2, and 3 hr after administration of insulin or IL-1β. Plasma ACTH concentrations (line) were measured in trunk blood of the same rats. Note the dissociation of CRF and AVP turnover in response to IL-1β.

Quantitative Immunocytochemistry

Detailed studies in various biological models have demonstrated a linear relationship between peptide concentration and immunostaining intensity (31, 35, 36). The advantage of quantitative immunocytochemistry over neurochemical techniques is the potential for determining changes in peptide content in specific brain structures that are too small to dissect for microanalysis (e.g., AVP systems in the zona interna and zona externa of the median eminence) (31). For quantitative evaluation of immunostaining intensities in biological preparations, care must be taken in standardizing (1) the fixation procedure, (2) the immunocytochemical procedures, and (3) the instrumental conditions of the quantitative analysis. For reasons of standardization, we prefer to use immersion fixation rather than perfusion fixation of biological tissues. Variation in thickness of cryostat sections can be limited by the use of an electrically driven cryostat (Dittes, Heidelberg, Germany). Incubation of sections should be performed under standardized conditions (with respect to incubation time, antibody dilution, wash procedures, etc.) and all sections of one experiment should be treated simultaneously. In our laboratory, we have successfully used the following protocol: brain tissues are immersed for 2 hr in 10 ml of an ice-cold solution containing the appropriate fixative. After fixation the tissues are rinsed in 5% sucrose dissolved in sodium phosphate or Tris-HCl buffer (pH 7.4) for 18 hr at 4°C. For quantification, tissue sections of up to 25 animals are embedded together in a cryomold containing OCT compound. Cryostat sections are mounted on object slides coated with gelatin/chrom alum and processed for immunocytochemistry. Briefly, tissue sections are incubated with primary antisera in PBS or Tris-HCl buffer containing 0.3% Triton X-100 (v/v) at 4°C in a humid atmosphere. After rinsing, the sections are incubated with fluorescein isothiocyanate (FITC)-conjugated second antibodies binding to the primary antibodies in buffer for 1 hr at room temperature. After rinsing, sections are embedded in a solution of buffer and glycerol (3 : 1) and stored at 4°C.

Although quantitative analysis of immunostaining intensity of signals obtained after the peroxidase–anti-peroxidase technique can be performed as well, we prefer quantitative determination of fluorescence intensities because measurements in biological and nonbiological models with different types of fluorimeters have generated the most reliable data with respect to neuropeptide concentrations (28–32, 35, 36). In addition to static microfluorometry, which is used in most of our studies, scanning microfluorometry can be used for quantitative evaluation of changes in neuronal networks (cf. Ref. 37). Figure 7 shows a simplified scheme of a static fluorimeter. For orientation and selection of the object, low-intensity violet light is used to prevent photodecomposition of the fluorophores. Measurement of short duration

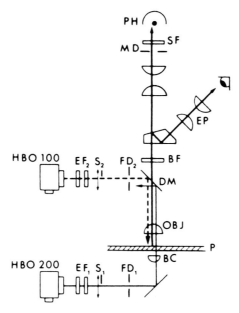

FIG. 7   Diagram of a static microfluorimeter (MPV II; Leitz). HBO 100 and HBO 200, high-pressure mercury lamps; EF_1 and EF_2, excitation filters (two Sp425, 2 mm BG3, 1 mm LP 395); S_1 and S2, electrically controlled shutters; FD_1 and FD_2, field diaphragms; DM, dichroic mirror (TK 455); OBJ, objective; P, preparation; BC, bright-field condensor; BF, barrier filter (LP 455); EP, eye piece; MD, measuring diaphragm; SF, selection filter; PH, photomultiplier tube.

(approximately 1 sec via electrically controlled shutters) are performed under conditions that give optimal image contrast between the fluorescence and background (nonspecific fluorescence). Static microfluorometry is limited because objects under study must be selected by the operator and must be manipulated by hand into the measuring field. It is therefore conceivable that, to facilitate unbiased and random sampling, coded preparations should always be used. Microfluorometry using a static microfluorimeter can be performed only on relatively large areas comprising numerous nerve terminals (CRF or AVP in the median eminence). For measurements at the level of individual varicosities scanning microfluorimeters should be used.

In summary, quantitative immunocytochemistry is a valuable tool for the measurement of experimentally induced changes in neuropeptide stores in cell bodies, terminals, and networks. In addition, the technique can be used to determine changes in concentrations of monoamines and second messengers in tissue sections (35, 37, 38).

Acknowledgments

We thank Dr. E. Kawashima (Glaxo, Geneva, Switzerland) and Dr. J. McKearn (Montsano, St. Louis, MO) for the generous gifts of recombinant IL-1β preparations and corresponding antisera, H. Nordsiek for reproducing the figures, and the Royal Dutch Academy of Sciences for financial support.

References

1. J. J. Oppenheim, E. J. Kovacs, K. Matsushima, and S. K. Durum, *Immunol. Today* **7,** 45 (1986).
2. F. Berkenbosch, R. H. Derijk, A. Del Rey, and H. O. Besedovsky, *Adv. Exp. Med. Biol.* **274,** 303 (1990).
3. R. H. Derijk and F. Berkenbosch, *Int. J. Neurosci.* **59,** 91 (1991).
4. L. Remvig, J. Vibe-Peterson, M. Svenson, C. Enk, and K. Bendtzen, *Allergy* **46,** 59 (1991).
5. J. W. Larrick, *Immunol. Today* **10,** 61 (1989).
6. S. P. Eisenberg, R. J. Evans, W. P. Arend, E. Verderber, T. Brewer, C. H. Hannum, and R. C. Thompson, *Nature (London)* **343,** 341 (1990).
7. F. Berkenbosch, D. A. W. Wolvers, and R. H. Derijk, *J. Steroid Biochem. Mol. Biol.* **4,** 639 (1991).
8. R. H. Derijk, N. Van Rooijen, F. J. H. Tilders, H. O. Besedovsky, A. Del Rey, and F. Berkenbosch, *Endocrinology (Baltimore)* **129,** 330 (1991).
9. P. Salacinski, J. Hope, C. McLean, V. Clement-Jones, J. Sykes, J. Price, and P. J. Lowry, *J. Endocrinol.* **81,** 131P (1979).
10. A. E. Bolton and W. M. Hunter, *Biochem. J.* **133,** 529 (1973).
11. J. G. Cannon, J. W. M. Van der Meer, S. Endres, G. Lonnemann, and C. A. Dinarello, *Leukocyte Biol.* **8,** 373 (1988).
12. S. J. Hopkins and M. Humphreys, *J. Immunol. Methods* **133,** 127 (1990).
13. J. G. Ratcliffe and C. R. W. Edwards, *in* ''Radioimmunoassay Methods'' (K. E. Kirkham and W. M. Hunter, eds.), p. 502. Churchill-Livingstone, Edinburgh, 1971.
14. F. Berkenbosch, I. Vermes, and F. J. H. Tilders, *Endocrinology (Baltimore)* **115,** 1015 (1984).
14a. R. H. Derijk and F. Berkenbosch, *Am. J. Physiol.* **263,** 1092 (1992).
14b. R. H. Derijk, P. J. L. M. Strijbos, N. Van Rooijen, N. J. Rothwell, and F. Berkenbosch, *Am. J. Physiol.* (in press) (1993).
15. N. Van Rooijen, *Res. Immunol.* **143,** 215 (1992).
16. H. Fleisch, *Handb. Exp. Pharmacol.* **83,** 441 (1988).
17. I. Claassen, N. Van Rooijen, and E. Claassen, *J. Immunol. Methods* **134,** 153 (1990).
18. N. Van Rooijen, *Res. Immunol.* **143,** 177 (1992).
19. C. D. Dijkstra, E. A. Dopp, P. Joling, and G. Kraal, *Immunology* **54,** 589 (1985).
20. J. W. A. M. Van Oers and F. J. H. Tilders, *Endocrinology (Baltimore)* **128,** 496 (1991).

21. J. W. A. M. Van Oers, F. J. H. Tilders, and F. Berkenbosch, *Endocrinology (Baltimore)* **124,** 1239 (1989).
22. F. J. H. Tilders, J. W. A. M. Van Oers, A. White, F. Menzaghi, and A. Burlet, "Circulating Regulatory Factors and Neuroendocrine Function" (J. C. Porter and D. Jezova, eds.), p. 135. Plenum Press, New York, 1990.
23. G. Scatchard, *Ann. N.Y. Acad. Sci.* **51,** 660 (1949).
24. C. P. Barsano and G. Baumann, *Endocrinology (Baltimore)* **124,** 1101 (1989).
25. J. E. Roulston, *J. Immunol. Methods* **63,** 133 (1983).
26. V. Van Heyningen, D. J. H. Brock, and S. Van Heyningen, *J. Immunol. Methods* **62,** 147 (1983).
27. R. S. Farr, *in* "Methods in Immunology and Immunochemistry" (C. A. William and M. W. Chase, eds.), p. 66. Academic Press, New York, 1971.
28. F. Berkenbosch, J. van Oers, A. Del Rey, F. Tilders, and H. Besedovsky, *Science* **238,** 524 (1987).
29. D. M. Gibbs, *Fed. Proc., Fed. Am. Soc. Exp. Biol.* **44,** 203 (1985).
30. F. Berkenbosch, D. C. E. de Goey, A. Del Rey, and H. O. Besedovsky, *Neuroendocrinology* **50,** 570 (1989).
31. F. Berkenbosch, D. C. E. De Goeij, and F. J. H. Tilders, *Endocrinology (Baltimore)* **125,** 28 (1989).
32. F. Berkenbosch and F. J. H. Tilders, *Brain Res.* **442,** 312 (1988).
33. H. Gainer, Y. Peng Loh, and Y. Saine, "Peptides in Neurobiology" (H. Gainer, ed.), p. 271. Plenum, New York, 1977.
34. D. C. Parish, E. M. Rodriquez, S. D. Birkett, and B. T. Pickering, *Cell Tissue Res.* **220,** 809 (1981).
35. F. Berkenbosch, J. De Vente, J. Schipper, and H. W. M. Steinbusch, "Monoaminergic Neurons: Lightmicroscopy and Ultrastructure" (H. W. M. Steinbusch, ed.), p. 167. Wiley, London, 1987.
36. F. Berkenbosch, E. A. Linton, and F. J. H. Tilders, *Neuroendocrinology* **44,** 338 (1986).
37. J. Schipper and F. J. H. Tilders, *Brain Res. Bull.* **9,** 69 (1982).
38. J. de Vente, J. Garssen, F. J. H. Tilders, H. W. M. Steinbusch, and J. Schipper, *Brain Res.* **411,** 120 (1987).

[13] *In Vivo* and *in Vitro* Methods for Studying Effects of Cytokines on Adrenocorticotropic Hormone, Arginine Vasopressin, and Oxytocin Secretion

Junichi Fukata, Hajime Segawa, Yoshiyuki Naito, Norihiko Murakami, Hiromasa Kobayashi, Osamu Ebisui, Takeshi Usui, and Hiroo Imura

Introduction

It has been recognized that cytokines, which were originally isolated from lymphocytes and monocytes and identified as immunomediators, have a broad spectrum of actions as factors involved in various kinds of cell-to-cell communication. Among the cytokines identified so far, interleukin 1α (IL-1α), IL-1β, IL-6, tumor necrosis factor α (TNF-α), and interferons have been reported to be major cytokines induced during the early inflammatory processes and affecting various neuroendocrine functions, especially stimulation of activities in the hypothalamic–pituitary–adrenal (HPA) axis. These cytokines are, therefore, presumed to be mediators of acute-phase responses to infectious challenge (1). There have been, however, considerable controversies among researchers, particularly with respect to the mechanisms of action of cytokines in neuroendocrine modulations. Some of the discrepancies are possibly due to differences in the methodologies employed in the experiments. In *in vivo* experiments, a cascade of events induced by cytokines must be carefully considered, because neuroendocrine functions may be modified as a second effect. For example, blood osmolarity, blood volume, and blood pressure, which may change after cytokine challenge, can influence secretion of arginine vasopressin (AVP) and possibly oxytocin (OT). Data acquired by *in vitro* (artificial) systems should also be assessed carefully as to their physiological significance. The purpose of this article, therefore, is to describe *in vivo* and *in vitro* systems that have been used in the study of the effects of several cytokines on pituitary hormone secretion, especially that of adrenocorticotropic hormone (ACTH), AVP, and OT, and also to present some data obtained using these methods as examples.

Methods in Neurosciences, Volume 16

Cytokines

Recombinant human interleukin 1α (rhIL-1α), rhIL-1β, recombinant rat interleukin 1α (rrIL-1α), rrIL-1β, and rhIL-2 were obtained from Otsuka Pharmaceutical Co., Ltd. (Tokushima, Japan). The rat IL-2 used is a product of Collaborative Research, Inc. (Bedford, MA) purified from concanavalin A-stimulated rat splenocyte culture. Recombinant human IL-6 was donated by T. Kishimoto and T. Hirano (Osaka University, Japan) and by Ajinomoto Co., Ltd. (Tokyo). Recombinant human tumor necrosis factor α (rhTNF-α), rhIL-4, rhIL-5, and rhIL-8 were gifts from Dainippon Pharmaceutical Co., Ltd. (Osaka), Ono Pharmaceutical Co., Ltd. (Osaka), Suntory, Ltd. (Osaka), and Sandoz-Forshungs Institute (Wien, Austria), respectively.

Assessment of Effects of Cytokines on Pituitary Hormone Secretion in Vivo

Animals

Rat
Adult male rats of the Wistar strain, weighing 300–350 g, are used in all the experiments. The rats are housed in an environmentally controlled room under controlled temperature conditions ($25 \pm 1°C$) on a 12-hr light, 12-hr dark cycle (lights on at 0800 hr). Laboratory chow and water are provided *ad libitum*. Several days before blood sampling, the rats are anesthetized with pentobarbital and implanted with a chronic intraatrial silastic cannula through the jugular vein. The other end of the cannula is passed underneath the skin of the neck and secured to the skull with screws and acryl cement, and then filled with heparin. After the operation, the rats are allowed to recover in individual housing cages. On the day before blood sampling, each cannulated rat is placed in a specially designed sampling box, and its venous cannula is connected to a plastic syringe via a polyethylene tube leading to the outside of the box through a stainless steel spring attached to the top of the box. Under these conditions, the rats are otherwise unrestricted and have free access to laboratory chow and water during the experimental period.

On the morning of the experiment, blood samples (0.6 ml for ACTH and 0.6 ml or less for AVP or OT determination; one sample per hormone assay) are withdrawn into heparinized syringes through the venous cannula before (-15 and 0 min) and 15, 30, 60, and 120 min after the injection of cytokines, which are usually diluted in 0.5 ml or less of 0.9% saline containing 0.1% bovine serum albumin, or vehicle through the same intraatrial cannula. Blood samples are immediately cooled on ice and centrifuged, and the separated plasma samples are stored at $-20°C$ until hormone extraction. The red blood cells are suspended in normal saline and returned to the rat after each sampling.

In addition to measuring the hormone levels in the blood, several indices possibly related to the cytokine-induced neuroendocrine changes are evaluated in a separate group of rats. To assess the pyrogenic activity of cytokines, we administer the peptides to be tested either intravenously (iv) or intraperitoneally (ip) and measure the change in rectal temperature with an electronic thermometer (model CTM-303; Terumo Co., Tokyo) (2). Plasma osmolarity is also monitored during the sampling period by measuring the freezing point with an osmometer (model OM-801; Vogel GMBH, Giessen, Germany), using serum specimens. Arterial blood pressure is measured via a PE-50 polyethylene catheter, which is placed in the abdominal aorta through the femoral artery and connected to the pressure transducer under pentobarbital anesthesia or in an unanesthetized condition.

Rabbit

New Zealand White rabbits, weighing 2.5–3.0 kg, are used for the experiment. To obtain plasma samples from unrestrained, freely moving rabbits, the intraatrial cannula is inserted as in the rat model described above. The surgery, however, must be carried out more carefully than in rats. First, a diluted pentobarbital solution (1% in normal saline), which is used to avoid local phlebitis, is injected into an ear vein at the initial dose of 2 ml/kg. An appropriate depth of anesthesia can be maintained with supplemental anesthetic (0.4 ml/kg) every 30–40 min. Sterile conditions should be carefully maintained during the operation. After the skin on the right lateral neck and head is shaved and disinfected, a small incision is made in the skin, and sterile silastic tubing (medical grade, 0.025-in. and 0.060-in. o.d.; Dow Corning Corp., Midland, MI) is inserted via the exposed external jugular vein into the right atrium. After backflow of blood is confirmed, the catheter is secured in the right position and the skin is sutured back together. The other end of the catheter, which is passed underneath the skin of the neck, is advanced via a small incision in the disinfected skin on the skull, and is secured to the skull with screws and acryl cement. The cannula is then filled with heparin. After surgery, appropriate antibiotics should be administered for at least 3 days.

To continuously obtain cerebrospinal fluid (CSF) from freely moving rabbits, several kinds of devices are used. Figure 1A illustrates each of them, and the left half of Fig. 1B shows the devices assembled on the skull. Surgery to implant the devices usually follows the venous cannulation. First, a wide area of the head of the rabbit is shaved, and the head is positioned horizontally, using a stereotaxic holder. After disinfection and opening of the skin locally, a hole is drilled on the sagittal midline at two-fifths of the distance between the bregma and the lambda suture behind the bregma. A guide cannula installed with a stylet is placed in the hole vertically to 12 mm below the surface of the skull. Successful cannulation is indicated by spontaneous CSF flow after removal of the stylet. Increasing the intracranial pressure by pushing on the thoracic cavity of the rabbit may make verification of the successful cannulation easier. Then the CSF sampling cannula, a venous cannula, and a cannula protector are secured to the skull with acryl cement and stainless steel screws. Successful operation can allow CSF and plasma sampling for a month or even longer.

Sampling of CSF and plasma should begin after a recovery period of at least 1 week. Each rabbit is housed individually in a specially designed sampling cage for rabbits, which is well ventilated, controlled under the same light–dark schedule as the breeding room, and allows steady CSF and plasma sampling from unanesthetized animals with minimum restriction of their movement (Fig. 1C). Cerebrospinal fluid is continuously aspirated by a peristaltic pump at 160 μl/hr, which is less than half of the reported rabbit CSF production rate (3), and collected every 30 min in cooled sampling tubes. To avoid mixing of the CSF in the sampling catheter, 5 μl of air is injected into the sampling needle from its lateral cannula every 30 min. The dead space within the PE-20 polyethylene tubing occupies less than 200 μl, and both AVP and OT in rabbit CSF appear to be stable for at least 2 hr at room temperature. Rectal temperature, plasma osmolarity, and arterial blood pressure are monitored as in the rat experiment.

Hormone Assays

Plasma ACTH levels are determined after silicic acid extraction by radioimmunoassay (RIA), using anti-ACTH rabbit antiserum (West) provided by the National Pituitary Agency of the NIDDK. Plasma AVP levels are determined by RIA, using AVP RIA kits (Mitsubishi Yuka Co., Ltd., Tokyo) after extraction with a Sep-Pak C_{18} cartridge. To measure plasma OT levels, rabbit samples are extractd as for AVP and subjected to RIA, using anti-OT rabbit serum (4) and synthetic OT (Peninsula Laboratories, Belmont, CA) as the standard and tracer labeled with ^{125}I by lactoperoxidase. Rat plasma OT levels are measured in unextracted plasma by using the same RIA system. Recovery rates of ACTH, AVP, and OT by these extraction procedures are 88, 90, and 80%, respectively, and their minimal detectable concentrations are 25, 0.6, and 5 pg/ml, respectively.

Cerebrospinal fluid AVP levels in the rabbit are quantitated without extrac-

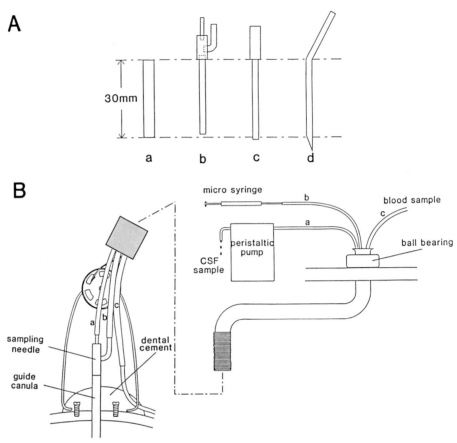

FIG. 1   A system to study the effects of interleukins on arginine vasopressin and oxytocin levels in plasma and cerebrospinal fluid (CSF) of conscious, freely moving rabbits. (A) Devices to collect CSF continuously from a freely moving rabbit; devices are made of 19-, 22-, or 27-gauge stainless steel tubing and 22-gauge stainless steel wire. a, A guide cannula made from 19-gauge stainless steel tubing cut to 30 cm in length; b, a sampling needle made from 19-, 22-, or 27-gauge stainless steel tubing. A 30-mm length of 22-gauge tubing and a 10-mm length of 27-gauge tube are set into either end of a piece of 10-mm long 19-gauge tubing, as illustrated. After insertion of another piece of 22-gauge tubing, which is curved, into the lateral hole of the central 19-gauge piece, the entire device is soldered; c, a cap made of 22-gauge stainless steel wire covered with 19-gauge stainless steel tubing; d, a stylet made from a 22-gauge injection needle. All the devices should be autoclaved before use. (B) *Left:* Devices assembled on the rabbit skull. The joint between the guide cannula and the sampling needle is tightly connected with the appropriate silicone tubing. In a breeding cage, the needle cap (c) is set in place of the sampling needle. A cannula protector is made from a 12-cm length of appropriate steel wire. The wire is bent into a U shape and soldered to the swivel snap at the top of the curve. *Right:* The

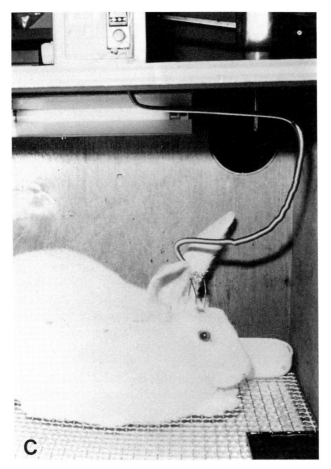

FIG. 1 (*continued*)

devices assembled at the top of the sampling cage. All the cannulas are led to the outside of the cage via a stainless steel wire connected between the cannula protector of the rabbit skull and a Z-shaped piece of aluminum tubing attached to the center of the ceiling. A ball bearing system attached to the aluminum shaft at the top of the cage permits the assembly to turn around freely. a, Cannula (PE-20) for CSF sampling; b, cannula (PE-50) for periodic addition of air; c, cannula for venous sampling. (C) A rabbit in a sampling cage with sampling equipment.

tion by RIA, using anti-AVP rabbit serum donated by N. W. Kasting (University of British Columbia, Vancouver, Canada) and AVP obtained from Peninsula Laboratories. Arginine vasopressin is labeled similarly to OT. Cerebrospinal OT levels are also measured without extraction, using the same RIA used to measure plasma OT levels.

Effects of Cytokines on Plasma Hormone Levels

Using these assay systems, the effects of cytokines on ACTH, AVP, and OT levels can be tested in rats and rabbits.

As shown in Fig. 2 (5), rhIL-1β, rhIL-1α, and rrIL-1β [Met(0)-rrIL-1β] were almost equally effective in increasing plasma ACTH levels; about 30 min after bolus iv injection, each of these cytokines increased plasma ACTH to its peak level; minimal effective doses of these cytokines ranged from 0.1 to 0.01 μg/rat. On the other hand, although rhIL-1α showed a similar time course, its effect was about 10 times weaker than that of the other recombinant IL-1s tested. Recombinant human IL-6 and rhTNF-α also showed similar increases in plasma ACTH levels; their lowest effective doses were 1.0–0.1 and 0.5–0.1 μg/rat, respectively. Recombinant human IL-3, rhIL-4, rhIL-5, and rhIL-8 showed no effects on rat plasma ACTH levels even when 10 μg of the substance per rat was injected. Cytokine-induced ACTH release can be further analyzed by the same system. For example, we attempted to neutralize plasma corticotropin-releasing hormone (CRH) or AVP after cytokine administration. As shown in Fig. 3 (6), rhIL-6-induced plasma ACTH elevation was completely abolished in rats pretreated with an anti-rat/human CRH rabbit serum. The stimulatory effect of IL-6 was partially but significantly attenuated by the similar infusion of an anti-AVP rabbit serum. The ACTH-releasing activities of chemically modified cytokines can also be assayed in these rats, and the data acquired may indicate where the neuroendocrinologically active domain is located within the native molecule (2).

The effects of cytokines on plasma AVP or OT levels can be tested by basically the same system, with some preliminary modifications. That is,

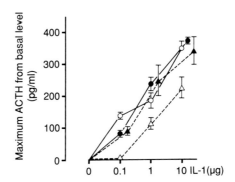

FIG. 2 Comparative potencies of recombinant human and rat IL-1 in increasing plasma ACTH levels in rats. The highest plasma ACTH level observed over 2 hr after iv injection of each cytokine is shown. ○, rrIL-1α; ●, Met(0)-rrIL-1β; △, rhIL-1α; ▲, rhIL-1β. [A portion of the data is from Naito et al. (5).]

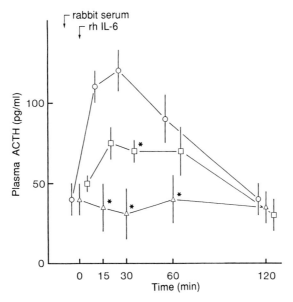

FIG. 3   Recombinant human IL-6-induced changes in plasma ACTH levels in rats. To neutralize plasma CRH or AVP, an anti-rat/human CRH rabbit serum that binds 25.6 μg of rat/human CRH or sufficient anti-AVP rabbit serum to bind 0.7 μg of AVP under *in vitro* conditions was injected 10 min before infusion of 5 μg of IL-6. As the control, the same volume of normal rabbit serum was similarly infused. Each point represents the mean ± SEM of ACTH determination in five rats. ○, Normal rabbit serum; △, anti-rat/human CRH rabbit serum; □, anti-AVP rabbit serum; *$p < 0.05$, compared to rats treated with normal rabbit serum. Statistical analysis was performed by analysis of variance and subsequent Bonferroni method. [Modified from Naitoh *et al.* (6).]

arterial blood pressure and serum osmolarity should be checked to assess the mechanisms of the cytokine effects. In the absence of changes of these parameters in rats, iv infusion of rhIL-1α or rhIL-1β was observed to stimulate plasma AVP and OT levels (Fig. 4), whereas rhIL-6 even at doses as high as 10 μg lacked these effects. The AVP-secreting activity of rhIL-1β was also observed in the rabbit system (Fig. 5). Considering the thermostatic effect of AVP in the brain, the measurement of AVP concentrations in the brain after the administration of thermogenic cytokines is of interest. As shown in Fig. 6, our system is stable enough to permit observation in the rabbit of the distinct diurnal rhythm of AVP in CSF that has been reported in other species (7). Experiments employing this system to determine how cytokines affect AVP or OT levels in CSF are now underway.

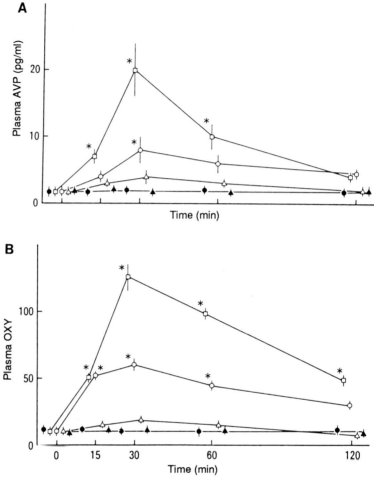

FIG. 4   Effects of interleukins on plasma AVP levels (A) and on OT levels (B) in rats. Cytokines were injected intravenously at time 0. □, 10 μg of rhIL-1β; ○, 1 μg of rhIL-1β; △, 0.1 μg of rhIL-1β; ▲, 10 μg of rhIL-6; ●, vehicle. Each point represents the mean ± SEM of five rats. *$p < 0.05$, compared to vehicle group. [Data from Naito et al. (4).]

Animal models are also useful in the biochemical or histochemical observation of changes in the tissue content of hypophysiotropic hormones or their mRNA levels (8–11). CRH, AVP, and OT levels in rat pituitary portal plasma after IL-1 injection have been studied (12), and a push–pull perifusion technique has also been applied to study CRH release after IL-1 administration (13).

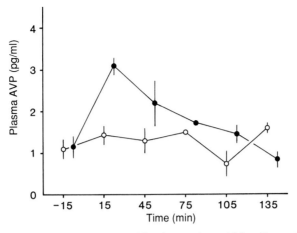

FIG. 5   Plasma AVP levels in plasma of freely moving rabbits. Recombinant human
IL-1β (0.5 μg/kg) (●) or vehicle (○) was injected intravenously at time 0. AVP levels
at 15 min were significantly higher in the rhIL-1β-treated rabbits than in vehicle-
treated rabbits.

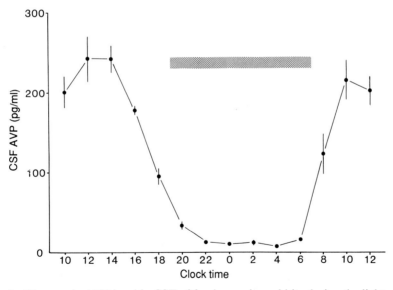

FIG. 6   Changes in AVP level in CSF of freely moving rabbits during the light–dark
cycle. The shaded bar indicates the dark period.

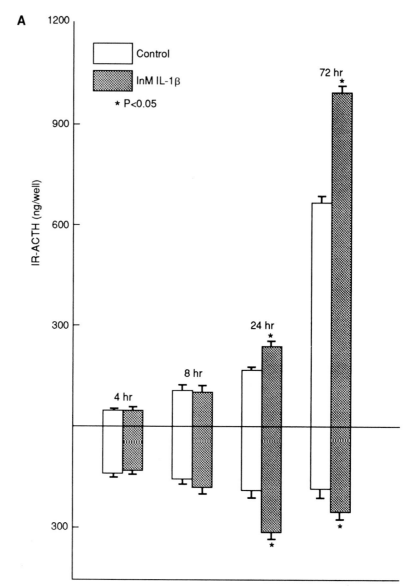

FIG. 7   Effects of human IL-1β on the synthesis and release of ACTH from AtT-20 cells. (A) Changes in ACTH levels in medium (above the horizontal line) and cells (below the horizontal line) during incubation with rhIL-1β. (B) Dot hybridization analysis of POMC mRNA levels in mouse AtT-20 cells after rhIL-1β treatment. [Data from Fukata *et al.* (16).]

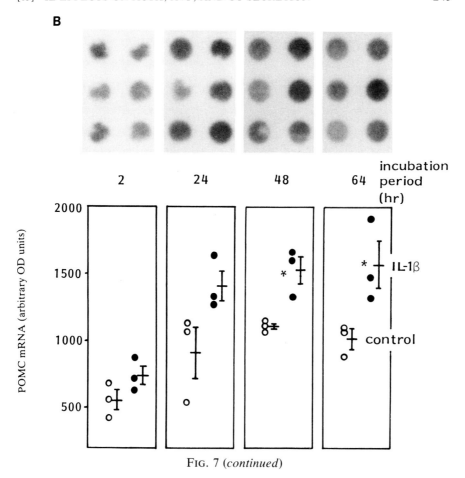

FIG. 7 *(continued)*

Assessment of Cytokine Action on Pituitary Hormone Secretion *in Vitro*

Several kinds of *in vitro* culture systems for analyzing the mechanism of cytokine action on pituitary hormones have been introduced. Studies of direct effects of cytokines on pituitary hormone synthesis and secretion, using primary cultures of normal pituitary cells (12, 14), dispersed adenoma cells (15), or hormone-producing cell lines (16), along with studies of IL-1 receptors (17), have been conducted. Indirect effects on pituitary function via the hypothalamus can also be examined by measuring hypothalamic hormone release from excised hypothalamic tissues (18), or by monitoring the neuronal activities of hypothalamic cells *in vitro* (19).

Pituitary Cell Culture

A mouse pituitary adenoma cell line, AtT-20, can easily be used to study the effects of cytokines on ACTH and other proopiomelanocortin (POMC)-derived peptide synthesis (16). A subclone, AtT-20/D16v, is grown in Dulbecco's modified Eagle's medium (DMEM) supplemented with 10% fetal calf serum, penicillin G (50 units/ml), and streptomycin sulfate (50 μg/ml) at 37°C in a humidified atmosphere of 5% CO_2 : 95% air. In an experiment in which ACTH levels are measured, cells are disseminated in 24-well plates at a density of 0.5–1.0 $\times$ 10^5 cells/well. After 2–3 days of incubation, the wells in which cells have grown to 60–80% confluency are rinsed and maintained in sterile DMEM supplemented with 0.2% bovine serum albumin, ascorbic acid ($2.5 \times 10^{-4} M$), bacitracin (50 μg/ml), and antibiotics. The growth rate of the cells is assessed by quantitating the incorporation rate of [^{3}H]thymidine into the cells. Adrenocorticotropic hormone levels are measured by RIA. To quantitate POMC mRNA levels, the cells are cultured in 35-mm dishes with cytokines. Cytoplasmic dot hybridization or Northern blot hybridization analysis is carried out with a ^{32}P-labeled 1.1-kbp fragment of human POMC gene excised with *Sma*I as a probe (16). As shown in Fig. 7, rhIL-1β, which induced no significant changes during the first several hours, increased ACTH levels both in media and cells after 24 hr of incubation. This effect of IL-1β appeared to be a consequence of direct stimulation of ACTH synthesis, because significant increases in POMC mRNA levels in these cells were observed. Recombinant human IL-1α and rhIL-6 also showed similar effects on the cell line (16).

Enzymatically dispersed pituitary tissues, cultured as monolayer cells under conditions similar to those used for AtT-20 cells, can also be used to test cytokine actions. Recombinant human IL-1α, rhIL-1β, or rhIL-6 showed little stimulatory effect on ACTH release from dispersed rat pituitary cells during a period of time comparable to that used in the AtT-20 cell experiment (12, 14). The cytokines showed a suppressive effect on CRH-stimulated ACTH release after 2–3 days of incubation (20).

Hypothalamic Tissue Culture

Studies employing RIA systems have demonstrated that cytokines stimulate CRH secretion from hypothalamic slices or blocks into the incubation medium (18). A direct effect of IL-1β on hypothalamic neurosecretory neurons, as shown in Fig. 8, was observed by Li *et al.* (19), who used an intracellular recording technique. A part of coronal section (400 μm) of the adult rat hypothalamus, which was identified as a portion of the supraoptic nucleus (SON), was perfused with medium containing rhIL-1β at a rate of 2 ml/min at 36°C, and membrane potentials were recorded. Recombinant human IL-1β depolarized the membrane and caused an increased firing rate in a majority of the cells tested. The effect persisted even during synaptic uncoupling with

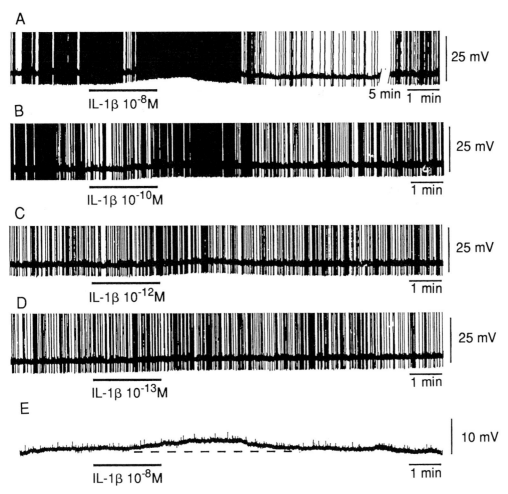

FIG. 8   Cytokine-induced depolarization of rat SON neurons *in vitro*. (A–D) Effects of rhIL-1β at 10^{-8}, 10^{-10}, 10^{-12}, and 10^{-13} M. (E) Depolarization by 10^{-8} M rhIL-1β during 10^{-6} M tetrodotoxin perfusion. Horizontal bars indicate period during which interleukin was added. [Data from Li *et al.* (19) with permission.]

tetrodotoxin, suggesting that rhIL-1β exerts a direct excitatory effect on SON neurons themselves.

Comments

Using either *in vivo* or *in vitro* systems, much information has accumulated about cytokine effects on neuroendocrine functions. Concerning cytokine-stimulated ACTH release, it is generally accepted that the acute ACTH secretion observed after cytokine challenge is due to increased secretion of CRH from the hypothalamus. However, the mechanism behind the phenomenon is controversial. For example, it has still not been conclusively determined whether IL-1α and IL-1β have the same potency in affecting ACTH secretion, mainly because many experiments reported so far employed human recombinant cytokines in rodent systems. There are considerable interspecies variations in the amino acid structure of ILs, and only one amino acid substitution has been reported to markedly change the bioactivity of interleukins (21). Considering that the two subtypes of IL-1 receptor identified so far have different affinities for IL-1α and IL-1β molecules, it is of value to compare the effects of the two types of IL-1 in a homologous bioassay system. We attempted to study the effect of recombinant rat IL-1β (rrIL-1β) in rats as shown in Fig. 2, but the rrIL-β we used has an additional methionine residue in its N-terminal structure. Therefore the result of that experiment is still not conclusive. With respect to other cytokines, differences between natural and synthesized proteins in glycosylation should also be considered. Cellular mechanisms in the brain intervening between cytokines and neurosecretory cells must also be carefully analyzed, because a single domain of a cytokine molecule might not necessarily be responsible for all the pleiotropic effects of the particular cytokine on the brain (2).

Acknowledgments

This work was supported by grants from the Ministry of Education, Science, and Culture, and from the Science and Technology Agency, Japan, and by a grant from the Yamanouchi Foundation for Research on Metabolic Disorders.

References

1. H. Imura, J. Fukata, and T. Mori, *Clin. Endocrinol. (Oxford)* **35,** 107 (1991).
2. Y. Naito, J. Fukata, Y. Masui, Y. Hirai, N. Murakami, T. Tominaga, Y. Nakai, S. Tamai, K. Mori, and H. Imura, *Biochem. Biophys. Res. Commun.* **167,** 103 (1990).

3. H. M. Kaplan and E. H. Timmons, "The Rabbit: A Model for the Principles of Mammalian Physiology and Surgery," p. 136. Academic Press, New York, 1979.

4. Y. Naito, J. Fukata, K. Shindo, O. Ebisui, N. Murakami, T. Tominaga, Y. Nakai, K. Mori, N. W. Kasting, and H. Imura, *Biochem. Biophys. Res. Commun.* **174**, 1189 (1991).

5. Y. Naito, J. Fukata, T. Tominaga, Y. Masui, Y. Hirai, N. Murakami, S. Tamai, K. Mori, and H. Imura, *Biochem. Biophys. Res. Commun.* **164**, 1262 (1989).

6. Y. Naito, J. Fukata, T. Tominaga, Y. Nakai, S. Tamai, K. Mori, and H. Imura, *Biochem. Biophys. Res. Commun.* **155**, 1459 (1988).

7. S. M. Reppert, W. J. Schwartz, and G. R. Uhl, *Trends Neurosci.* **10**, 76 (1987).

8. F. Berkenbosch, J. van Oers, A. del Rey, F. Tilders, and H. Besedovsky, *Science* **238**, 524 (1987).

9. T. Suda, F. Tozawa, T. Ushiyama, T. Sumitomo, M. Yamada, and H. Demura, *Endocrinology (Baltimore)* **126**, 1223 (1990).

10. Y. Naito, J. Fukata, S. Nakaishi, Y. Nakai, Y. Hirai, S. Tamai, K. Mori, and H. Imura, *Neuroendocrinology* **51**, 637 (1990).

11. N. Murakami, J. Fukata, T. Usui, Y. Naito, T. Tominaga, Y. Nakai, Y. Masui, K. Nakao, and H. Imura, *J. Pharmacol. Exp. Ther.* **260**, 1344 (1992).

12. R. Sapolsky, C. Rivier, G. Yamamoto, P. Plotsky, and W. Vale, *Science* **238**, 522 (1987).

13. H. Watanabe, S. Sasaki, and K. Takebe, *Neurosci. Lett.* **133**, 7 (1991).

14. J. Fukata, Y. Naitoh, T. Usui, S. Nakaishi, H. Kohmoto, T. Tsukada, Y. Nakai, and H. Imura, *Abstr. Int. Cong. Endocrinol. 8th,* Abstr. No. 01-18-995 (1988).

15. W. B. Malarkey and B. J. Zvara, *J. Clin. Endocrinol. Metab.* **69**, 196 (1989).

16. J. Fukata, T. Usui, Y. Naitoh, Y. Nakai, and H. Imura, *J. Endocrinol.* **122**, 33 (1989).

17. H. Kobayashi, J. Fukata, T. Tominaga, N. Murakami, M. Fukushima, O. Ebisui, H. Segawa, Y. Nakai, and H. Imura, *FEBS Lett.* **298**, 100 (1992).

18. S. Tsagarakis, G. Gillies, L. H. Rees, M. Besser, and A. G. Grossman, *Neuroendocrinology* **49**, 98 (1989).

19. Z. Li, K. Inenaga, S. Kawano, H. Kannan, and H. Yamashita, *NeuroReport* **3**, 91 (1992).

20. J. Fukata, O. Ebisui, N. Murakami, H. Kobayashi, H. Segawa, S. Muro, Y. Naito, T. Tomimaga, Y. Nakai, Y. Masui, and H. Imura, "Stress and Reproduction," p. 39. Raven Press, New York, 1992.

21. G. Ju, E. Labriola-Tompkins, C. A. Campen, W. R. Benjamin, J. Karas, J. Plocinski, D. Biondi, K. L. Kaffka, P. L. Kilian, S. P. Eisenberg, and R. J. Evans, *Proc. Natl. Acad. Sci. U.S.A.* **88**, 2658 (1991).

[14] *In Vivo* and *in Vitro* Models for Evaluating Effects of Interleukin 1 on Hypothalamic–Pituitary–Gonadal Axis

Pushpa S. Kalra and Satya P. Kalra

Introduction

Bidirectional communication between the immune and neuroendocrine systems has gained increased recognition in recent years. Hypothalamic hormones, whose primary function is to regulate the release of pituitary hormones, have been shown to influence the secretion of immune factors from macrophages (1). The cytokines interleukin 1 (IL-1) and IL-6, secreted by activated macrophages in response to an immune challenge, are the chemical messengers that constitute a regulatory link in the opposite direction to alter hypothalamic–pituitary secretions.

Whether peripheral IL-1 secreted by immune cells can penetrate the blood–brain barrier is still the subject of debate. However, there is convincing evidence that both IL-1 and IL-1-binding receptors are present in the hypothalamus (2–6). *In situ* hybridization studies have confirmed the production of IL-1β in the brain. Although IL-1β mRNA expression was low or nondetectable in the brain of nonstimulated rats, abundant IL-1β mRNA was found following stimulation by lipopolysaccharides and interferon γ (7–9), suggesting that endogenous production of IL-1 may occur in response to cerebral trauma or immune challenge.

In the brain, IL-1 functions as a neuromodulator/neurotransmitter with multiple effects, including induction of fever, slow-wave sleep, anorexia, and stimulation of prostaglandin E_2 and catecholamines. The hormonal effects of IL-1 include modulation of the hypothalamo–pituitary–adrenal (HPA) axis (10, 11) and the hypothalamo–pituitary–gonadal (HPG) axis (12).

Pituitary gonadotrophs are the source of luteinizing hormone (LH) and follicle-stimulating hormone (FSH). These two gonadotropins control gonadal function, which includes secretion of steroids and inhibin by gonads and follicle growth, ultimately leading to ovulation in the female and spermatogenesis in the male. The secretion of pituitary gonadotropins is, in turn, regulated by hypothalamic luteinizing hormone-releasing hormone (LHRH), a decapeptide released in an episodic fashion into the fenestrated capillaries of the hypophysial portal system in the median eminence (ME) for transporta-

Methods in Neurosciences, Volume 16

tion to the pituitary gonadotrophs to stimulate the release of LH and FSH. Cytokines can, therefore, act at several levels in the hypothalamo–pituitary axis to affect the secretion of pituitary gonadotrophs. A number of laboratories have evaluated the effects and mode of action of cytokines on pituitary gonadotropin secretion (13–16). The following section describes a variety of experimental protocols employed by us in male and female rats to systematically evaluate the effects of the cytokine, IL-1, on pituitary LH and hypothalamic LHRH release (17–19).

Effect of IL-1 on Luteinizing Hormone Release

Peripheral and Central Action

Peripheral Action

Circulating IL-1 can modulate LH secretion by acting directly at the level of pituitary gonadotrophs in two ways. It can directly inhibit or stimulate the release of LH or it can modify the LH-stimulating action of incoming hypothalamic LHRH. To evaluate the effects of IL-1 on LH secretion, intact or gonadectomized rats are employed. Rats are implanted with intraatrial cannulas 1 day before the experiment. Interleukin is diluted in sterile saline on the day of experiment. A blood sample is withdrawn via the intraatrial cannula into a heparinized syringe before the intravenous injection of either vehicle (control) or vehicle containing IL-1. Thereafter, blood samples are withdrawn at intervals for 2–4 hr. Plasma harvested from blood samples is assayed for LH by radioimmunoassay (RIA). Because LH secretion in intact rats is in the low basal range, it would be possible to detect the stimulatory effects of cytokines on LH release, but the inhibitory effects of cytokines are not generally discernible in intact rats. To evaluate the inhibitory effects on LH release, rats are gonadectomized and allowed to recover for 2–3 weeks to stabilize episodic LH hypersecretion. In this long-term gonadectomized model, one can evaluate the time course of decrease in LH release and the impact on the component(s) of LH episodes by withdrawing blood samples at 5-min intervals or less for a period of 2–3 hr after intravenous injection of cytokines. Standard statistical procedures are employed to evaluate the impact of IL-1 on various parameters of LH episodes (20–23). The volume of blood samples can be altered to accommodate gonadal steroid measurements, if desired. We have failed to detect any effects of intravenously administered IL-1α or IL-1β on LH release (17).

Effects of IL-1 on Luteinizing Hormone Release from Pituitary in Vitro

Techniques that utilized either hemipituitaries or dispersed pituitary cells in culture have been employed to demonstrate the effects of cytokines on LH release from pituitary gonadotrophs (16, 24, 25). The use of pituitary halves, instead of dispersed pituitary cells, has the advantage of an intact pituitary architecture so that paracrine effects, if any, are not disrupted. Pituitary halves are preincubated for 2 hr in 1.0 ml of Earle's balanced salt (Flow Laboratories, Inc., McLean, VA) solution containing 0.1% glucose and 0.1% bovine serum albumin (BSA) at 37°C under an atmosphere of 95% O_2/5% CO_2. Conditioned media from the third hour of incubation are collected for estimation of basal release, and during the fourth hour medium is supplemented with 10^{-8} M IL-1α or IL-1β. For the interaction of cytokines with LHRH similar experimental protocols are used. Hemipituitaries or dispersed pituitary cells are cultured for various period of time with either the cytokine alone or with LHRH (10^{-11}–10^{-8} M). The LH responses induced by cytokines alone or together with LHRH are then compared to controls and to basal release rates to determine the interaction, if any, between the two peptides. Our results showed no direct effects of the cytokine on LH release from hemipituitaries in culture (P. S. Kalra and S. P. Kalra, unpublished observations).

Central Action

The central action of cytokines on LH release can be studied either by intracerebroventricular (icv) injection of IL-1 or by microinjection into discrete hypothalamic sites. Therefore, the experimental design involves placement of permanent, stainless steel cannulas into the third or lateral cerebroventricles or aimed at various sites in the hypothalamus 1–2 weeks before the day of the test. As described above, it is possible to evaluate the effects of central injection of IL-1 on basal LH secretion in intact rats or on episodic LH secretion in gonadectomized rats. An example depicted in Figure 1 shows that icv injection of IL-1β gradually suppresses LH release by inhibiting pulsatile LH release in castrated male rats. The frequency of LH episodes decreased to 1.6 ± 0.2 vs 2.9 ± 0.5 pulses/90 min in controls and pulse amplitude decreased to 0.9 ± 0.3 vs 1.7 ± 0.3 ng/ml.

In addition, two experimental designs have been employed to determine the action of cytokines on the spontaneously occurring preovulatory LH surge on proestrus in cycling rats or the ovarian steroid-induced LH surge in ovariectomized rats (17).

Proestrous Rats

Adult female rats are implanted with an icv cannula in the lateral or third ventricle of the brain (see details below). Estrous cyclicity is documented by daily examination of vaginal lavage. A blunt-end medicine dropper con-

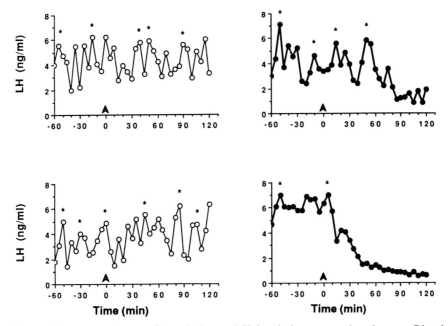

FIG. 1   Representative profiles of plasma LH levels in castrated male rats. Blood samples were withdrawn at 5 min via an intraatrial cannula for 60 min before and for 120 min after the icv administration of 3 μl of saline (left) or 100 ng of IL-1β (right) at time 0 (arrowheads). Interleukin 1β decreased plasma LH levels by suppressing the frequency and amplitude of LH pulses. *, LH peaks identified by CLUSTER analysis.

taining a drop of saline is inserted into the vagina; the saline is gently pumped into the vagina, withdrawn, and transferred to a microscope slide to examine cells under a microscope. The day of estrus is characterized by a predominance of large cornified, irregular shaped cells. This is followed by 2 or 3 days of metestrus and diestrus, when the vaginal lavage contains a preponderance of small leukocytes. Large, round cells with prominent nuclei in the vaginal lavage are characteristic of proestrus. The day of proestrus should be preceded by 2 days of diestrus (leukocytes) and followed by 1 day of estrus (cornified cells). At least two to three consecutive estrous cycles are documented before the rats are used for experimentation. The intraatrial cannula is implanted on the morning of proestrus in rats anesthetized with ether. Barbiturates block the LH surge and should not be used as anesthetics. In rats maintained on a controlled light schedule with lights on from 0500 to 1900 hr, the increase in the rate of LH secretion predictably occurs between 1400 and 1600 hr and peak levels are observed between 1600 and 1800 hr.

A blood sample is withdrawn just before IL-1 or saline is administered by the icv route. Thereafter, additional blood samples can be withdrawn at 1- or 2-hr intervals until 2000 hr for examination of the effects of cytokines on the preovulatory surge of LH in the plasma. To examine the occurrence of ovulation, rats are killed on estrus morning. The oviducts are carefully removed, and placed between two microscope slides that are pressed together gently and examined under a microscope. Ova are clearly visible in the cumulus mass and can be counted.

Experiments involving proestrous rats can be tedious and cumbersome, involving daily examination of vaginal lavage for 2–3 weeks and a limited number of rats on proestrus may be available on any given day. An alternative procedure utilized by Rivier and Vale (14) was to synchronize estrous cycles by two subcutaneous (sc) injections of 2 μg of [D-Tyr^6,Pro^9,Net]GnRH (gonadotropin-releasing hormone) at 0900 and 1400 hr in rats at random stages of the cycle. This treatment caused 80% of the rats to display estrus (cornified cells in the vaginal lavage) on the following morning. These synchronized rats were then utilized on the day of proestrus after monitoring two regular 4-day estrous cycles. Whether this treatment with a GnRH agonist alters any neuroendocrine event is not known; however, there were differences in the effects of IL-1β on ovulation. Whereas administration of IL-1β on proestrus inhibited the LH surge both in rats with spontaneous cycles (P. S. Kalra and S. P. Kalra, unpublished results) and those with synchronized cycles (14), ovulation was not inhibited in the former (Fig. 2).

Steroid-Induced Luteinizing Hormone Surge

An alternative, well-characterized procedure that has gained widespread acceptance is to induce the LH surge with steroids in ovariectomized (ovx) rats. Adult female rats are ovariectomized and receive an icv cannula. After a 7- to 10-day recovery period, rats are injected sc with 30 μg of estradoil benzoate (EB) dissolved in 0.1 ml of sesame oil at 1000 hr. Forty-eight hours after EB injection, 2 mg of progesterone (P) in 0.1 ml of sesame oil is injected sc at 1000 hr. This treatment schedule induces a robust, proestrous-type LH surge starting at 1400 hr and lasting for 4–5 hr. Therefore a blood sample is withdrawn before icv IL-1 or saline injection at 1300 hr. Blood samples are withdrawn thereafter at 1- or 2-hr intervals until 1800 hr for LH measurements (17).

Mode of Action

Our results indicated that central, but not systemic, injections of IL-1 readily inhibited the episodic LH secretion in gonadectomized rats and blocked the preovulatory and ovarian steroid-induced LH surges in ovx rats (17, 19). These results raised two questions with respect to the mode of action of

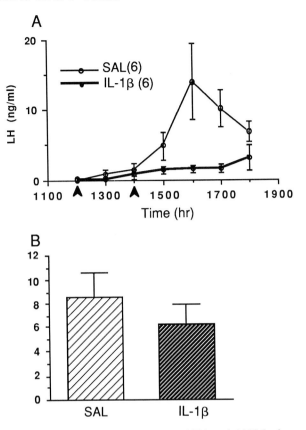

FIG. 2   (A) The icv administration of IL-1β at 1200 and 1400 hr in proestrous rats inhibited the preovulatory LH surge that normally occurs in the afternoon as seen in saline (SAL)-injected rats. However, ovulation was not significantly inhibited in these rats as depicted by the number of ova counted in the oviducts on the following morning of estrus (B).

IL-1 in inhibiting LH release. It is possible that inhibition of LH release is a consequence of suppression of hypothalamic LHRH release. Alternatively IL-1 may activate other neural systems within the hypothalamus that are inhibitory to LHRH.

Effects of IL-1 on Hypothalamic Neuropeptidergic Systems That Inhibit Luteinizing Hormone-Releasing Hormone–Luteinizing Hormone

To determine whether the effects of IL-1 on LHRH–LH release are mediated by activation of neuropeptidergic signals that in turn may inhibit LHRH and

LH release, we examined the involvement of two inhibitory peptidergic systems. The endogenous opioid peptides (EOP), including β-endorphin, comprise a peptidergic neural network in the hypothalamus that inhibits LHRH and pituitary LH release (26, 27). Interestingly, endotoxins and IL-1 stimulate release of proopiomelanocortin (POMC)-derived peptides in blood and cerebrospinal fluid (CSF) (1, 28, 29) and stimulate POMC mRNA levels in the pituitary (30). To examine the possibility of EOP involvement in mediating the IL-1-induced suppression of the LH surge we used a pharmacological approach to block the endogenous opioid receptors (18).

The general opioid receptor antagonist, naloxone, was employed at a dose that, on its own, does not further stimulate the LH surge induced by P in estrogen-primed ovx rats. Naloxone hydrochloride (2 mg/0.6 ml of saline/hr), infused intravenously for 2 hr starting immediately after the central administration of IL-1α or IL-1β, countered the IL-1-induced suppression of the LH surge in response to P (18) and also prevented the IL-1-induced inhibition of LH secretion in castrated male rats (19). Similarly, Rivier and Vale (14) reported a reversal of IL-1-induced blockade of ovulation by preimplanting proestrous rats with naloxone pellets.

The three classes of EOP, β-endorphin, enkephalins, and dynorphins, inhibit LHRH–LH release via selective activation of μ, δ, and κ opioid receptor subtypes, respectively. In view of the possibility that opioid receptor subtypes may be differentially activated under different physiological and pathophysiological conditions, pharmacological blockade of selective opioid receptor subtypes can be used to identify the opioid receptor subtype involved in mediation of IL-1 inhibition of LH release. Norbinaltorphimine dihydrochloride or naltrindole hydrochloride (10 nmol) was administered icv 1 hr before IL-1β to selectively block κ and δ receptors, respectively (31, 32). For blockade of μ_1 receptors, a long acting antagonist, β-funaltrexamine hydrochloride (4.8 nmol; 33), was administered icv, 24 hr before IL-1β injection. The results showed that only the latter antagonist prevented the IL-1β-induced inhibition of LH release in castrated male rats, thereby suggesting that the μ opioid receptors are involved in the inhibitory LH response of IL-1β (19).

The putative involvement of hypothalamic corticotropin-releasing factor (CRF) activation in mediating the suppressive effects of IL-1 on LH release was also examined by pharmacological blockade of hypothalamic CRF receptors in castrated male rats (19). The CRF receptor antagonist, α-helical CRF (9–41) (Bachem Fine Chemicals, Torrance, CA), was administered (100 μg/3 μl saline) icv before IL-1β administration. Another approach to block CRF action was passive immunoneutralization by icv administration of a specific CRF antibody (rC70; gift of W. Vale, Salk Institute, La Jolla, CA). Blockade of endogenous CRF activity by either of these approaches failed to block the IL-1-induced suppression of LH release in castrated male rats, suggesting that activation of hypothalamic CRF by IL-1 may not be responsible for suppressing release of reproductive hormones in response to IL-1β.

Stereotaxic Procedures

Because IL-1 is effective only if administered directly into the brain, rats are implanted with permanent cannulas in the cerebral ventricles several days before the experiment. Interleukin 1 is effective when injected into either the lateral or third ventricle of the brain.

Third Ventricle Cannulation

Stainless steel tubings of various thickness are purchased in 6- or 12-in. lengths from Small Parts, Inc. (Miami, FL). We have devised a holder to hold the cannula in the stereotaxic apparatus by fitting a length of 22-gauge tubing inside a 5-cm length of 18-gauge steel tubing so that it extends 5 mm below the tip of the outer tubing (Fig. 3). The upper end of these two tubings is bent to form an L that will hold the assembled tubings securely in position. Fit this holder in the frame of the stereotaxic apparatus (Trentwell's, Inc., Southgate, CA), ensuring that it is completely vertical.

The cannula consists of three pieces of stainless steel tubing: a 5-mm piece of 18-gauge tubing (guide cannula), an 18-mm length of 22-gauge tubing (cannula), and a 32-mm piece of 26-gauge tubing (stylet). Fit the stylet inside the 22-gauge tubing so that it extends 0.5 mm beyond the lower tip, bend the upper extension of the 26-gauge tubing to an L (Fig. 3).

Rats anesthetized with sodium pentobarbital [40 mg/kg, intraperitoneal (ip)] are placed in a stereotaxic apparatus with the incisor bar adjusted to 5.0 mm above the ear bar. Make an incision on the skin to expose the skull and identify the interaural line. Mark a point 6.4 mm anterior to the interaural line on the sagittal suture. Drill three small holes around this point at a distance of approximately 2–3 mm. Insert small machine screws into these holes (1/8-in. machine screws; Small Parts, Inc.) to anchor the cement and cannula. Place the 5-mm guide cannula on the cannula holder, drill a small window at the 6.4-mm anterior area to expose the superior sagittal sinus, then lower the stereotaxic holder so that the guide cannula just touches the exposed dura on the superior sagittal sinus. Cover the exposed brain surface with gelfoam and cement the 5-mm guide cannula to the skull and screws with acrylic dental cement (TRIM, powder and liquid; Harry J. Bosworth Co., Skokie, IL). Allow cement to dry and harden and lift up the cannula holder, leaving the 18-gauge guide cannula affixed to the skull. Insert the 26-gauge stylet in the guide cannula to gently pierce the superior sagittal

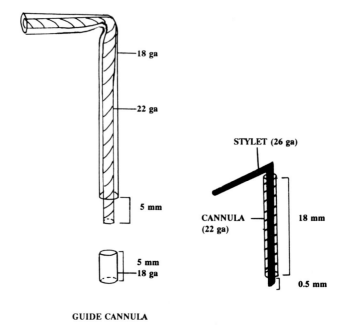

STYLET (26 ga)

CANNULA (22 ga)   18 mm

0.5 mm

18 ga

22 ga

5 mm

5 mm
18 ga

GUIDE CANNULA

FIG. 3   Diagrammatic representation of the stereotaxic cannula holder and cannula components for cannulation of the third ventricle of the brain. See text for details.

sinus, which will cause bleeding. Remove and replace the stylet within the 22-gauge cannula and insert both into the guide cannula and part way into the brain. With the aid of forceps and a ruler (graduated in millimeters), carefully push the cannula into the brain so that exactly 5 mm of cannula remains exposed above the guide cannula (the cannula is inserted into the brain to a depth of 8 mm). Wait at least 15 min before removing the stylet and examine the cannula for CSF efflux. If not, then gently raise and/or lower the cannula a fraction of a millimeter at a time (avoid excessive up and down movement, which may cause brain damage) to initiate CSF flow. Cement the cannula in place, leaving approximately 2 mm exposed. When dry, insert the stylet, point the bent "handle" of the stylet caudally and cement the end to the dried cement to hold the stylet in place until the day of the experiment.

Lateral Ventricle Cannulation

The stereotaxic holder for the lateral ventricle cannula consists of three pieces of stainless steel tubing: a length of 26-gauge tubing fitted inside a

5-cm long 22-gauge tubing such that it extends 14.5 mm below the tip. This assembly is fitted inside an 18-gauge tube such that this outer 18-gauge tubing extends 5 mm from the lower tip of the middle 22-gauge tube (Fig. 4). This assembly will leave the inner 26-gauge tubing extending 9.5 mm beyond the outer 18-gauge tubing. The upper end of the assembly is crimped and bent to an L shape to hold all three pieces securely without any vertical movement. The lateral ventricle cannula is made of a 14-mm long 22-gauge tubing with an inner 26-gauge stylet that extends 0.5 mm at the lower end and 15 mm at the upper end, which is bent to an L.

Install the holder in a stereotaxic frame, remove the stylet from the cannula, and fit the cannula onto the holder. The 26-gauge inner tubing of the holder will extend 0.5 mm beyond the end of the cannula. Adjust the incisor bar to −3.3 mm to hold the rat's skull in a horizontal position.

Place the rat, anesthetized with sodium pentobarbital, in the stereotaxic apparatus, expose the skull, and identify the interaural line. Locate and mark the skull at 8.2 mm anterior to the interaural line and 1.3 m lateral to the midline. Drill one hole in the skull at this spot for the cannula and another two holes approximately 2 mm rostral and caudal to it. Insert anchoring machine screws in these two holes. Lower the cannula until it just touches the dura, note the vertical scale on the stereotaxic apparatus, and lower the cannula an additional 3.5 mm into the brain. Pack gelfoam around the cannula and cement the cannula in place along with the anchoring machine screws. When dry, raise the holder and insert the stylet in the cannula. After 15 min,

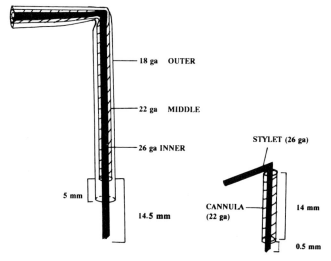

FIG. 4   Diagrammatic representation of the stereotaxic cannula holder and cannula with stylet for cannulating the lateral ventricle of the brain. See text for details.

remove the stylet to verify CSF efflux. Reinsert the stylet and cement the tip of the L to the existing cement.

Intracerebroventricular Injection

The injection assembly consists of an 18- to 20-in. length of PE-20 tubing (Clay Adams, Div. of Becton-Dickinson, Parsippany, NJ), one end of which is attached to a 50-μl Hamilton syringe. Insert a piece of 26-gauge steel tubing at the other end such that exactly 14 mm of steel tubing is exposed for lateral ventricle injections and 18 mm is exposed for third ventricle injections.

About 1 hr before the start of the experiment, cut the cemented end of the stylet with wire cutters, and remove the stylet. Observe the cannula periodically for CSF efflux and reinsert the stylet when CSF is detected. The tubing and syringe injection assembly is prefilled with sterile saline. Draw up an air bubble in the tubing (4–5 μl on the syringe), then draw up the test solution, which has been prepared to deliver the desired dose in 2–3 μl. Larger volumes (5–10 μl) can be injected into the lateral ventricle. Gently hold the rat, remove the stylet, and insert the steel tubing at the tip of the injection tubing into the cannula until the PE-20 tubing is flush with the end of the rat cannula. This ensures that the tip of the steel tubing reaches the lower end of the rat cannula. Gently and slowly inject 3 μl, wait a few seconds before withdrawing the tubing, then replace the stylet in the cannula to prevent backflow of CSF.

Intraatrial Cannulation

To avoid the effects of surgical and anesthetic stress, the intraatrial cannula is installed 1 day before the scheduled day of experiment, except in proestrous rats, which are cannulated on the morning of verified proestrus. The procedure used by us is a modification of that described by Harms and Ojeda (34). The cannula consists of a 20-cm length of silastic tubing (0.025 in. i.d. × 0.047 o.d.; Dow Corning, Midland, MI), one end of which is passed through two small holes in a small rectangle (1 × 2 cm) of silastic sheeting (8 × 6 × 0.02 in.; Dow Corning, Midland, MI). The sheet is then folded over and sealed into place with silastic medical adhesive, silicon type (Dow Corning), at a distance of 35 mm from one end of the tubing. When the adhesive is dry (24 hr) the sheet is trimmed to a small semicircle to eliminate sharp corners and jagged edges. The 35-mm length of tubing is trimmed before use to an appropriate length suitable for the size of the rat (29–30 mm for <300 g body weight; 31 mm for 300–400 g, and 32 mm for >400 g body weight).

The rat is anesthetized with ether and a longitudinal skin incision is made on the neck over the area of the right jugular vein. The vein is freed from surrounding tissue by gentle teasing and ligated with silk suture approximately 1 cm rostral to the pectoralis muscle. Another loop of silk suture is passed around the jugular vein near the pectoralis muscle and loosely knotted. The cannula tubing is filled with saline and a syringe is attached to the long end. The jugular vein is nicked with small, sharp scissors between the two ligatures and the small end of the cannula is slipped into the vein. The tubing is carefully pushed into the vein toward the heart up to the level of the silastic sheet. Blood is gently withdrawn with the syringe to verify cannula placement and pushed back in. The loose knot is then tightly secured, holding the cannula in place in the vein. The silastic sheet is secured to the pectoralis muscle with another suture. The syringe is removed and the tubing end is exteriorized to the dorsal neck region of the rat through a large 16-gauge needle. Knot the end of the cannula and suture the skin incision. The entire procedure can be completed in 5–10 min and the rat recovers rapidly from anesthesia.

Blood Withdrawal

At least 1 hr before the start of the experiment, the free end of the exteriorized cannula is attached to a length of similar tubing. A 50-cm long piece of silastic tubing is fitted to a 1.0-ml syringe at one end with a 22-gauge hypodermic needle and a 22-gauge piece of stainless steel tubing is fitted into the other end; this collection assembly is filled with heparinized saline. The knot on the exteriorized rat cannula is cut and the collection tubing is attached to it by slipping the steel tubing into the cut end. Blood is withdrawn gently and approximately 0.5 ml of heparinized saline is pushed into the cannula. The tubing is then draped outside the cage and allowed to hang freely with the syringe attached. This procedure does not require anesthesia or handling of the rat. Blood samples can be withdrawn into heparinized syringes from outside the cage at appropriate intervals without disturbing the rat. To ensure stability of blood volume in the rat, an equal amount of saline is injected after withdrawal of each blood sample. Plasma is stored frozen at $-20°C$ until hormone analysis.

For frequent blood withdrawal for the analysis of LH pulses, the outer length of cannula is attached to the "pull" end of tubing attached to a P3 peristaltic pump (Pharmacia, Piscataway, NJ), which has been precalibrated to withdraw blood at the rate of 100 μl/5 min. This allows continuous withdrawal of blood at a constant rate without disturbing the rat. These same pumps can be used for iv infusions at a constant rate over several hours when the "push" end of the pump tubing is attached to the intraatrial cannula in the rat.

Neuropeptide Release

Effects of IL-1 on Luteinizing Hormone-Releasing Hormone

Hypothalamic LHRH release *in vivo* may be determined by utilizing the push–pull perfusion technique or microdialysis with the cannula tip aimed at the ME or anterior pituitary, or by measuring LHRH levels in the cannulated hypophysial portal veins (35–39). However, the feasibility of these techniques to determine the effects of IL-1 on LHRH release is questionable because IL-1 may reduce the rate of LHRH release to nondetectable levels, as measured by RIA. Furthermore, IL-1 must be administered directly into the brain via icv cannulas, which would physically limit the placement of the additional push–pull cannula or microdialysis probe. In view of these limitations, we elected to use short-term incubations of the medial basal hypothalamus to determine the basal rate of LHRH release in the presence of IL-1. Ovariectomized rats injected sc with 30 μg of EB and 15 mg of P were decapitated 48 hr later. The medial basal hypothalamus–preoptic area (MBH-POA) was rapidly dissected and incubated *in vitro* in Kreb–Ringer bicarbonate buffer (KRB; see method below). The basal release rate of LHRH was assessed in two 30-min incubation periods. Incubation for an additional 30-min period in the presence of IL-1α or IL-1β (0.1, 1.0, or 10.0 nM) resulted in significant declines in LHRH efflux as compared to the basal release rate (17).

Extending these studies further, it was noted that suppression of LHRH release by 10 nM IL-1α or IL-1β was not detected in similar incubations of the microdissected ME, which is rich in LHRH-containing nerve terminals and is outside the blood–brain barrier. This lack of effectiveness of IL-1 on LHRH release from the ME, in contrast to its effectiveness in suppressing LHRH release from the entire MBH-POA, suggested that IL-1 may not have a direct effect on LHRH release from nerve terminals. It further supported the concept of a site of action within the blood–barrier, as was suggested by the ineffectiveness of sytemic IL-1 administration on the steroid-induced LH surge (17), and supported the possibility that IL-1 may activate other neural systems within the hypothalamus that are inhibitory to LHRH release.

Endogenous opioid involvement in IL-1-induced suppression of LHRH release was examined in *in vitro* incubations of the MBH-POA. The IL-1α- and IL-1β-induced suppression of LHRH release from the MBH-POA was prevented by the simultaneous addition of naloxone hydrochloride to the incubation medium at a concentration of 100 μg/ml, which does not stimulate LHRH release (Fig. 5).

In Vitro Static Incubations

The medium for incubation consists of KRB buffer (118 mM NaCl, 4.7 mM KCl, 2.5 mM CaCl$_2$, 1.18 mM KH$_2$PO$_4$, 1.18 mM MgSO$_4$, 25 mM NaHCO$_3$) supplemented with 0.01% BSA, 0.2% glucose, and 0.003% bacitracin (Sigma, St. Louis, MO). The KRB is gassed with 95% O$_2$/5% CO$_2$ for 10 min and the pH is adjusted to 7.4 with 1 N NaOH. A depolarizing solution, to stimulate neuropeptide release, contains a higher K$^+$ concentration in KRB with the

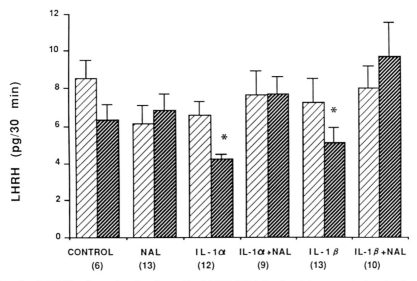

FIG. 5   LHRH release *in vitro* from the MBH-POA in short-term static incubations. Hypothalami of ovx rats, pretreated with estrogen and progesterone, were preincubated for 60 min, then basal LHRH release was assessed for 30 min (lighter bars). During the next 30 min, designated test period (darker bars), the hypothalami were incubated in KRB alone (control), naloxone hydrochloride (NAL, 100 μg/ml), IL-1α (10 nM), IL-1β (10 nM), or a combination of IL-1 and NAL. Addition of IL-1α or IL-1β significantly suppressed LHRH efflux (*$p < 0.05$ vs respective release during the basal period). Coincubation with the opoid antagonist NAL prevented this suppression. [Reproduced from Ref. 18 (Kalra *et al.*, Endogenous opioid peptides mediate the Interleukin-1-induced inhibition of the release of luteinizing hormone (LH)-releasing hormone and LH. *Endocrinology*, 1990, **127**, 2381–2386) with permission. © The Endocrine Society.]

proportion of NaCl adjusted isoosmotically (e.g., to prepare a 45 mM KCl solution, reduce NaCl from 118 to 77.7 mM); BSA, glucose, and bacitracin are added in the same concentrations as in KRB.

Rats are killed by decapitation and the brain is rapidly removed. A block of neural tissue encompassing the MBH-POA is dissected out and placed in ice-cold KRB. The MBH-POA block is bounded caudally by the mammillary bodies, laterally by the lateral sulcus, and rostrally by the rostral border of the optic chiasm. The tissue is cut to a depth of 1 mm and generally weighs 25–30 mg. The tissue is halved sagittally and the two halves placed in the well of a 24-well polystyrene tissue culture plate (Becton Dickinson) in 250 μl of KRB. The plate is incubated at 37°C in a Dubnoff metabolic shaking incubator with exposure to 95% O_2/5% CO_2 and constant shaking at 60 cycles/min. The tissue is preincubated for two 30-min periods to stabilize the rate of LHRH efflux. During this period the medium is discarded and fresh KRB is added at 30-min intervals. This is followed by a 30-min incubation period to assess basal release. Varying concentrations of IL-1α or IL-1β (1 pM to 10 nM) in KRB are added for an additional 30-min test period; control wells receive fresh KRB alone. In an initial study we serially added increasing concentrations of IL-1 for a total incubation period of 4 hr. However, this method is not recommended because LHRH release from control tissue, incubated in KRB alone, was significantly reduced after 3 hr (17). Finally, the tissue is incubated for 30 min in KRB containing 45 mM KCl to stimulate neuropeptide release as an index of tissue viability. The conditioned medium is collected every 30 min in polystyrene tubes placed in an ice-water bath. The samples are lyophilized (SpeedVac concentrator; Savant, Farmingdale, NY) and stored at -20°C until analysis of LHRH by RIA. Lyophilization eliminates the need to acidify the samples for storage and to neutralize before analysis. The amounts of LHRH released during the test period are compared to the basal amounts released during the preceding 30-min period and also to the amount released in control wells by analysis of variance (ANOVA), paired t test, or Student's t test, as appropriate.

In studies to assess the *in vitro* release of other neuropeptides (CRF and β-endorphin) we have utilized tissue slices for incubations. The MBH-POA is rapidly dissected as described above and sliced sagittally at 300 μm in a McIlwain tissue chopper (Brinkman/Mickle Instruments Co., Westbury, NY). Tissue slices from two MBH-POA are preincubated and incubated in 400 μl of KRB as described above. The conditioned medium is aliquoted (100 μl for each neuropeptide), lyophilized, and stored at -20°C until analysis of CRF, β-endorphin, and LHRH by appropriate RIAs. This procedure has the advantage of greater exposure of neural surface to test substances. Coincubating slices from two hypothalami reduces individual variability and adequate amounts of neuropeptides are released that can be easily quantitated. Thus several neuropeptides can be simultaneously measured. Tissue viability is retained as determined by stimulation of neuropeptide release by a high K^+ concentration (P. S. Kalra, unpublished results).

In Vitro Perfusion System

An alternative technique to assess neuropeptide release *in vitro* is the perfusion method, during which fresh medium is continuously pumped over the tissue (40). The basic apparatus consists of a multiple microchamber module (MMCM; Endotronics, Coon Rapids, MN), which incorporates a peristaltic pump, a solid metal block maintained at 37°C by pumping warmed water through it, and a compartment that houses six incubation chambers. Neural tissue is placed in the 0.5-ml capacity incubation chambers, which are enclosed by small circles of wire gauze at the top and bottom to restrain the tissue as the medium continuously flows through the chambers. The flow rate of the medium is controlled by precalibrating the peristaltic pump to the desired speed. As the medium is pumped through the tubing that zigzags across the heating block it is warmed and aerated before entering the bottom of the incubation chamber containing the tissue. The medium exits from the top of the incubation chamber after bathing the tissue and is collected at 5- to 10-min intervals with the aid of an automatic fraction collector. Fractions are stored at 4°C until completion of the experiment, then lyophilized and stored at −20°C until analysis.

The MBH-POA is dissected, halved sagittally, or sliced at 300 μm and placed in incubation chambers. The tubings and chambers are prefilled with Earle's balanced salt solution, pH 7.4, supplemented with 5 mM glucose, 1 mM bacitracin, and 0.1% BSA. In earlier studies (40), we incubated 6 MBH-POAs per chamber (12 halves); however, subsequent studies show that perfusion of one MBH-POA per chamber with a flow rate of 200 μl/10 min released detectable amounts of LHRH by RIA (41).

The advantage of continuous flow of the medium is that hypothalamic secretions are rapidly removed, presumably simulating the conditions of secretion *in vivo,* and release rates can be estimated at short intervals. However, this "advantage" may be a self-defeating limitation in the examination of IL-1 effects, because we suspect that IL-1 causes sequential changes in hypothalamic peptides that interact to eventually inhibit the activity of LHRH neurons. Another limitation is the considerable interchamber variability noted with the perfusion technique, necessitating inclusion of controls (tissue perfused with medium alone) in each set of six perfusions. Because only six perfusions can be performed in a day, the experimental design must be balanced to simultaneously study the different experimental and control groups. Additionally, substantial quantities of the test substances are needed for continuous perfusion of tissues for 30–60 min, which can be prohibitively expensive. Addition of test substances to the tissue is complicated by the lack of direct access to tissue because once started, the perfusion apparatus and chambers should not be opened. In contrast, the static incubation method allows direct access of test substances to tissue when medium is changed every 30 min, tissue is exposed to the test substance for an exact period, and small quantities of the test substance suffice. A comparison of the static and continuous perfusion techniques reveals that, in our hands, the former is the method of choice for investigating neuropeptide release *in vitro*.

Hormone Analyses

Luteinizing Hormone

Plasma levels of LH are measured by the double-antibody RIA technique, utilizing antiserum to rat LH prepared in rabbits and purified rLH for standards (LH RP-2) available from the National Pituitary Agency of NIADDK (National Institutes of Diabetes and Digestive and Kidney Diseases). The tracer is rat LH iodinated with ^{125}I by the chloramine-T method (purchased from Hazelton Washington, Vienna, VA). The second antibody to precipitate the antigen–antibody bound complex is rabbit anti-gamma globulin prepared in sheep. Plasma samples (25 μl) and LH standards (range, 5 to 600 pg) are brought up to 200 μl with phosphate-buffered saline (PBS; 0.1 M sodium phosphate, 0.15 M NaCl, and 0.01% merthiolate), pH 7.5, containing 1% BSA. Diluted antiserum [1 : 30,000 in PBS with 0.5 M disodium ethylenediaminetetraacetate (EDTA) and 2% normal rabbit serum (NRS)] is added (50 μl/tube) and tubes are incubated for 48 hr at 4°C. ^{125}I-Labeled LH, diluted in assay buffer to 20,000 cpm/50 μl, is added and the tubes are incubated for 24 hr at 4°C before addition of the second antibody. After an additional 24-hr incubation, the tubes are centrifuged for 30 min at 3000 rpm. The supernatant is aspirated and the pellet is counted in a γ counter. Luteinizing hormone levels in the samples are calculated by extrapolation from the standard curve following logit-log transformation. Plasma samples are analyzed in duplicate and all samples from one experiment are measured in a single assay to avoid interassay variability.

Luteinizing Hormone-Releasing Hormone

The LHRH RIA utilizes the antiserum EL-14 (supplied courtesy of Drs. M. Kelly and W. E. Ellinwood, Oregon Health Science University, Portland).

Synthetic LHRH for standards and radioiodination is purchased from Peninsula Laboratories (Belmont, CA). The LHRH is iodinated with ^{125}I, utilizing the chloramine-T method, and the tracer is purified on a QAE Sephadex A-25 (Pharmacia/LKB) column with 0.1 M borate buffer containing 0.1% gelatin. Lyophilized incubation samples are redissolved in an equivalent volume of distilled water and the volume brought up to 300 μl with PBS with 0.01% merthiolate and 1% BSA (see LH assay buffer, above). Standards (range, 0.2 to 80 pg) are similarly prepared in tubes containing lyophilized KRB. One hundred microliters of antiserum (diluted 1 : 120,000) in PBS–EDTA–2% NRS is added and the tubes incubated for 48 hr at 4°C. ^{125}I-Labeled LHRH (10,000 cpm/100 μl) is then added and the incubation continued for an additional 48 hr. Antigen–antibody bound complex is precipitated by the addition of 1.5 ml of cold 95% ethanol and centrifugation at 2400 rpm for 20 min. The supernatant is aspirated and radioactivity in the precipitate is counted in a γ counter.

The LHRH content in the whole hypothalamus, the microdissected ME-ARC, or micropunched hypothalamic nuclei can be quantitated by the same RIA. Homogenize the tissue in 0.1 N HCl, freeze, thaw, centrifuge, and discard precipitate. If protein content is to be measured, reserve an aliquot before centrifugation. The supernatant is carefully neutralized to pH 7.4–7.6 with 1 N NaOH, using a small pencil electrode for the pH meter. Centrifuge again to remove precipitated proteins, then estimate the LHRH content in aliquots of the supernatant by RIA. The LHRH concentrations are expressed in terms of either tissue weight or per unit of protein in the homogenate [measured by the Lowry method with protein estimation dye from Bio-Rad (Richmond, CA)]. The tissue levels of other neuropeptides are similarly measured with specific RIAs following acid extraction.

Steroid Hormones

The inhibition of LHRH–LH release by IL-1 *in vivo* results in reduced release of gonadal steroids. Circulating levels of estradiol (E$_2$) and P in the female and testosterone (T) in the male are quantitated by RIA following extraction of plasma with anhydrous diethyl ether for E$_2$ and T and with isooctane for P, which selectively extracts progestins and not the corticoids. The use of specific antisera (commercially available) precludes the need to isolate the steroids by column chromatography. However, if the amount of plasma sample is limited, Sephadex LH-20 column chromatography is used to purify several steroids from the same ether-extracted sample. Tritiated steroids (E. I. Du Pont-New England Nuclear, Wilmington, DE) are used as tracers and the antigen–antibody complex is separated from the free ^{3}H-labeled steroid with dextran-coated charcoal solution (42, 43). Bound radioactivity in the supernatant is counted in a liquid scintillation counter and amounts of steroid in the samples are extrapolated from the standard curve following logit-log transformation. The limit of detectability is 5 pg/tube for the steroids and 0.5–1.0 ml of plasma is extracted for estradiol; smaller amounts (0.1–0.2 ml) can be used for P and T estimations.

Summary

To assess the effects of IL-1 on the HPG axis, we employed a variety of techniques as outlined above (17–19). These results showed that the cytokine, IL-1, inhibits pituitary LH secretion in castrated male rats as well as the steroid-induced and preovulatory surges of LH in female rats. Although both IL-1α and IL-1β were potent inhibitors of LH release, the β subtype was relatively more effective. This inhibition did not occur at the level of pituitary gonadotrophs, but was due to inhibition of hypothalamic LHRH release. Additionally, our data suggested that LHRH-containing nerve terminals in the ME are not the direct targets of IL-1. Our *in vivo* and *in vitro* studies tested the possibility that IL-1 activated those intervening hypothalamic peptidergic systems that are inhibitory to LHRH. Of the two inhibitory peptidergic systems examined, our results showed that endogenous opioids and not CRF were responsible for suppression of LHRH–LH secretion and μ opioid receptors probably were engaged by the opioids released in response to IL-1.

Acknowledgments

Original work incorporated in this article was supported by a grant from the NIH (HD 11362). We are grateful to Ms. Sally McDonell for secretarial assistance and to Mr. Kenneth Quirk for technical assistance. Human recombinant IL-1α and IL-1β was generously provided by Eli Lilly Company (Indianapolis, IN).

References

1. A. Kavelaars, F. Berkenbosch, G. Croiset, R. E. Ballieux, and C. J. Heijnen, *Endocrinology* (*Amsterdam*) **26**, 759 (1990).
2. C. D. Breder, C. A. Dinarello, and C. B. Saper, *Science* **140**, 321 (1988).
3. R. M. Lechan, R. Toni, B. D. Clark, J. G. Cannon, A. R. Shar, C. A. Dinarello, and S. Reichlin, *Brain Res.* **514**, 135 (1990).

4. G. Katsuura, P. E. Gottschall, and A. Arimura, *Biochem. Biophys. Res. Commun.* **156,** 61 (1988).

5. W. L. Farrar, P. L. Kilian, M. R. Ruff, J. M. Hill, and C. B. Pert, *J. Immunol.* **139,** 459 (1987).

6. T. Takao, D. E. Tracey, W. M. Mitchell, and E. G. De Souza, *Endocrinology (Baltimore)* **127,** 3070 (1990).

7. C. E. Bandtlow, M. Meyer, D. Lindholm, M. Spranger, R. Heumann, and H. Thoenen, *J. Cell Biol.* **111,** 1701 (1990).

8. G. A. Higgins and J. A. Olschowka, *Mol. Brain Res.* **9,** 143 (1991).

9. J. I. Koenig, *Prog. NeuroEndocrinImmunol.* **4,** 143 (1991).

10. A. Bateman, A. Singh, T. Kral, and S. Solomon, *Endocr. Rev.* **10,** 92 (1989).

11. A. J. Dunn, *Progr. NeuroEndocrinImmunol.* **3,** 26 (1990).

12. S. P. Kalra and P. S. Kalra, *in* "Hormones and Gynecological Endocrinology" (A. R. Genazzani and F. Petraglia, eds.), p. 321. Parthenon Publishing Group Ltd., Park Ridge, NJ, 1992.

13. C. Rivier and W. Vale, *Endocrinology (Baltimore)* **124,** 2105 (1989).

14. C. Rivier and W. Vale, *Endocrinology (Baltimore)* **127,** 849 (1990).

15. Y.-T. Feng, E. Shalts, L. Xia, J. Rivier, C. Rivier, W. Vale, and M. Ferin, *Endocrinology (Baltimore)* **128,** 2077 (1991).

16. E. W. Bernton, J. E. Beach, J. W. Holaday, R. C. Smallridge, and H. G. Fein, *Science* **128,** 519 (1987).

17. P. S. Kalra, A. Sahu, and S. P. Kalra, *Endocrinology (Baltimore)* **126,** 2145 (1990).

18. P. S. Kalra, M. Fuentes, A. Sahu, and S. P. Kalra, *Endocrinology (Baltimore)* **127,** 2381 (1990).

19. J. J. Bonavera, S. P. Kalra, and P. S. Kalra, *Brain Res.* (in press) (1993).

20. J. D. Veldhuis and M. L. Johnson, *Am. J. Physiol.* **250,** E486 (1986).

21. G. R. Merriam and K. W. Wachter, *Am. J. Physiol.* **243,** E310 (1982).

22. J. F. Gitzen and V. D. Ramirez, *Life Sci.* **38,** 17 (1986).

23. R. V. Gallo, *Neuroendocrinology* **30,** 122 (1980).

24. J. E. Beach, R. C. Smallridge, C. A. Kinzer, E. W. Bernton, J. W. Holaday, and H. G. Fein, *Life Sci.* **44,** 1 (1989).

25. B. L. Spangelo, A. M. Judd, P. C. Isakson, and R. M. McLeod, *Endocrinology (Baltimore)* **125,** 575 (1989).

26. S. P. Kalra and P. S. Kalra, *Neuroendocrinology* **38,** 418 (1984).

27. C. A. Leadem and S. P. Kalra, *Neuroendocrinology* **41,** 342 (1985).

28. D. B. Carr, R. Bergland, A. Hamilton, H. Blume, M. Kasting, M. Arnold, J. B. Martin, and M. Rosenblatt, *Science* **217,** 845 (1982).

29. A. Kavelaars, F. Berkenbosch, G. Croiset, R. E. Ballieux, and C. J. Heijnen, *Endocrinology (Baltimore)* **126,** 759 (1990).

30. S. L. Brown, L. R. Smith, and J. E. Blalock, *J. Immunol.* **139,** 3181 (1987).

31. P. S. Portoghese, M. Sultone, and A. E. Takemori, *Life Sci.* **40,** 1287 (1987).

32. P. S. Portoghese, M. Sultone, and A. E. Takemori, *Eur. J. Pharmacol.* **146,** 185 (1988).

33. S. J. Ward, P. S. Portoghese, and A. E. Takemori, *J. Pharmacol. Exp. Ther.* **220,** 494 (1982).

34. P. G. Harms and S. R. Ojeda, *J. Appl. Physiol.* **36,** 391 (1974).

35. J. E. Levine and M. T. Dufy, *Endocrinology* **122,** 2211 (1988).
36. D. E. Dluzen and V. D. Ramirez, *J. Endocrinol.* **107,** 331 (1985).
37. J. E. Levine and K. D. Powell, *in* "Methods in Enzymology" (P. M. Conn, ed.), Vol. 168, p. 166. Academic Press, San Diego, 1989.
38. D. K. Sarkar, S. A. Chiappa, and G. Fink, *Nature (London)* **264,** 461 (1976).
39. M. Ching, *Neuroendocrinology* **34,** 279 (1982).
40. P. S. Kalra, W. R. Crowley, and S. P. Kalra, *Endocrinology (Baltimore)* **120,** 178 (1987).
41. C. P. Phelps, P. S. Kalra, and S. P. Kalra, *Brain Res.* **515,** 208 (1990).
42. P. S. Kalra and S. P. Kalra, *Acta Endocrinol. (Copenhagen)* **85,** 449 (1977).
43. P. S. Kalra and S. P. Kalra, *Endocrinology (Baltimore)* **111,** 24 (1982).

[15] Methodological Evaluation of Sites and Mechanisms of Action Involved in Neuroendocrine Effects of Cytokines

Akira Arimura and Paul E. Gottschall

Introduction

Ample evidence has accumulated suggesting the presence of a bidirectional interaction between the neuroendocrine system and immune system. Although the suppressive effects of glucocorticoid on immune function have been known for many years, more recent evidence indicates that other agents of the nervous system and neuroendocrine system may influence immune function as well. Pituitary hormones and many neuropeptides have been shown to affect the activity of the immune system. In addition, neural circuits innervate the thymus, lymph nodes, bone marrow, and spleen and may influence immune function through the effects of classic neurotransmitters. The most important recent finding in this research field may be the observation that the immune system can exert a regulatory role over the neuroendocrine system via cytokines that are elaborated from immune cells. The polypeptide cytokines, including interleukin 1 (IL-1), tumor necrosis factor (TNF), interferon, and interleukin 6 (IL-6) have been shown to alter neuroendocrine function either via the central nervous system (CNS) or through a direct action on endocrine cells. Thus the immune system may serve a sensory function for transmitting information of infection and inflammation that the sensory components of the nervous system cannot recognize (1). Furthermore, receptors for these cytokines have been demonstrated in the CNS and in endocrine tissues. Despite these advances, information regarding how the immune signal carried in the circulation by cytokines is transmitted to and affects the neuroendocrine system is still limited. This article describes selected methods for investigating the site and mechanisms of action of cytokines on the neuroendocrine system—their pitfalls and limitations as well as their advantages. The studies performed in our laboratory have emphasized the effects of IL-1 on the hypothalamic–pituitary–adrenal axis; however, the methods described in this article regarding IL-1 may also be employed for studying the effects of other cytokines on the secretion of various pituitary hormones.

Selected Methods for Determining Primary Site of Action of Blood-Borne Cytokines on Neuroendocrine Function

The most widely used method for studying the direct action of a bioactive substance on the anterior pituitary may be the technique of primary culture of rat pituitary cells. Primary monolayer culture of pituitary cells was first employed for examining the hormone-releasing or release-inhibiting effects of various hypophysiotropic factors (2). Because monolayer pituitary cell cultures consistently respond to the classic hypophysiotropic hormones with the release of or the release inhibition of the respective pituitary hormone in a dose-dependent manner, the method has been considered the most reliable, specific, and convenient bioassay for substances that affect pituitary cells by a direct action. Therefore the method has been used extensively as a tool for screening the natural and synthetic releasing or inhibiting factors that affect secretion of anterior pituitary hormones, but it has also been employed for studying cellular mechanisms such as the synthesis and secretion of hormones and processes such as cell signaling. Although there are disadvantages, this *in vitro* method is considered the most dependable tool for studying the direct action of cytokines on pituitary cells. This method was employed for studying the direct effects of IL-1 on hormone secretion from the anterior pituitary cells.

Preparation of Primary Monolayer Rat Anterior Pituitary Cell Cultures

Male Sprague-Dawley rats weighing 250–300 g (Charles River Breeding Laboratories, Wilmington, MA) are used as pituitary donors. The rats are sacrificed, the pituitaries removed, the posterior lobes removed with fine forceps, and the anterior lobes halved. The collected anterior lobe halves are washed in sterile, isotonic N-2-hydroxyethylpiperazine-N'-2-ethanesulfonic acid (HEPES) buffer and enzymatically dispersed with collagenase type II (Worthington Biochemical, Freehold, NJ) and DNase II (Sigma Chemical Co., St. Louis, MO) (2, 3). Following dispersion, a modified version of the culture and experimental protocol can be utilized (4). The cells are collected by centrifugation and washed three times by resuspension in Dulbecco's modified Eagle's medium (DMEM) supplemented with 10% horse serum, 2.5% heat-inactivated fetal calf serum, and 1% antibiotic–antimycotic solution (GIBCO-Bethesda Research Laboratories, Grand Island, NY). An aliquot of the cell suspension is counted with a hemacytometer and the remaining suspension diluted with serum-supplemented DMEM so that 1 ml of cell suspension contains a density of 1.5×10^5 cells. One-milliliter aliquots are plated in 24-well tissue culture plates (Falcon; Becton Dickinson, Oxnard, CA) and the plates incubated at 37°C in a water-saturated atmosphere of 95% air, 5% CO_2 for 3–4 days.

Prior to the experiment, the cultured anterior pituitary cells are routinely incubated for 2 hr in serum-free DMEM with two changes of the medium. The cells are then incubated for 3 hr in 0.5 ml of HEPES-buffered (25 mM) DMEM containing test materials. Ascorbic acid (2.5 × 10^{-4} M) and 0.25% bovine serum albumin (BSA) are added to the medium during assay incubation in order to prevent possible oxidation and adsorption of the test samples, respectively. At the end of each test incubation period, the medium is collected separately from each well and used immediately (or frozen at −70°C) for adrenocorticotropic hormone (ACTH) determination by radioimmunoassay, because of the relative instability of ACTH. The medium can be stored at −20°C until assayed for other pituitary hormones. The viability of the cells following completion of the experimental protocol is consistently greater than 95%, as determined by trypan blue exclusion (5).

Direct Effect of Cytokines on Anterior Pituitary Hormone Secretion

Numerous *in vitro* studies have been carried out to address whether cytokines directly stimulate the secretion of ACTH and other hormones. However, the results are confusing and seem to vary from laboratory to laboratory. The original and most provocative report was that murine interleukin 1 (IL-1), a cytokine produced by activated monocytes and other cells, stimulated ACTH release from mouse ACTH-secreting pituitary tumor cells (AtT-20) (6), suggesting that IL-1 may be a tissue corticotropin-releasing factor (CRF), a hypothesis originally proposed by Brodish (7). If IL-1 is indeed a tissue CRF, IL-1 should stimulate ACTH release not only from the AtT-20 cell line, but also from primary cultures of rat pituitary cells. In our laboratory, however, neither human recombinant IL-1α nor IL-1β (obtained from Immunex Corp., Seattle, WA; 1 × 10^8 thymocyte mitogenesis U/mg protein) at concentrations ranging from 0.01 to 10 nM stimulated ACTH release in the *in vitro* rat pituitary assay system (2, 3). Adrenocorticotropic hormone release was slightly, yet significantly, increased by 100 nM IL-1β, but not by IL-1α at the same concentration. Synthetic CRF increased ACTH release in a dose-dependent manner at concentrations ranging from 0.001 to 1 nM (Fig. 1). As shown in Table I, IL-1β failed to alter the secretion of any other pituitary hormones, including growth hormone (GH), prolactin, follicle-stimulating hormone (FSH), and luteinizing hormone (LH). Two other laboratories also reported that IL-1 had no effect on ACTH secretion in primary culture of rat pituitary cells (8, 9).

A controversial report on the direct action of IL-1 on pituitary cells came

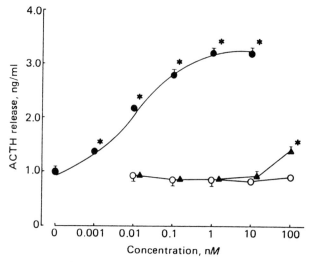

FIG. 1   Dose–response effects of synthetic rat hypothalamic CRF (●), recombinant human IL-1α (○), and IL-1β (▲) on ACTH release in monolayer male rat pituitary cell culture during a 3-hr incubation period. Each point represents the mean ± SEM of four replicate cultures. *$p < 0.01$ compared to basal levels. [Reproduced from Uehara *et al.* (3) with permission from S. Karger AG, Basel.]

TABLE I   Effects of IL-1α and IL-1β on Secretion of Growth Hormone, Prolactin, Follicle-Stimulating Hormone, and Luteinizing Hormone from Male Rat Pituitary Cells in Primary Culture[a]

Concentration (nM)	GH release (ng/ml)	PRL release (ng/ml)	FSH release (ng/ml)	LH release (ng/ml)
Control	438 ± 13	1472 ± 55	14.6 ± 1.6	23.7 ± 0.2
IL-1α				
0.01	428 ± 38	1513 ± 65	13.6 ± 0.8	24.5 ± 1.6
0.10	425 ± 25	1454 ± 39	13.1 ± 0.5	24.4 ± 0.5
1.00	398 ± 16	1398 ± 39	14.8 ± 1.5	22.3 ± 0.9
10.00	458 ± 33	1453 ± 31	13.8 ± 1.1	21.9 ± 1.3
100.00	485 ± 29	1525 ± 31	12.1 ± 1.1	24.8 ± 1.0
IL-1β				
0.01	418 ± 24	1457 ± 63	14.2 ± 1.0	23.9 ± 1.1
0.10	445 ± 31	1520 ± 60	14.4 ± 1.4	24.8 ± 1.3
1.00	492 ± 38	1540 ± 48	12.1 ± 0.8	23.6 ± 1.3
10.00	470 ± 31	1519 ± 25	11.0 ± 0.4	23.8 ± 2.1
100.00	499 ± 48	1560 ± 72	13.8 ± 0.5	23.5 ± 1.0

[a] All incubations were carried out for 3 hr. Each value represents the mean ± SEM of four replicate cultures. [Reproduced from Uehara *et al.* (3) with permission from S. Karger AG, Basel.]

from Bernton and colleagues (10). These authors reported, using monolayer culture of female rat pituitary cells, that recombinant human IL-1β stimulated the secretion of ACTH, LH, GH and thyroid-stimulating hormone (TSH). Increased hormone secretion into culture supernatants was found with IL-1 concentrations ranging from 10^{-12} to 10^{-9} M. Prolactin secretion by the monolayers was inhibited by similar doses of IL-1. Because these concentrations of IL-1 are within the range reported for IL-1 in serum, it was suggested that IL-1 generated peripherally by mononuclear immune cells may act directly on the anterior pituitary to modulate hormone secretion in $vivo$. That these changes in pituitary hormone secretion were indeed due to IL-1 itself was supported by the abolishment of these effects after incubation of the IL-1 with an antibody raised against human recombinant IL-1. The discordance of these results obtained by different laboratories, which used similar in $vitro$ methods, cannot be immediately explained. Nevertheless, apparently minor differences in experimental procedures and IL-1 preparations might yield different results. Differences in the sex of the donor animals, the strain of rats, the culture conditions (including the isolation protocol and the concentrations of fetal calf serum, which contains a significant amount of estrogen), and the duration of cytokine exposure might affect the responsiveness of the pituitary cells. However, in most of the experiments described above, the cultured pituitary cells responded appropriately to the physiological releasing factors with the secretion of the respective pituitary hormones. Therefore, a factor that is likely to yield discordant results might be the different cytokine preparations used by different laboratories. Even though the cytokine used by different investigators is provided from the same source, it is possible that different lots of the recombinant preparations have varying degrees of contamination with endotoxin. It is also possible that the effect of endotoxin is enhanced in the presence of cytokine. Thus, abolishment of the hormone-releasing activity of the cytokine after incubation with antibody may not necessarily serve as undisputed evidence that the effect is indeed due to the cytokine itself. If the stimulatory effect found in $vitro$ is indeed the result of a direct action of the cytokine, its injection would also stimulate the release of the pituitary hormone in rats in which the release of endogenous releasing hormones is pharmacologically (11) or surgically blocked (12) or in which the activity of the endogenous releasing hormones is nullified by immunoneutralization (8, 13). It should be noted that primary cell culture with rat anterior pituitary cells is a sensitive and specific method for investigating the secretion of pituitary hormones, but the cultured pituitary cells are vulnerable to toxic substances, which may result in the release or leak of hormones into the culture medium. Extracts of tissues other than the hypothalamus, such as stomach, elicit ACTH release when tested in primary cultures of rat pituitary cells (14). However, the greatest CRF activity purified from the extracts shown in $vitro$ could not be demonstrated in $vivo$ with pharmacologically blocked rats (14), although these pharmacologically blocked rats did respond to synthetic CRF. If IL-1 releases multiple hormones through direct action on the pituitary (10), secretion of these multiple hormones should also increase *in vivo* in animals in which the release of endogenous releasing hormones is suppressed or their actions nullified by an antiserum or an antagonist. Therefore the releasing activity demonstrated *in vitro* with monolayers of pituitary cells must be reconfirmed in *in vivo* experiments, before a decisive conclusion is drawn.

In our laboratory and others, IL-1-induced ACTH release *in vivo* has been completely or considerably suppressed by immunoneutralization of endogenous CRF by administration of CRF antiserum to the animals prior to IL-1 injection (8, 13). Because the IL-1 preparation used in these experiments failed to alter the release of pituitary hormones *in vitro,* these results support the view that the primary site of action of IL-1 on acute ACTH release is in the brain, and not directly on the pituitary.

In Vivo Method for Studying Site and Mechanism of Action of Cytokines on Neuroendocrine Function

For studying the physiological action of cytokines on the neuroendocrine system, it is recommended that conscious and freely moving animals be used, because anesthetics clearly interfere with neural transmission in the brain. Administration of cytokines as well as sampling blood for determination of circulating pituitary hormones must be made without stressing the animals. Accordingly, the animals are implanted with an indwelling venous catheter for injection of the test substances or collecting blood. In our laboratory, young adult, male CD rats, 280–300 g in body weight (Charles River Breeding Laboratories), are routinely used. They are housed at a constant room temperature of 23°C with a 12-hr light–dark cycle (lights on at 06:00 hr). Food and water are available *ad libitum*. It is recommended that all experiments be conducted at around the same time of the day. Our experiments are conducted between 0900 and 1200 hr for studying the hypothalamic–pituitary–adrenal axis.

When studying the effect of cytokines on GH secretion, it is recommended that samples of blood be drawn frequently over an extended period because of the nature of spontaneous pulsatile secretion of GH. GH response to a GH-releasing stimulator is greater during the peak than the trough of circulating GH levels. Furthermore, it is important to establish a dose–response relationship. Growth hormone secretion is controlled by GH-releasing factor (GRF) and somatostatin, which inhibits the secretion. It is possible that cytokines influence the secretion of both hypothalamic peptides, but the threshold may vary, resulting in varying effects on GH release depending on the dosage.

An indwelling catheter filled with heparin solution (50 U/ml in saline) (Silastic tubing, i.d. 0.6 mm, o.d. 1.2 mm; Dow Corning, Midland, MI) can be implanted into the jugular vein so that the tip of the catheter enters the right atrium. In our laboratory, this procedure is carried out under ether anesthesia 1 day before the experimental procedures. After surgical implantation, rats are housed individually. Otherwise, the rats will bite each other's cannula tubing. On the day of the experiment, a tubing extension with syringe is attached to the catheter, and cages are placed in a quiet room for 2 hr to allow animals to adapt to these conditions. Test samples are injected intravenously (iv) through the intraatrial cannula, and blood samples (1.0 ml) are withdrawn into heparinized syringes from the same cannula at the appropriate times following the injection of each sample. Blood samples are centrifuged, and plasma is separated for hormone determination. The red blood cells are resuspended in physiological saline and returned to each animal before the withdrawal of the next sample in order to maintain the blood volume (3, 13, 15). Excessive blood loss results in elevated levels of ACTH and IL-6 levels (G. Komaki *et al.*, unpublished observations).

Using this animal preparation, the temporal pattern of plasma ACTH levels was determined after iv injection of IL-1 (16). As shown in Fig. 2 (16), iv injection of IL-1β increased plasma ACTH levels in a dose-dependent manner. The peak levels were observed 10 min postinjection of IL-1β at a dose of 100 or 1000 ng/100 g of body weight. At 60, 120, and 180 min, plasma ACTH fell to levels that were not different from the corresponding control values.

Whether IL-1-induced ACTH release is mediated by hypothalamic CRF can be examined by immunoneutralization of endogenous CRF by a CRF antibody. Five hundred microliters of the undiluted rabbit antiserum or an equivalent purified IgG against CRF is injected iv through the implanted atrial catheter, and then IL-1 is injected iv 30 min later. Figure 3 shows the temporal pattern of blood ACTH levels after iv IL-1, which was injected 30 min after iv injection of normal rabbit serum or anti-CRF serum. Preinjection of 0.5 ml of anti-CRF serum completely prevented IL-1-induced ACTH release (13). A similar finding was also reported by other laboratories (9).

The effect of cytokines on the secretion of other pituitary hormones has been studied in several laboratories (see other chapters in this volume, [24], [26], and [27]), but the results are conflicting (17). Whether altered hormone secretion after administration of cytokine is mediated by the respective releasing or inhibiting hormone may be examined in a similar design, using an antiserum to the respective hypothalamic hypophysiotropic hormone.

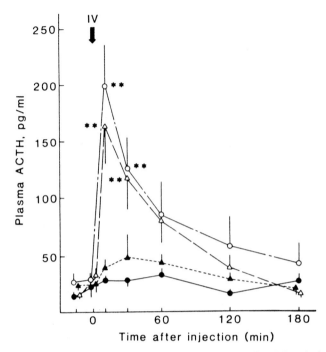

Fig. 2   Effect of iv administration of IL-1β on plasma ACTH levels in conscious rats. Arrow indicates the time of iv administration of IL-1β or saline solution (0.5 ml/rat). The number of rats used is indicated in parentheses: ●, saline (9); ▲, IL-1β, 10 ng/100 g (8); △, IL-1β, 100 ng/100 g (8); ○, IL-1β, 1000 ng/100 g (8). Each point represents the mean ± SEM. **$p < 0.01$ compared to saline-injected control values. [Reproduced from Ref. 16 (G. Katsuura, P. E. Gottschall, R. R. Dahl, and A. Arimura, *Endocrinology*, 1988, **122**, 1773) with permission. © The Endocrine Society.]

Microinjection of Cytokines into Cerebroventricle or a Specific Area in Brain

If the primary site of action of cytokines for anterior pituitary hormone secretion is in the brain, then central administration of the cytokine should be more effective than systemic administration. Therefore a smaller dose of cytokine, which does not alter pituitary hormone secretion when injected iv or intraperitoneally (ip), may induce a significant response when injected into the cerebroventricle or in a critical site in the brain. Although experiments can be conducted in conscious animals, the central administration of cytokines must be made with a minimum of stress to the animals.

In our laboratory, the rat is placed on a stereotaxic instrument (David Kopf Instruments, Tujunga, CA) under sodium pentobarbital anesthesia (50

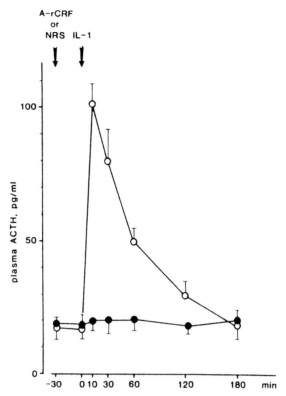

FIG. 3   Effect of immunoneutralization of endogenous CRF on the elevation of plasma ACTH levels induced by IL-1β. ○, NRS plus IL-1β; ●, A-rCRF plus IL-1β. Each point represents the mean ± SEM of ACTH determination from six animals. NRS, Normal rabbit serum; A-rCRF, rabbit antiserum against rat CRF. [Reproduced from Ref. 13 (A. Uehara, P. E. Gottschall, R. R. Dahl, and A. Arimura, *Endocrinology*, 1987, **121**, 1581) with permission. © The Endocrine Society.]

mg/kg body weight, ip). The incisor bar is adjusted until the height of lambda and bregma skull points are equal. The flat-skull position is achieved when the incisor bar is lowered 3 mm below horizontal zero. Stereotaxic coordinates are determined in preliminary studies according to the atlas of Paxinos and Watson (18). The anterior (A), lateral (L), and ventral (V) coordinates are measured from the interaural, midline, and skull surface, respectively. A stainless steel guide cannula (27 gauge; Plastics One, Roanoke, VA), 15 mm in length with a guard ring outside the guide cannula 2 mm from the bottom tip, is implanted on the skull surface and secured in place with dental cement at an appropriate position according to the stereotaxic coordinates. The bottom tip of the guide cannula is thus located 2 mm below the skull surface and does not penetrate the dura mater. Animals are allowed a 7-day postsurgery recovery period and are handled daily for the 3 days before the experiment. Further experimental procedures, such as implantation of an intraatrium catheter, are performed the day before the experiment. For intracerebroventricular (icv) injection, an injection cannula (30 gauge) is connected with a Hamilton microsyringe by polyethylene tubing (PE-20) at the point 13 mm plus the ventral coordinate for a desired area from the bottom tip so that the end of the polyethylene tubing is seated at the top of the guide cannula when inserted in the brain. The injection cannula is inserted through the guide cannula to place the tip in the desired area and a 5-μl (for icv) or 1-μl (for a specific area of brain tissue) sample in 0.9% saline is injected over 10 sec while the conscious animals are gently held. The cannula is held in place for 5 to 10 more seconds and is slowly removed. This procedure in itself is not stressful to the animals, that is, it does not increase circulating ACTH. However, it is recommended that it be assured whether saline injection alone does not increase blood ACTH levels. This animal preparation is useful for studying not only the central site of action of cytokines, but also for investigating the neurotransmitter systems that are involved in the transmission of the neuronal signal(s) elicited by circulating cytokines.

Figures 2 and 4 show representative plasma ACTH responses after iv or icv injection, respectively, of human recombinant IL-1β in conscious rats (16). Neither iv nor icv injection of 0.9% saline altered plasma ACTH levels. Because different preparations of cytokines have various specific bioactivities, the dosage should be stated as units per kilogram, or the specific activity of the recombinant preparation should be stated. The human recombinant preparation of IL-1β used in our laboratory for most of the experiments described here (unless otherwise stated) was obtained from Cistron (Pine Brook, NJ) and has a specific activity in excess of 10^6 thymocyte mitogenesis units/mg protein. Today, human recombinant preparations are often nearly 100-fold more potent. Intracerebroventricular injection of 3 ng of IL-1β significantly increased plasma ACTH levels. Even 0.3 ng of cytokine tended to increase plasma ACTH. On the other hand, 100 ng/100 g body weight of the cytokine was required for a significant increase in plasma ACTH levels when injected iv. Intravenous injection of 1000 ng/100 g IL-1β induced a maximal response with a pronounced elevation of plasma ACTH levels at 10 and 30 min after injection, but plasma ACTH levels fell at 60 min postinjection. Injection of 30 ng of IL-1β icv raised plasma ACTH levels at 10 min, reaching peak values between 30 and 60 min postinjection, and plasma ACTH levels remained elevated for 2–3 hr after injection. In this experiment, pretreatment with indomethacin, a cyclooxygenase inhibitor, completely prevented the ACTH response induced by either iv or icv injection of IL-1β, suggesting that the metabolites of arachidonic acid generated by cyclooxygenase, possibly prostaglandins, play a key role in transmission of the im-

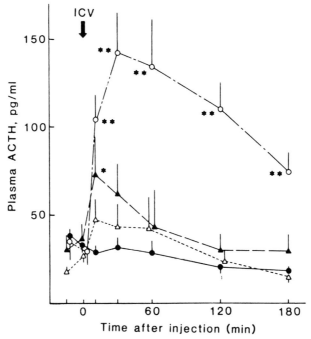

FIG. 4   Effect of icv administration of IL-1β on plasma ACTH levels in normal rats. Arrow indicates the time of icv administration of IL-1β or saline solution (5 μl/rat). The number of rats used is indicated in parentheses: ●, saline (12); △, IL-1β, 0.3 ng (8); ▲, IL-1β, 3 ng (8); ○, IL-1β, 30 ng (8). Each point represents the mean ± SEM. **p<0.01 compared to saline-injected control.   [Reproduced from Ref. 16 (G. Katsuura, P. E. Gottschall, R. R. Dahl, and A. Arimura, *Endocrinology*, 1988, **122**, 1773) with permission. © The Endocrine Society.]

mune signal to the ACTH-releasing element, possibly CRF neurons. Indomethacin failed to prevent the ACTH response to immobilization stress (15). Because IL-1β was considerably more potent in stimulating ACTH release when injected icv compared to iv, it strongly suggests that the brain is the primary site of action of IL-1β.

In Vivo Method for Studying Critical Sites in Brain for Cytokine-Induced ACTH Release

Discrete areas in the brain through which immune signals are transduced and transmitted to CRF neurons in the paraventricular nucleus (PVN) can also be investigated in conscious animals with similar animal preparations as described in the preceding section. Although the site or sites of entry of blood-borne cytokines into the brain is still in dispute, it was suggested that the circulating cytokines would enter the brain through the site where the blood–brain barrier is absent, such as circumventricular organs, including the organum vasculosum of the lamina terminalis (OVLT), subfornical organ (SFO), median eminence, pineal body, and area postrema. The febrile response to systemic injection of pyrogen was altered by placement of lesions in the anteroventral area of the third ventricle and the OVLT (19, 20). Brain lesions can be made with a radio-frequency generator (Becton-Dickinson, Rutherfold, NJ). Current (2 mA) is passed through a single electrode (26 gauge) with a 0.2-mm noninsulated tip that is stereotaxically placed into the target area of the brain. The duration of passage of current should be adjusted so that an appropriate size of lesion is made. It is convenient to test the current conditions beforehand, using freshly prepared egg white, directly inspecting the extent of coagulation of the egg white with different current durations. For example, a 20-sec current duration was used for OVLT and SFO lesions and a 10-sec current duration was used for bilateral preoptic area lesions. The reference electrode is placed into an area of subcutaneous tissue in the nucchal area. In sham-operated rats, the electrode is inserted into the area for the same period of time without passage of current.

Destruction of neurons can also be achieved by microinjection of kainic acid (21). For instance, rats are placed on the stereotaxic instrument under pentobarbital anesthesia and kainic acid (0.3 or 3 μg) in 1 μl of 0.9% saline is slowly injected into the desired area, such as the OVLT, or 0.5 μl is injected into the preoptic area (POA) bilaterally (15). Microinjection is made via an injection cannula (30 gauge) connected to a Hamilton microsyringe by polyethylene tubing (PE-20).

Experiments may be performed 1–3 weeks after placement of the lesion by radio-frequency current or kainic acid microinjection. The site and size of the lesioned area are verified by standard histological techniques. After the experiment, the brain is fixed, and cut at 50 μm on a cryotome, and sections are mounted serially and stained with cresyl violet. To demonstrate the area of diffusion of the 1-μl solution that was injected, 1 μl of horseradish peroxidase is injected through the needle, and the section is stained by diaminobenzidine (Sigma Chemical) and counterstained by cresyl violet. The control sham-operated animals that have been injected with saline in the same regions may have a similar needle track and area of diffusion of the solution. In contrast to radio-frequency-induced lesions, the extent of a kainic acid lesion is not defined by a region of actual tissue ablation.

Although experiments involving placement lesions in the brain of animals yield interesting results, their interpretation may not always be made with ease. Radio-frequency-induced lesions damage all tissues, including neurons, astroglia, and blood vessels, the latter two tissues regenerating during the postlesion period. Permeability of the vascular wall may be altered after the lesion, temporarily destroying the blood–brain barrier (22) and allowing substances in the circulation to reach the brain readily. The state of increased vascular permeability persists for 19 days and then returns to normal (22). Although damaged neurons do not regenerate, astroglia proliferate to repair the damaged tissues. It is known that astrocytes are the target cells for IL-1, and IL-1 has been shown to stimulate proliferation of astroglia (23), induce the synthesis and release of prostaglandin (24), and stimulate the production of IL-6 (25–27). Kainic acid destroys neuronal cell bodies, but not neuronal fibers. It also stimulates proliferation of astroglia that lasts for 27 days (28). In our laboratories, placement of a lesion in the OVLT of rats by radio frequency or kainic acid resulted in an enhanced ACTH response to IL-1β iv 1 week after lesion. Three weeks after lesion, the ACTH response to IL-1β iv returned to normal in rats that underwent radio-frequency-induced lesion, but remained enhanced in those that received microinjection of kainic acid (15). These findings suggested that neuronal cell structures, both cell bodies and fibers, in the OVLT may not be required for an IL-1-induced ACTH response because, although radio frequency destroyed these neuronal structures, the ACTH response remained augmented 1 week after the lesion. These findings support the possibility that IL-1β acts on nonneuronal components, probably astrocytes, in the OVLT, and astrocytes that had proliferated in response to the lesion release a larger amount of a mediator resulting in an enhancement of ACTH release. Unlike the OVLT, placement of a lesion in the POA either by radiofrequency or kainic acid suppressed the ACTH response to IL-1β iv (15). The decreased response that followed POA lesion suggested that the neuronal elements essential for the ACTH response to IL-1β had been destroyed. In other words, the neuronal structures in the POA, especially kainic acid-sensitive cell bodies, may play a critical role in the transmission of the immune signal to CRF neurons (15).

It is known that astrocytes synthesize and release prostaglandins, an effect that is possibly mediated by IL-1 (24, 29). We have shown that IL-1β stimulates release of prostaglandin E_2 (PGE$_2$) from rat astrocyte cultures but not from neuron cultures (24). Whether PGE$_2$ production in the OVLT stimulated by blood-borne IL-1β plays a critical role in transmission of the immune signal to the CRF neurons was investigated by microinjection of indomethacin into the OVLT. Microinjection of indomethacin indeed significantly suppressed the ACTH response to IL-1β iv, compared with the rats injected with saline in the same region of the brain (15). Because the POA is located in close proximity to the OVLT, we speculated that prostaglandins diffused or were transported through an interstitial channel to the POA from the OVLT. The wide spaces, not found elsewhere in the brain, that surround the capillaries in the OVLT and other circumventricular organs may be a specialized "pool" for the mixing and rapid interstitial distribution of chemical substances such as prostaglandins. It was reported that although ion concentrations in the brain cell microenvironment of interstitial fluid may be viewed as stable over long periods of time, neuronal function is associated with short-term variations in interstitial fluid composition (30). There are also changes in the concentrations of other chemical components, including classic neurotransmitters, prostaglandins, peptides, and others (30). Evidence is now accumulating that these dynamic variations are not "noise" but that they represent meaningful signals to neighboring neurons and glial cells (30). Accordingly, immune signals may be carried to neighboring cells, such as from the OVLT to the POA, or even over longer distances by prostaglandins circulating within the isolated milieu of the brain behind the blood–brain–barrier. It is possible that the neurons in the POA respond directly to prostaglandins or indirectly via classic neurotransmitter interneurons. Microinjection of prostaglandins, in particular PGE_2, into the POA induced ACTH release. Furthermore, a prostaglandin antagonist (SC-19220, at 1 μg/ml; G. D. Searle, Skokie, IL) microinjected into the POA completely blocked the ACTH response to IL-1β iv in rats (15). These findings may substantiate the view that the target cells for PGE_2 involved in IL-1-induced ACTH release are present in the POA.

Microinjection of antagonists or neurotransmitter synthesis inhibitors into discrete areas of the brain can be used for studying the involvement of these neurotransmitters and their target neurons in the transmission of circulating immune signals to various neuroendocrine cells in the brain. It is generally accepted that central monoaminergic systems play an important role in the regulation of CRF and ACTH secretion, although the specific role of individual aminergic systems has remained somewhat controversial (31–34). It was suggested that both noradrenergic and adrenergic systems are important for CRF release (34). If catecholaminergic pathways are indeed essential for transmission of immune signals to CRF neurons in the PVN, depletion of catecholamines by inhibiting its synthesis in the critical area of the brain may suppress or abolish IL-1-induced ACTH release. This possibility is discussed in article 12 by Dunn in Vol. 17.

Microperfusion Methods for Determining Neurotransmitters in Discrete Areas of Brain Involved in Transmission of Immune Signals

Direct evidence for stimulation of the release of prostaglandins and other neurotransmitters in a discrete area of the brain following IL-1 iv can be determined in conscious rats by a microdialysis technique (35–37) or a push–pull method (38, 39). In particular, the microdialysis approach is rapidly gaining recognition as a powerful tool for measuring neurotransmitter release in specific brain areas. A probe that mimicks the function of blood capillaries is used to "eavesdrop" on the activities of cells. The probe consists of a thin steel shaft connected to a semipermeable membrane. As fluid is continuously pumped through the probe, low molecular weight compounds (depending on the permeability cut-off) flow through the semipermeable membrane from the extracellular space according to their concentration gradients. Aliquots of the effluent are collected in tubes by a fraction collector. Neurotransmitter (or other agents) release can then be quantitatively determined in the perfusate/dialysates to give an estimate of its original concentration in the extracellular fluid, provided that the relative exchange rate is known. Conversely, a substance added to the perfusate flows into the extracellular fluid along its particular concentration gradient.

The microdialysis probe used in our laboratories is illustrated in Fig. 5. One end of a 1-cm piece of acetate cellulose dialysis tubing (200-μm o.d., 180-μm i.d., minimal molecular weight cut-off of 50,000) is sealed with epoxy resin (40, 41). Fused silica tubing is used for both the inlet and outlet lines (inlet, 150-μm o.d., 30-μm i.d.; outlet, 150-μm o.d., 50-μm i.d.). The inlet line is inserted into the dialysis tubing and placed alongside the outlet line

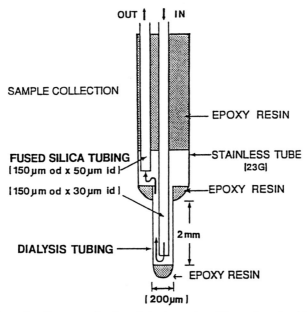

FIG. 5 Schematic diagram of microdialysis probe. [Reproduced with permission from Komaki *et al.* (40).]

in a thin-walled 23-gauge stainless steel tube (1.5 cm) so that approximately 2 mm of the dialysis membrane is exposed. Both ends of the 23-gauge steel tubing are sealed with epoxy resin. On the day of the experiment, the inlet line is connected with a 57-cm length of fused silica tubing (150-μm o.d., 75-μm i.d.) which extends to a gas-tight Hamilton syringe (1 ml) in the microinfusion pump (CMA/100; Carnegie Medicine AB, Stockholm, Sweden). The outlet line is connected with 57 cm of polyethylene tubing (PE-10) for sample collection. Individual rats are implanted with an indwelling jugular catheter as described above, and placed in a stereotaxic instrument (David Kopf Instruments). The skull is exposed and a small hole is drilled to implant the microdialysis probe into the desired brain area, following the coordinates in the rat brain atlas of Paxinos and Watson (18). The dialysis probe is lowered through the hole in the skull. Seven to eight minutes is taken for lowering the probe 1 mm into the site to minimize the damage to the brain induced by the probe. If the probe must be advanced into the pituitary gland through the dura for collecting hypophysiotropic hormones transported through the hypophysial portal veins from the median eminence, a probe specially designed to protect the vulnerable tip by a tungsten wire should be used (42). The dialysis device is fixed with dental cement to a screw on the skull. After surgery, animals are housed in individual cages. Twenty to 24 hr after surgery, the inlet and outlet tubings of the probe are connected for infusion and sampling, respectively. A saline-filled silicone tubing extension is also connected to the implanted jugular vein catheter, so that the rat can move freely in the cage. The dialysis probe is perfused with artificial cerebrospinal fluid (CSF) (124 mM NaCl, 5 mM KCl, 25 mM NaHCO$_3$, 5 mM D-glucose, 2 mM CaCl$_2$, pH 7.4), containing 0.5% bovine serum albumin.

The perfusion rate is determined beforehand by immersing the probe into the solution of a known concentration of the substance of interest to determine the flow rate that results in the largest quantitative recovery of the substance in the perfusate/dialysate. The recovery rate for PGE$_2$ *in vitro* is defined as the percentage of the ratio between the concentration of PGE$_2$ in the perfusate and the concentration of PGE$_2$ in the solution in which the probe was immersed. In our laboratory, for PGE$_2$, the recovery varied depending on the flow rate, ranging from 1.34% for a flow rate of 4.8 μl/min to 5.54% for a flow rate of 1.2 μl/min. Recovery of PGE$_2$ at any flow rate was not altered by different concentrations of PGE$_2$ in the external solution. Generally, the slower the flow rate, the greater the recovery of PGE$_2$ in the perfusate (40). Therefore, for determining PGE$_2$ in the extracellular fluid, the perfusion was initiated at a constant flow rate of 1.2 μl/min.

Two hours after the initiation of perfusion, the perfusate was collected every 20 min into tubes in a fraction collector maintained at 4°C, and the samples were immediately stored at -80°C until assayed for PGE$_2$ by commercial kit radioimmunoassay. After collecting three 20-min fractions for determining the basal concentration of PGE_2, recombinant human IL-1β (Otsuka Pharmaceutical Corp., Tokushima, Japan; 2×10^7 U/mg protein) was injected iv. Twenty-minute fractions of perfusate were collected for an additional 260 min. To examine the effect of indomethacin on prostaglandin E_2 release from specific loci, such as the OVLT or the PVN, artificial CSF containing indomethacin (1 mM) was perfused through the dialysis tubing from 10 min before to 180 min after IL-1β injection. On completion of the experiment, animals were anesthetized with pentobarbital and perfused with saline via the ascending aorta followed by 10% formaldehyde for fixation of the tissue. The location of dialysis probe was verified histologically in 50-μm coronal brain sections stained with cresyl violet.

The mean basal levels of PGE_2 in various areas of the rat brain determined by microdialysis at our laboratories after correction for recovery were as follows: OVLT, 0.51 ± 0.04; medial POA, 0.48 ± 0.05; PVN, 0.35 ± 0.05; hippocampus, 0.33 ± 0.03; CSF in lateral ventricle, 0.24 ± 0.03 ng/ml (40). In this study, injection of IL-1β iv induced a significant increase in PGE_2 levels in all the areas examined. Prostaglandin E_2 levels in the OVLT and the medial part of the medial POA increased in the first 20 min, an effect that was more rapid and of greater magnitude compared to the PGE_2 response in the PVN, hippocampus, or CSF. Furthermore, inclusion of indomethacin in the perfusate abolished the IL-1β-induced PGE_2 response in the OVLT, but the suppressive effect in the PVN was not statistically significant. Representative data of PGE_2 levels in OVLT are illustrated in Fig. 6. These findings suggest that the OVLT is a site where the initial biochemical response to blood-borne IL-1β occurs, resulting in activation of cyclooxygenase. Increased concentrations of PGE_2 in the PVN, hippocampus, and CSF after IL-1β iv may at least partly be due to PGE_2 that diffused from or was transported from other areas of the brain (40). The microdialysis method is a powerful tool for *in vivo* determinations not only of prostaglandins, but also of other neurotransmitters in specific loci in the brain.

The push–pull perfusion device originally developed by Gaddum (39) may have an advantage in terms of recovery of the substances from the extracellular fluid, especially when the molecular size or property of the compounds does not permit rapid diffusion of the molecule across the semipermeable membrane of the microdialysis probe. Using this method, a specific area of the brain is directly perfused and the same amount of interstitial fluid in the perfused area is withdrawn for the quantitative determination of substances. However, the push–pull method has serious problems, such as extreme pressure changes leading to flow obstructions and tissue damage. Pressure changes caused by tissue resistance leads to the accumulation of liquid or to erosion in the perfused region and, therefore, the success of a perfusion

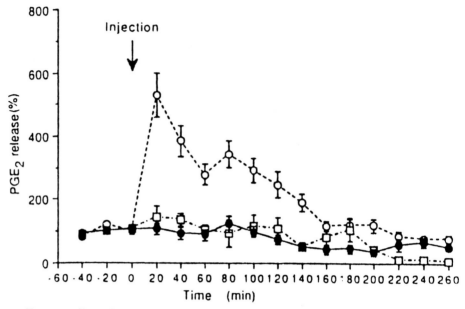

FIG. 6   Effect of IL-1β on PGE$_2$ release in OVLT perfused with artificial cerebrospinal fluid with or without indomethacin (Idm, 1 mM). Replacement solution containing Idm started 10 min before and ended at 180 min after the IL-1β injection. Arrow indicates the time of iv injection of IL-1β or saline solution. The number of rats used is indicated in parentheses: ○, IL-1β (5); □, Idm plus IL-1β (5); ●, saline (4). Each point represents the mean ± SEM and values are expressed as a percentage of respective basal PGE$_2$ levels (average of three fractions collected before injection). [Reproduced with permission from Komaki *et al.* (40).]

system lies largely in maintaining a constant pressure in the tissue. This requirement is not fulfilled by systems in which precision delivery and withdrawal mechanisms are matched to force a constant flow through a closed circulation path, because unbuffered pressure changes result from the changing resistance of the tissue, such as swelling. These problems have been discussed elsewhere (43, 44).

In Vivo Method for Determining Hypothalamic Hypophysiotropic Hormones in Hypophysial Portal Blood

The effect of cytokines on the release of hypophysiotropic hormones can be investigated *in vivo* by determining respective releasing or inhibiting hormone levels in the hypophysial portal blood. The original technique for collecting the hypophysial portal blood was described by Porter (45), and modified by other investigators, including us (46). In our laboratory, adult male rats of the CD strain (Charles River Breeding Laboratories), weighing 300–400 g, are anesthetized with urethane (150 mg/100 g body weight, ip). Each animal is secured in the supine position on an operating board, and the ventral surfaces of the hypothalamus and anterior pituitary are exposed by the parapharyngeal approach as described by Porter (45). Then 2 mg of sodium heparin is administered iv and, throughout the remaining period of the experiment, physiological saline containing sodium heparin (1 mg/ml) is infused into the jugular vein at a rate of 0.02 ml/min. Following the parapharyngeal surgery, the pituitary stalk is cut at the point closest to the junction with the pituitary gland, and then the pituitary is removed from the fossa. About 30 min after hypophysectomy, PE-60 polyethylene tubing (0.03-in. i.d.) held by a micromanipulator is placed over the stump of the pituitary stalk. The hypophysial portal blood is collected through the tubing in a microfraction collector (46) with a negative pressure by a Harvard withdrawal pump (Dover, MA). The microfraction collector is held in the arm of a metallic container, which is filled with dry ice so that the fraction collector is kept cold throughout the experiment. The space surrounding the glass vials (6 × 50 mm; Kimble Products Division, Owens-Illinois, Inc., Toledo, OH) in the collector is reduced by adding saturated sodium chloride solution, which also serves as an antifreeze. The PE-100 polyethylene tubing filled with saturated saline is immersed in the sodium chloride solution in the air-tight microfraction collector and the other end is connected to the withdrawal pump. The portal blood is collected directly into glass vials containing 0.5 ml of 2 N acetic acid through the PE-60 polyethylene tubing, when somatostatin in the blood is determined. The acidified whole blood is extracted twice with 80% acetone, followed by washing with organic solvent, which consists of ethyl acetate and anhydrous ether (3 : 1, v/v). The aqueous layer is evaporated by nitrogen gas flow and kept at −20°C until assayed for somatostatin. The recovery of added somatostatin after extraction averaged 83%. The volume of hypophysial portal blood is estimated by using the dry weight of the precipitate after extraction (47). The portal blood may be collected in tubes that do not contain acetic acid and the plasma is separated by centrifugation. Extraction is then performed with a standard C_{18} cartridge for determining the concentration of the desired hypophysiotropic hormone by the appropriate radioimmunoassay (48). Using such an animal preparation, CRF and vasopressin levels in the hypophysial portal blood in urethane-anesthetized rats were found to rise after iv injection of IL-1, indicating that IL-1 activates the adrenocortical axis at the level of the brain via increased release of hypothalamic CRF and vasopressin (8). The limitations of this technique for determining levels of hypophysiotropic hormones in the portal blood are that the samples are collected under anesthesia and that the animals are surgically stressed. The surgical procedure, which damages the tissue itself, may increase circulating cytokines. Furthermore, anesthesia may interfere with the neural transmission of the signal in the brain. Therefore results determined by this procedure, in particular negative findings, may sometimes be difficult to interpret.

Glial Cell Culture to Identify Cytokine-Responsive Cells in CNS

In an effort to further support the evidence obtained *in vivo* that prostaglandins may be a primary mediator of the action of IL-1 in the brain, an astroglial cell culture system was developed, generally according to previously published procedures (49). Using this system, it may be determined if glial cells produce prostaglandin in response to IL-1 (24) or any other cytokine. For this culture, timed pregnant rats are obtained from Charles River Breeding Laboratories and astrocyte cultures are prepared from the brains of 1-day-old rats. The pups are sacrificed by CO_2 inhalation, the carcasses dipped in 70% ethanol, and the heads are removed with sterile scissors. All further procedures are performed aseptically. The skin is opened along the midline of the head and folded back, the skull is opened with two cuts laterally and peeled anteriorly. The brain is taken from the head with a spatula, the cerebellum removed (it is very small at birth and consists of two small lobes) and discarded, and the brains are placed into sterile phosphate buffer (137 mM NaCl, 5.4 mM KCl, 0.17 mM Na_2HPO_4, 0.22 mM KH_2PO_4, 5.5 mM glucose, 59 mM sucrose). The meninges are carefully and fully removed from the brains to minimize contamination of the cultures with fibroblasts. The whole brains are washed several times with buffer and cut with a sterile razor blade into 1-mm^3 pieces. The pieces of brain are then washed several times with buffer, and placed into a 50-ml conical tube with 20 ml of buffer containing 0.03% ethylenediaminetetraacetic acid (EDTA), 0.25% trypsin (Sigma type III), and 200 μg of deoxyribonuclease II (DNase). The tube is incubated in a 37°C water bath for 12 min, and it is vortexed every 4 min. At the end of the incubation the remaining larger fragments are allowed to sediment by gravity for 1–2 min, and the cells are pipetted off into a new 50-ml tube. The remaining fragments are discarded. The solution is diluted with an equal volume of culture medium [DMEM containing 10% horse serum, 2.5% fetal bovine serum, and 1% antibiotic–antimycotic solution (GIBCO-Bethesda Research Laboratories)] and the cells are sedimented by centrifugation at 800 g. Fibrous material that is associated with the cell pellet must not be discarded. Pipette off the clear-looking culture medium, dilute with fresh culture medium to 40 ml, and centrifuge again. The cells should be washed with fresh culture medium a third time, and by this time the fibrous material will not be present, and a firm pellet is obtained. Total cell number is determined and the cells are diluted with culture medium to a concentration of 1×10^6 cells/ml. Ten milliliters of the medium containing the cells is added to 100-mm culture dishes that had been previously coated with poly-L-lysine (Sigma; 100 μg/ml sterile water). Typically, our recovery is 1×10^7 cells/brain. The plates are incubated in a CO_2 incubator for 7 days with a medium change on day 3 or 4. The cells are removed from the 100-mm plates by washing once with phosphate buffer (see above) and incubating for several minutes with phosphate buffer containing 0.25% trypsin and 0.03% EDTA. The cells are recovered by washing two times with culture medium, and plated into the appropriate container. For prostaglandin and interleukin 6 measurements in our laboratory, the cells are diluted to 2–10 $\times$ 10^5 cells/ml and inoculated into 24-well culture plates (poly-L-lysine coated) at 1 ml/well. The density of inoculation will determine the contamination of oligodendrocytes, the small, phase-dark cell growing on top of the bed of type I astrocytes. In general, the cells are used after an additional 7- to 10-day growth period. Inoculation of 1×10^6 cells/ml results in a culture of cells that are 95% immunohistochemically positive for glial fibrillary acidic protein.

For measurement of the prostaglandin response to IL-1, the wells of 24-well plates are washed twice with serum-free DMEM and the sample containing IL-1 (or any other test substance) is diluted in 0.5 ml of DMEM containing 25 mM HEPES buffer and 0.1% bovine serum albumin (BSA). The plates are incubated for the appropriate period at 37°C in 5% CO_2, 95% air, and medium is removed from the wells and stored frozen (-70°C) until assay.

Using such an assay system, it was shown that addition of IL-1β to primary cultured astrocytes resulted in a dose-dependent rise in PGE_2 release during a 3-hr period. However, IL-1β was ineffective in stimulating PGE_2 release from neurons in culture. Thus these results, along with data from *in vivo* studies showing that the ACTH response to IL-1β was abolished by PGE_2 synthesis inhibitors or a PGE_2 antagonist, provide support for the notion that PGE_2 plays an obligatory role in the response to IL-1β (24). In addition, it appears unlikely that IL-1 acts directly on neurons and the response may be mediated by glial cells. Involvement of central PGE_2 in the IL-1-induced febrile response has been suggested by many investigators (see other chapters in this volume and in Volume 17).

Interestingly, the prostaglandin response to IL-1β in astrocytes appeared to be regulated by several neuropeptides. Angiotensin II appeared to act synergistically with IL-1 in stimulating PGE_2 production, whereas CRF and somatostatin significantly inhibited the response (24). More recently, we and others have found that IL-1β stimulates the release of IL-6 in rat astrocytes cultured with the cytokine for 6 hr. Interleukin 1-induced IL-6 release appears to be augmented by the neuropeptide pituitary adenylate activating polypeptide (PACAP) and, like the response in macrophages, is inhibited by the synthetic glucocorticoid dexamethasone (at least under short-term culture conditions) (P. E. Gottschall and A. Arimura, unpublished observations).

Summary, Conclusions, and Future Studies

Based on the evidence presented here, which has combined the methods of brain microinjection, brain lesion, brain microdialysis, and the culture of brain astrocytes, we believe a working hypothesis may be developed for the involvement of the OVLT, astrocytes, and PGE_2 in IL-1-stimulated ACTH release. On activation, circulating monocytes produce and release the cytokine, IL-1β. Interleukin 1β in the blood penetrates the fenestrated endothelia of the OVLT and enters the perivascular spaces, where it binds and activates cell surface receptors for IL-1 on local astrocytes. In response to IL-1, these astrocytes produce PGE_2, which diffuses (or is transported) into the interstitial spaces toward its target neurons in the POA. Prostaglandin E_2 binds specific neuronal receptors in the POA, activating neurons that send processes to CRF-producing perikarya in the PVN. The activation of CRF neurons in the PVN stimulates the release of CRF from the nerve terminals in the median eminence. Corticotropin-releasing factor, released into capillaries of the median eminence, traverses the hypophysial portal circulation and stimulates the pituitary corticotropes to release ACTH.

Clearly, this remains a working hypothesis and further studies must be performed to clarify such a mechanism. First, from several unpublished autoradiography experiments, it is not at all clear that IL-1 indeed crosses into the brain in the OVLT. However, using colloidal gold-labeled IL-1β, it has been reported that IL-1β binds to and is pinocytosed into endothelial cells in the region of the OVLT (50). Others have data suggesting a saturable transport mechanism for IL-1 into the brain (51; see also article 4 in this volume). Other than the lesion experiments, there is no good evidence that suggests that astrocytes located in this area are responsive to IL-1. Studies using electrophysiological techniques have indicated that there are IL-1-responsive neurons in the OVLT (T. Hori, personal communication), yet this result does not explain how ablation of the OVLT enhances the ACTH response to IL-1. Second, it is clear from such a hypothesis that prostanoids produced in the OVLT must travel a significant distance via the interstitial fluid from the OVLT to activate neurons in the POA. Third, interneuron(s) mediating such a response from the POA to the PVN may be chemically identified by pharmacological methods. Finally, prostaglandins may not be the only mediators involved in such a response, particularly in view of the fact that blockade of ascending noradrenergic projections to the hypothalamus inhibits IL-1β-stimulated ACTH release.

Acknowledgments

The studies described here were supported in part by a grant from the Office of Naval Research and research aid from Otsuka Pharmaceutical Company.

References

1. J. E. Blalock, *Yearb. Endocrinol.*, p. 15 (1987).
2. W. Vale and G. Grant, *in* "Methods in Enzymology" (B. O'Malley and J. Hardman, eds.), Vol. 37, p. 82. Academic Press, New York, 1975.
3. A. Uehara, S. Gillis, and A. Arimura, *Neuroendocrinology* **45,** 343 (1987).
4. M. D. Culler, T. Kenjo, N. Obara, and A. Arimura, *Am. J. Physiol.* **247,** E609 (1984).
5. M. J. Phillips, *in* "Dye Exclusion Tests for Cell Viability" (P. F. J. Kruse and M. K. Patterson, eds.), p. 406. Academic Press, New York, 1973.
6. B. M. R. N. J. Woloski, E. M. Smith, W. J. Meyer, G. M. Fuller, and J. E. Blalock, *Science* **23,** 1035 (1985).
7. A. Brodish, *Fed. Proc., Fed. Am. Soc. Exp. Biol.* **36,** 2088 (1977).
8. R. Sapolsky, C. Rivier, G. Yamamoto, P. Plotsky, and W. Vale, *Science* **238,** 522 (1987).
9. F. Berkenbosch, J. Van Oers, A. Del Rey, F. Tilders, and H. Besedovsky, *Science* **238,** 524 (1987).
10. E. W. Bernton, J. E. Beach, J. W. Holaday, R. C. Smallridge, and H. G. Fein, *Science* **198,** 519 (1987).
11. A. Arimura, T. Saito, and A. V. Schally, *Endocrinology (Baltimore)* **81,** 235 (1967).
12. S. M. McCann, R. Mack, and C. Gale, *Endocrinology (Baltimore)* **64,** 870 (1959).
13. A. Uehara, P. E. Gottschall, R. R. Dahl, and A. Arimura, *Endocrinology (Baltimore)* **121,** 1580 (1987).
14. A. Uehara, M. Minamino, M. H. Townsend, and A. Arimura, *Proc. Soc. Exp. Biol. Med.* **183,** 106 (1986).
15. G. Katsuura, A. Arimura, K. Koves, and P. E. Gottschall, *Am. J. Physiol.* **258,** E163 (1990).
16. G. Katsuura, P. E. Gottschall, R. R. Dahl, and A. Arimura, *Endocrinology (Baltimore)* **122,** 1773 (1988).
17. D. E. Scarborough, *Ann. N.Y. Acad. Sci.* **594,** 169 (1990).
18. G. Paxinos and T. Watson, "The Rat Brain in Stereotaxic Coordinates." Academic Press, New York, 1982.
19. J. T. Stitt, *J. Physiol. (London)* **368,** 501 (1985).

20. K. E. Cooper, *Annu. Rev. Neurosci.* **10,** 297 (1987).
21. J. Coyle, M. Molliver, and M. Kuhar, *J. Comp. Neurol.* **180,** 301 (1978).
22. I. Klatzo, A. Piraux, and E. J. Laskowski, *J. Neuropathol. Exp. Neurol.* **17,** 548 (1958).
23. D. Giulian, D. G. Young, J. Woodward, D. C. Brown, and L. B. Lachman, *J. Neurosci.* **8,** 709 (1988).
24. G. Katsuura, P. E. Gottschall, R. R. Dahl, and A. Arimura, *Endocrinology (Baltimore)* **124,** 3125 (1989).
25. T. Kasahara, H. Yagisawa, K. Yamashita, Y. Yamagucho, and Y. Akiyama, *Biochem. Biophys. Res. Commun.* **167,** 1242 (1990).
26. P. E. Gottschall, K. Koves, K. Mizuno, I. Tatsuno, and A. Arimura, *Am. J. Physiol.* **261,** E362 (1991).
27. P. E. Gottschall, I. Tatsuno, and A. Arimura, *Mol. Cell. Neurosci.* **3,** 49 (1992).
28. W. J. Nicklas, R. C. Duvoisin, and S. Berl, *Brain Res.* **167,** 107 (1979).
29. A. Fontana, F. Kristensen, R. Dubs, D. Gemsa, and E. Weber, *J. Immunol.* **129,** 2413 (1982).
30. C. Nicholson, *Neurosci. Res. Program Bull.* **18,** 177 (1980).
31. A. Negro-Vilar, C. Johnston, E. Spinedi, M. Valenca, and F. Lopez, *in* "Physiological Role of Peptides and Amines on the Regulation of ACTH Secretion" (W. F. Ganong, M. F. Dallman, and J. L. Robert, eds.), p. 218. N.Y. Acad. Sci., New York, 1987.
32. J. Axelrod and T. D. Resine, *Science* **224,** 452 (1984).
33. F. J. H. Tilders, F. Berkenbosch, I. Vermes, E. A. Linton, and P. G. Smelik, *Fed. Proc., Fed. Am. Soc. Exp. Biol.* **44,** 155 (1985).
34. A. Szafarczyk, F. Malaval, A. Laurent, R. Gibaud, and I. Assenmacher, *Endocrinology (Baltimore)* **121,** 883 (1987).
35. U. Ungerstedt and A. Hallström, *Life Sci.* **41,** 861 (1987).
36. K. M. Kendrick, *in* "Use of Microdialysis in Neuroendocrinology" (P. M. Conn, ed.), p. 229. Academic Press, San Diego, 1989.
37. J. E. Chastain, F. Samson, S. R. Nelson, and T. L. Pazdernik, *Neuroscience* **37,** 155 (1990).
38. A. Bayon, *in* "*In vivo* and *in vitro* Studies on Peptide Release" (A. A. Boulton, B. Baler, and Q. J. Pittman, eds.), p. 113. Humana Press, Clifton, NJ, 1987.
39. J. H. Gaddum, *J. Physiol. (London)* **155,** 1 (1961).
40. G. Komaki, A. Arimura, and K. Koves, *Am. J. Physiol. (Endocrinol. Metab.)* **25,** E246 (1992).
41. T. Kihara, I. Ikeda, and A. Matsushita, *Brain Res.* **519,** 44 (1990).
42. J. E. Levine and K. D. Powell, *in* "Microdialysis for Measurement of Neuroendocrine Peptides" (J. N. Abelson and M. I. Simon, eds.), p. 166. Academic Press, San Diego, 1989.
43. R. D. Myers, *Methods Psychobiol.* **2,** 169 (1972).
44. M. P. Honchar, B. K. Hartman, and L. G. Sharpe, *Am. J. Physiol.* **236,** R45 (1979).
45. J. C. Porter, *in* "Methods for Studying Pituitary–Hypothalamic Axis *in Situ*" (J. G. Hardman and B. W. O'Malley, eds.), p. 166. Academic Press, New York, 1975.

46. K. Chihara, A. Arimura, and A. V. Schally, *Endocrinology* (*Baltimore*) **104,** 1656 (1979).
47. K. Chihara, A. Arimura, and A. V. Schally, *Endocrinology* (*Baltimore*) **104,** 1434 (1979).
48. D. M. Gibbs and W. Vale, *Endocrinology* (*Baltimore*) **111,** 1418 (1982).
49. D. W. Clarke, F. T. Boyd, M. S. Kappy, and M. K. Raizada, *J. Biol. Chem.* **259,** 11672 (1984).
50. M. Hashimoto, Y. Ishikawa, S. Yokoto, F. Goto, T. Bando, Y. Sakakibara, and M. Iriki, *Brain Res.* **540,** 217 (1991).
51. W. A. Banks and A. J. Kastin, *Life Sci.* **48,** PL-117 (1991).

[16]   *In Vivo* and *in Vitro* Methods for Studying Effects of Tumor Necrosis Factor on Pituitary Cells

Alberto E. Panerai, Vittorio Locatelli, and Paola Sacerdote

Introduction

The observation that interleukin 1 could induce the release of pituitary hormones prompted several new studies on the *in vivo* and *in vitro* effects of other cytokines such as interleukin 2, interleukin 6, and, most recently, tumor necrosis factor α (TNF-α). The *in vitro* methods for the study of the endocrine effects of cytokines rely greatly on slight modifications of other widely employed methods. *In vivo* studies involve primarily the use of pharmacological tools to define the role of cytokines, for example, TNF-α, in the physiological modulation of the secretion of pituitary hormones. Our studies have dealt mainly with the effects of TNF-α on the *in vitro* release of growth hormone and β-endorphin (BE), and on the *in vivo* effects of growth hormone (GH) secretion.

Methods for *in Vitro* Experiments

Collection of Pituitaries

Pituitaries are obtained from male Sprague-Dawley CD rats (300–350 g body weight). After ether anesthesia, rats are decapitated and the skulls opened with two lateral cuts parallel to the sagittal commissure. The theca is removed and the brain is ablated with extreme care with a 5-mm flat, smooth-edged spatula to avoid damage to the gland pulling the tuberculum. When the base of the skull is exposed, a small forceps with curved arms is pushed through the tentorium on both sides of the gland and the tentorium is ablated, paying attention not to remove or damage the gland. With the same forceps, the whole gland is now removed from the sella turcica and placed in a small petri dish containing sterile F10 medium, keeping the excised tuberculum on top. The intermediate and anterior pituitaries are separated under a stereomicroscope with sterile forceps with thin, straight arms, using the different colors of the two parts of the gland as a guide. Alternatively, a small ($\frac{2}{3}$ mm)

Methods in Neurosciences, Volume 16

scalpel can be used for the same operation. The two parts of the pituitary are placed in different petri dishes containing sterile F10 medium.

Pituitary Cell Dispersion

Pituitaries are rinsed twice in 20 ml of F10 medium and transferred to new petri dishes. The medium is removed with a sterile pipette, and pituitaries are arranged in a square. Pituitaries are each minced 20 times in two directions (one 90° to the other) with a razor blade. When the pituitaries have been minced, 20 ml of F10 medium is added with a sterile pipette, and the tissue is transferred to a sterile 50-ml Erlenmeyer flask with plug, using a plastic sterile pipette. The tissue is allowed to settle, and the F10 medium is then removed with a sterile pipette. Tissues are rinsed twice with 10 ml of fresh F10 and after 10 min the final rinse is removed. Collagenase, previously prepared, is now added to the flask, which is subsequently closed with the plug. The flasks are incubated for 30 min in a water bath kept at 37°C, with gentle agitation. After 30 min, the medium is discarded and collagenase plus DNase is added to the flask and the cells are incubated for another 30 min in the 37°C bath. The medium is thereafter removed with a sterile pipette. Tissue is washed with Dulbecco's phosphate-buffered saline (PBS) medium free of Ca^{2+} and Mg^{2+}. Cells are now ready to be dissociated with fire-polished pipettes. As the solution containing individual cells becomes turbid it is allowed to settle and is transferred, with a plastic sterile pipette, to a 50-ml plastic centrifuge tube. The latter step is repeated until the tissue disappears completely. The solution containing the cells is filtered, in two aliquots, through a premoistened sterile cloth into two plastic 50-ml centrifuge tubes. Filters are then washed with another 25 ml of F10 medium in each tube and the tubes centrifuged at 200 g for 10 min. The supernatant is eliminated and the pellet, resuspended in 50 ml of F10 medium, is centrifuged again. The supernatant is removed and cells are resuspended in 50 ml of F10 medium; viability is controlled with trypan blue stain.

Pituitary Cell Culture

After counting, 2×10^5 cells are plated in a single cell suspension onto 24-well culture plates. The cells are incubated at 37°C in F10 medium supplemented with glutamine (0.2 g/liter), 10% horse serum, 4% fetal calf serum, and gentamycin (25 μg/ml) in a humidified environment of 5% CO_2 and 95% O_2. Cells are kept in culture as described above until the third day, when the medium is removed and the cells are washed twice with serum-free F10.

Usually 10 pituitaries are required for 1 experiment, and $1.5-2.0 \times 10^6$ cells/pituitary can be expected.

Pituitary Fragments

Anterior pituitaries are each divided into 8 fragments, and 16 fragments/vial are incubated in 1 ml of modified Krebs–Ringer bicarbonate buffer. Vials are incubated for 1 hr at 37°C in a Dubnoff metabolic shaker in an atmosphere of 98% O_2 and 5% CO_2. The medium is replaced with fresh medium and vials are incubated for another hour, and then the medium is collected (basal values). Medium is replaced with fresh medium containing either saline (vehicle) or the drug or peptide under investigation, and the incubation is continued for the time desired (e.g., 1 hr).

Experimental Protocol

After the second wash with serum-free F10, cells (2×10^5) are resuspended in the "experimental" medium, that is, they will be incubated in 1 ml of F10 medium containing 0.1% bovine serum albumin (BSA) (controls), or F10 experimental medium with different concentrations of TNF. Incubation is maintained for the chosen time (e.g., 4 hr) at 37°C; the medium is thereafter collected in tubes containing aprotinin (1000 kallikrein-inactivating units/ml) and ethylenediaminetetraacetic acid (EDTA) (2 mg/ml) and kept frozen at $-20°C$ until the measurement of the hormones and/or peptides is made. At least five wells/group were used in each experiment.

Alternative Methods

Cell Perfusion

After a 3-day preincubation, 2×10^7 cells are incubated with preswollen Cytodex-1 beads (Pharmacia-LKB Biotechnology, Bromma, Sweden) and perifused with F10, 20 mM N-2-hydroxyethylpiperazine-N'-2-ethanesulfonic acid (HEPES), and 0.1% BSA for 2 hr at a flow rate of 0.6 ml/min; 1-min fractions are collected for hormone assay.

Sample Preparation

This step is relevant only to studies dealing with small peptides, because the possibilities of cross-reactivities of antibodies (also monoclonal) are high, both with related molecules (e.g., proopiomelanocortin derivatives) and unrelated ones [e.g., β endorphin (BE) and interferons]. Moreover, peptides have little or no species specificity, and cross-reactivities can also exist with peptides present in the incubation media, for example, calf or horse serum; this possibility is improbable for growth hormone or prolactin, for which species-specific radioimmunoassays are used.

High-Performance Liquid Chromatography Analysis

To identify BE and separate it from cross-reacting immunoreactivities, for example, proopiomelanocortin and β-lipotropin, high-performance liquid chromatography (HPLC) analysis before radioimmunoassay is recommended. This procedure is not an important step in studies on the intermediate pituitary or the hypothalamus, in which over 95% of β-endorphin immunoreactivity is true β-endorphin, but it is important in the anterior pituitary, in which true β-endorphin immunoreactivity is a minor component when compared to β-lipotropin- and proopiomelanocortin-derived immunoreactivity.

The procedure presented was developed for β-endorphin, but the method and elution reagents can be easily applied to other peptides as described or with slight modifications. The first step in HPLC analysis is sample concentration. This is obtained on Sep-pak (Millipore, Bedford, MA) octadodecasilyl silica cartridges prewashed with 1% formic acid, saline, methanol, and again with 1% formic acid as the last step (1). Samples are loaded on cartridges with a maximum volume of 2 ml, and are eluted with increasing concentrations of methanol–1% formic acid in volumes of 1 ml at each step. β-Endorphin immunoreactivity (β-endorphin and β-lipotropin) normally elutes with 90% methanol. The fraction containing both β-endorphin and β-lipotropin is vacuum dried in a Savant centrifuging apparatus (Speed-Vac; Savant, Hicksville, NY). At the moment of analysis, samples are resuspended in water and injected in a double-pump HPLC apparatus equipped with a μBondapak C_{18} column (Millipore) (1). The elution is obtained in 20 min with a gradient from 25 to 45% CH_3CN in 0.01% HCl and a flow rate of 1.5 ml/min. Samples are collected every 30 sec and again vacuum dried before radioimmunoassay. Typically, the elution time is 13.40 min for β-lipotropin, 14.60 min for β-endorphin(1–31) (the complete β-endorphin sequence), and 17.40 min for N-acetyl-β-endorphin(1–31).

Gel Filtration

To measure the immunoreactivity detected with the BE antiserum, a pool of incubation medium can be loaded on a 2×100 cm G-50 medium Sephadex column. The column is eluted with 0.01 M phosphate-buffered saline, pH 7.4, at 15 ml/hr, and 3-ml fractions collected. After passing the sample, the column is calibrated with blue dextran, iodinated BE and β-lipotropin, and free iodine. Fractions are vacuum dried and run in the β-endorphin radioimmunoassay (2).

Radioimmunoassays

The β-endorphin antiserum used in these studies is obtained against a synthetic camel (identical to rat) β-endorphin–BSA glutaraldehyde conjugate and is, therefore, directed toward the C terminal of the peptide, as is also demonstrated by the 100% cross-reactivity with β-lipotropin and the low cross-reactivity with human BE (5%). A minor cross-reactivity is also observed toward equimolar Met-enkephalin (0.1%), but not with Leu-enkephalin, dynorphin, α-melanocyte-stimulating hormone (α-MSH), β-MSH, substance P, somatostatin, thyrotropin-releasing hormone, corticotropin-releasing hormone, neurotensin, vasopressin, bombesin, cholecystokinin, vasoactive intestinal peptide, insulin, follicle-stimulating hormone, luteinizing hormone, prolactin, growth hormone, morphine, naloxone, or the cytokines interleukin 1α or 1β, and tumor necrosis factor (2).

Radioimmunoassay is run as follows: 0.1 ml of medium or vacuum-dried samples resuspended in the radioimmunoassay buffer is added to 0.2 ml of phosphate-buffered saline containing BSA, the antiserum at an initial dilution of 1 : 12,000, and 0.1 ml (10,000 cpm) of radioiodinated peptide (2000 Ci/mmol; Cat. No. IM 162; Amersham, Arlington Heights, IL). The tubes are incubated for 24 hr, and then 1 ml of charcoal–dextran mixture (2 g of Norit-A, Serve, Heidelberg, Germany; 200 mg of dextran T 70, Pharmacia, Uppsala, Sweden; in 800 ml of radioimmunoassay buffer) is added, and free iodine in the pellet is counted after centrifugation at 1500 g for 20 min. Sensitivity of the method is 10 pg/tube and intraassay and interassay variation coefficients are 8 and 11%, respectively. Plasma growth hormone (GH) radioimmunoassay was performed by a double-antibody radioimmunoassay with materials provided by the NIDDK (Bethesda, MD). Results were expressed in terms of the NIH-2 standard rat GH RP-2. The minimum detectable value is 0.6 ng/ml, and intraassay variability is 6%. Interassay variation is avoided because all assays from a given experiment are assayed in a single radioimmunoassay.

Methods for *in Vivo* Experiments

Animals

In our studies we used infant (14-day-old) Sprague-Dawley CD rats. Animals arrived with their mothers, when 3 days old, in a standard litter of nine pups/mother, and were allowed to remain with dams until 1 hr before the experiments. Infant rats were chosen for several reasons, one being the possibility of using small amounts of tumor necrosis factor. The second, and most important, reason, is that 14-day-old rats have an imperfect blood–brain barrier that allows peripherally administered molecules to reach the central nervous system readily. In preliminary studies in adult rats, we in fact observed that the peripheral administration of TNF-α does not elicit endocrine or behavioral effects (3), whereas they are present after intracerebroventricular administration. The infant rat model can be usefully exploited in this kind of experiment, that is, when it is necessary to reach the central nervous system with peptides or bigger molecule, for example, antisera administered peripherally.

The study presented has been chosen to illustrate the use of pharmacological tools for the investigation of the mechanism of action of a substance, in this case a cytokine. In these studies blood is obtained after decapitation, collected into EDTA (2 mg/ml)-containing tubes, and plasma separated after centrifuging at 1500 g for 15 min. In this study, β-endorphin was not taken into consideration, because in the infant (but also adult) rat sufficient volumes of blood cannot be obtained to allow for plasma separation of β-endorphin from cross-reacting substances such as β-lipotropin (1).

The points to be elucidated with the *in vivo* study are (1) the dose response of the effect of TNF-α on GH release, (2) the time course of the effects of TNF-α on GH release, (3) the role of endogenous opioids in the effects of TNF-α on GH release, (4) the role of growth hormone-releasing hormone (GHRH) and somatostatin in TNF-α-induced GH release; and (5) the role of prostaglandins in TNF-α-induced GH release.

The time course and dose response of TNF-α on GH secretion were studied by administering TNF-α at doses of 0.1, 1.0, and 5.0 ng/kg subcutaneously. The study showed that doses of 1.0 and 5.0 ng of the cytokine induce a dose-related increase of GH that is evident only 4 hr after administration, thus suggesting an indirect effect of the cytokine.

The role of opioids in the GH-releasing effect of TNF-α has been excluded on the basis of the results of two experiments. In the first experiment, the synthetic enkephalin analog FK-33 824 (250 μg/g, sc) was administered 15 min before sampling to rats treated 4 hr previously with the cytokine. In these animals, GH secretion was higher after the administration of the cytokine and the opioid, thus suggesting different sites of action for the two. The lack of a role for opioids in the effect of TNF-α is further confirmed by the observation that the nonspecific opiate receptor antagonist naloxone (5 μg/g, sc) administered 15 min before sampling to rats treated 4 hr before with the cytokine does not affect its growth hormone-releasing effect (1.0 and 5.0 ng/kg, sc).

A possible mediation of the effect of TNF-α through the physiological stimulus of growth hormone secretion, that is, growth hormone-releasing hormone (GHRH), was assessed by evaluting the effect of the passive immunization toward somatostatin (growth hormone-inhibiting hormone), which is the physiological inhibitor of growth hormone release. This neuropeptide, in fact, counterbalances GHRH, and its suppression can unveil a possible effect of the cytokine on GHRH. Passive immunization toward somatostatin was obtained by injecting each rat with 200 μl of an antiserum against synthetic somatostatin and sampling 2 hr following this treatment. The antiserum toward somatostatin was obtained against the synthetic peptide with a procedure similar to the one used for β-endorphin. Cross-reactivities are also similar to those of the β-endorphin antiserum. The amount of somatostatin antiserum injected was previously calculated to inhibit approximately 1.2 μg of the peptide, that is, more than the amount found in a normal rat hypothalamus. In this experimental model, the TNF-α-mediated release of growth hormone is increased by the passive immunization by the antiserum that, in the 10-day-old rat, can freely cross the blood–brain barrier. The experiment suggests that TNF-α-induced growth hormone secretion is mediated by the stimulation of growth hormone-releasing hormone (GHRH).

However, it remains to be elucidated whether the effect of the cytokine on GHRH is a direct one. The last experiment attempts to elucidate this point, exploring whether prostaglandins, similar to what is observed for many effects of cytokines, might also mediate the endocrine effect of TNF-α. Rats treated 4 hr previously with TNF-α were administered 15 min before sampling with the prostaglandin synthesis inhibitor indomethacin (5 mg/kg, sc). Indomethacin induces a clear-cut blockade of the GH secretion induced by TNF-α, thus suggesting a role for prostaglandins in the endocrine effect of the cytokine.

Alternative Method

A method often used to study the secretion of pituitary hormones is the use of rats that have undergone the anatomical destruction of the mediobasal hypothalamus or complete hypothalamic deafferentation. The surgery must be conducted under general anesthesia in a stereotaxic apparatus and must be controlled histologically. The model allows the study of the effect of treatment on a pituitary that, although *in situ* in the living animal, is somehow comparable to an *in vitro* gland.

Materials

F10 medium: Purchased from Biochrom KG (Berlin, Germany) (Cat. No. F 0715)

Dulbecco's PBS (Ca^{2+}, Mg^{2+}-free medium: Purchased from Biochrom KG (Cat. No. L 1825)

Radioimmunoassay buffer (for 2 liters of buffer): 0.14 M PBS, 49.81 g of $Na_2HPO_4 \cdot 2H_2O$, 1.8 g of EDTA (25 mM), 10.0 g of BSA (0.5%)

Collagenase

    Collagenase (2.5 mg/ml) (Cat. No. 103-586; Boehringer, Mannheim, Germany) in F10 medium; total volume, 15 ml

    Collagenase (2.5 mg/ml) plus DNase (0.25 mg/ml) (Cat. No. 104-159; Boehringer) in F10 medium; total volume, 15 ml

Krebs–Ringer bicarbonate buffer: NaCl (118 mM), $MgSO_4$ (1.2 mM), KH_2PO_4 (1.2 mM), KCl (4.7 mM), $CaCl_2$ (1.0 mM), $NaCHO_3$ (10 mM), glucose (10 mM), HEPES (20 mM), BSA (0.1%, w/v)

Trypan blue: 0.5% solution (Cat. No. L 6323; Biochrom KG)

Three hundred microliters of the solution containing the dispersed cells is transferred with 0.5 ml of trypan blue solution and 0.2 ml of F10 to a test tube, mixed thoroughly, and allowed to stand for 10 min. With a Pasteur pipette a small aliquot of the solution is added to a hemacytometer chamber. Cells are counted (nonviable cells are blue), and cells per milliliter determined: Cells per milliliter = the average count per square × dilution factor × 10^4 (count 10 squares).

    FK 33 824 (Sandoz AG, Basel, Switzerland): A synthetic enkephalin analog with relative specificity for the μ opiate receptor (4)

References

1. A. E. Panerai, A. Martini, A. M. DiGiulio, F. Fraioli, C. Vegni, G. Pardi, A. Marini, and P. Mantegazza, *J. Clin. Endocrinol. Metab.* **57**, 537 (1983).
2. N. Ogawa, A. E. Panerai, S. Lee, G. Forsbach, V. Havlicek, and H. G. Friesen, *Life Sci.* **25**, 317 (1979).
3. M. Bianchi, P. Sacerdote, L. Locatelli, P. Mantegazza, and A. E. Panerai, *Brain Res.* **546**, 139 (1991).
4. M. Miki, M. Ono, and K. Shizume, *Endocrinology (Baltimore)* **114**, 1950 (1984).

[17] Determination of Direct Effects of Cytokines on Release of Neuropeptides from Rat Hypothalamus by an *in Vitro* Method

Ashley Grossman, Stylianos Tsagarakis, Marta Korbonits, and Alfredo Costa

Introduction

The hypothalamus is one region of the brain in which the presence of numerous and specialized cell nuclei allows the integration of various but essential biological functions. In addition to its well recognized role in regulating pituitary function, thermogenesis, metabolic rate, sexual behavior, food intake, and sleep, the hypothalamus has more recently also been considered as the site where the endocrine and immune systems interface. Moreover, an exceptionally complex organization of the mechanisms of peptide release from the hypothalamic nuclei has emerged over the past years. Hypophysiotropic neurons, traditionally thought to be under central nervous system (CNS) control by a variety of neural afferents, have been shown to provide an extensive network of intra- and extrahypothalamic collateral projections, in addition to those ending in the median eminence. Such anatomical evidence has substantiated the need for revising our view of the neuronal organization in the hypothalamus. The hypothalamic network was regarded as a system whereby serially wired neuronal chains were activated sequentially, thus leading to a common neurosecretory path. In this model, the major function of the neuroendocrine axes was one of amplification. However, such a model of simple serial organization is no longer satisfactory, and a more complex view of parallel organization (1) appears to be more appropriate. According to the latter concept, neural information might follow alternate pathways, resulting in a diverse matrix of neuropeptides combinations, each of which may lead to a different patterning of pituitary hormone secretion. One feature that adds further complexity and subtlety to such hypothalamic organization is the coexistence (costorage and corelease) of neuropeptides and/or neurotransmitters (2), which has been shown to be variable or "plastic" according to the endocrine milieu. Therefore, even if the same neuronal pathways are stimulated, differential responses may occur depending on the particular neurochemical environment.

Methods in Neurosciences, Volume 16

The rat hypothalamus, which resembles in many respects the human hypothalamus in structure and function, appears to be a suitable model for detailed research. As will be later apparent, methods used to study the rat hypothalamus *in vitro* differ to a considerable extent according to a number of factors, such as the age of the hypothalamus (fetal or adult), the type of incubation (acute or chronic systems), the specific perifusion techniques (incubation or continuous flow), and so on. The aim of this article is to describe in detail the specific *in vitro* acute incubation system of hypothalamic explants that has been in use for several years in our department. This system has proved to be a valid model for assessing the *in vitro* activity of the isolated hypothalamus. Although in theory it may apply to the investigation of any hypothalamic hormone, the technique was initially employed to evaluate the secretion of corticotropin-releasing hormone 41 (CRH-41), growth hormone-releasing hormone (GHRH), gonadotropin-releasing hormone (GnRH), and somatostatin (SRIF). The use of this system has enabled us to obtain insight into the effects exerted by classic neurotransmitters and other factors on the hypothalamic release of these regulatory hormones.

Following the early observations that the immune and endocrine systems may show reciprocal interactions, this technique has more recently been employed in the investigation of the direct effects of cytokines on the release of hypothalamic hormones. Our findings further suggested that some of the products from activated immunocytes may act as direct neurotransmitters within the hypothalamus.

In addition, the availability of specific assays for arginine vasopressin (AVP) and oxytocin prompted us to adapt the system such as to allow the study of posterior hypothalamic endocrine function and its relation to immune activity.

The specific technique used varies slightly according to the peptide to be investigated, mainly depending on the requirements of the specific assay; nevertheless, the general features remain identical. The advantages and limitations of this system are discussed in comparison to other *in vitro* methods, particularly insofar as the hypothalamic effects of cytokines are concerned.

Investigating Hypothalamic Hormone Release *in Vitro*

Cellular processes underlying hormone secretion from the hypothalamus are relatively difficult to study in the whole animal. On the other hand, knowledge of the nature of mechanisms that regulate hypothalamic function is indispensable for a complete understanding of endocrine homeostasis. Consequently, over the past few years, several investigators have begun to use isolated hypothalamic preparations to elucidate the physiological, pharmacological, and biochemical characteristics of the hypophysiotropic neurons. However, different approaches have been adopted by various research groups to maintain the hypothalamus *in vitro*. These techniques can be roughly divided into three major groups: (1) synaptosomal and other subcellular preparations, (2) tissue cultures (including short- or long-term maintenance of hypothalamic preparations), and (3) neuronal cell cultures. It is evident that the particular type of preparation chosen implies the use of different technical devices and dictates the time course of the experiments.

Synaptosomes are subcellular compartments that consist of synaptic vesicles, mitochondria, and soluble constituents, surrounded by a plasma membrane. They contain the bulk of neurotransmitters and many neuropeptides (3, 4), and are ideal for the study of molecular events that take place at nerve endings, because they offer minimal barriers to diffusion. Synaptosomal preparations are normally used within minutes to hours. Their major disadvantages are the marked heterogeneity and the nonspecific release of products, which may represent leakage from damaged membranes (5).

Tissue cultures imply the maintenance of hypothalamic material in the form of slices or fragments over a period of hours to days. In short-term cultures the tissue is either incubated or perifused in cerebrospinal fluid (CSF)-like medium. It is clear, however, that the choice of the most adequate system strictly depends on the specific neurosecretory process to be tested and on the sensitivity of the detection method employed. So far as survival of the hypothalamic preparation is concerned, a number of studies have attempted to maintain tissues in culture for more than 24 hr (6, 7). However, optimal survival requires the addition of serum, which contains ill-defined substances (hormones, neurotransmitters, and growth factors) and may therefore affect the neurosecretory process under investigation. Furthermore, oxygen consumption decreases after a period of several hours, unless hypothalamic preparations from fetuses or neonates are used (8), although it is unclear as to whether widespread cell degeneration occurs.

Hypothalamic neurons in culture are prepared by dispersing the tissue into individual cells by different procedures; cells are then plated on culture dishes and maintained in either serum-containing or defined medium (9). Alternatively, neurons can be cultured on a capillary membrane perifusion system (10). In the latter case, the composition of the medium can be repeatedly changed, and the secretion products frequently sampled, while still permitting the rapid exchange of nutrients and metabolites. Although fetal or neonatal tissues may be artificial insofar as they may not differentiate into adult hypothalamic cells and the physiological interconnectedness may be lost over time, these systems are useful for relatively long-term studies.

In Vitro System of Acute Explants

In vitro hypothalamic explants, coupled with indirect measurements (bioassays) or, more recently, with direct measurements [radioimmunoassay (RIA) and immunoradiometric assay (IRMA)] of peptides, have been used over the past 20 years by several authors, and have included both incubated and perifused hypothalami (minced or whole) and median eminence fragments (11–14). Until the development of these techniques, relatively little work had been undertaken toward improving the understanding of the regulation of the release of hypothalamic hormones by direct measurements. The system described here was developed by Lengyel *et al.* (15), based on a technique originally devised by Jones and colleagues (16), to (a) establish the characteristics of peptide secretion *in vitro,* using specific RIAs, (b) identify the nature of the immunoreactive forms released *in vitro* by chromatographic techniques, (c) investigate the direct/indirect effects of various classic neurotransmitters, putative neurotransmitters, and neuromodulators on hypothalamic secretion, and (d) characterize the particular receptors involved, by using specific agonist and antagonist drugs.

Animals

Male Wistar rats, specific pathogen free, with a mean age of 80 days and body weight in the range of 200–300 g, are used for the experiments. Such rats are thus gonadally mature young adults. They are kept at four per cage and housed under conditions of constant temperature (18°C) and humidity (50%), with a lighting schedule from 04.00 to 17.00 hr. Animals are on a balanced diet for rodents and given free access to water and food. They are usually allowed to acclimatize to our facility for at least 4 days before being used for experiments.

Decapitation and Brain Removal

Rats are gently removed from their cages and decapitated, using a dedicated guillotine, within 15 sec by authorized investigators. Operations are invariably performed between 09.00 and 10.00 hr, to minimize any variation due to the circadian rhythms of hypothalamic hormone secretion. To remove the brain from the skull, one blade of a thick pair of scissors or rongeurs is placed into the foramen magnum and two horizontal cuts are made along the dorsolateral border of the calvarium. Then the dorsal calvarium is gently lifted and removed, care being taken that the meninges do not adhere to the skull vault, and a scissor cut is made between the olfactory bulb and the cerebral cortex, transecting the olfactory and optic nerves. Finally, the brain is carefully pulled out backward from the cranial vault, and the brainstem transected.

Hypothalamic Dissection

The brain is placed with its ventral surface upward, and the well-demarcated hypothalamic area is dissected within the following limits: the posterior border of the optic chiasm, the anterior border of the mamillary bodies, and the lateral hypothalamic sulci. The depth of the fragment is chosen according to the peptide whose secretion is to be investigated. Thus, in the case of CRH-41, the depth of the fragments is approximately 2 mm, in order to include the paraventricular nucleus (PVN), the principal source of hypothalamic CRH-41, which is located close to the third ventricle. For SRIF, GnRH, and GHRH, a depth of approximately 1 mm allows the inclusion of the relevant cell nuclei, which have a more anterior and inferior position than in the PVN. A depth of 3 mm is chosen for studies on AVP and oxytocin, for which the high posterior hypothalamic nuclei are to be included. The hypothalamic blocks obtained are then entirely bisected by a longitudinal incision through the midsagittal plane, using a surgical blade. The total dissection time is usually less than 2 min from decapitation; and approximately 30 min elapse between sacrificing the first animal and the completion of this stage (using 8–16 animals), during which time the tissue is placed in vials containing ice-cold incubation medium.

Some experiments are performed on the isolated median eminence, in which the hypophysiotropic hormones have their highest concentration. The median eminence contains a large number of nerve terminals in close proximity to the primary capillary bed of the portal system, from which they are released (17). In experiments on the median eminence, a dissecting microscope is required, through which the area of interest is easily recognized and then cut and removed.

Static Tissue Incubation

The freshly dissected hypothalamic halves (or the median eminences) are placed in sterile polyethylene vials containing a saline-based medium, such as Earle's balanced salt solution (EBSS), supplemented with 0.2% human serum albumin, 60 μg of ascorbic acid/ml to prevent oxidation, and 100 kallikrein-inactivating units (kIU) of aprotinin/ml to prevent peptide degradation by hypothalamic peptidases (Table I). Other enzyme inhibitors may be used, but they should be assessed for their interaction with the specific assays in use; for example, we found that bacitracin interfered with our RIA for CRH-41. The pH of the medium is 7.4, and the osmolality is within the range 290–300 mOsm/kg. The number of hypothalami incubated in each vial is usually one (two halves), and the volume of medium added is 400 μl. In the case of CRH-41 two hypothalami (four halves) are incubated in one vial, in 500 μl of EBSS, in order for the basal release to be measurable in our RIA. We always maintain the paired halves in the same vial, because the anatomical location of the PVN is quite close to the midline, and there is a high probability of unequal distribution of CRH-41-containing neurons in the two halves, resulting in a great variability of release between different incubation vials.

In the case of studies on the median eminence, three are incubated in 500 μl of EBSS, as described for intact hypothalami.

Vials are kept in a water bath at 37°C and gassed in an atmosphere of O_2/CO_2 (95%/5%), at a 1-liter/min flow rate. The shaking pace of the water bath machine is usually 130 strokes/min.

Sampling Procedure

The first part of experiments is referred to as the preincubation period. Previous studies have shown that peptide secretion is elevated during the first minutes of incubation, gradually decreasing thereafter; the release of

TABLE I   Concentrations of Constituents and Additives in Incubation Medium[a]

Constituents	Concentration (mg/ml)	Additives	Amount
NaCl	680	Ascorbic acid	60 μg/ml
KCl	40	Human serum albumin	0.5% (w/v)
$CaCl_2 \cdot 7H_2O$	36	Aprotinin	100 kIU/ml
$MgSO_4 \cdot 7H_2O$	20		
$NaH_2PO_4 \cdot 2H_2O$	15.8		
$NaHCO_3$	220		
D-Glucose	100		

[a] Earle's balanced salt solution (EBSS).

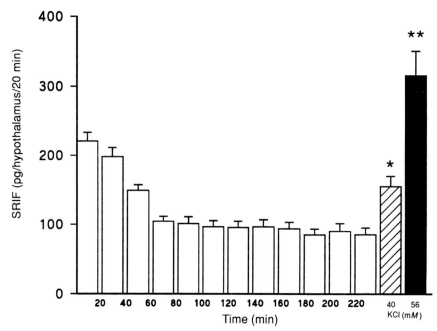

FIG. 1   Spontaneous secretion of somatostatin (SRIF) from hypothalami incubated over 240 min. The effect of 40 and 56 mM KCl is also shown. Each bar represents the mean ± SEM of concentrations from 10 to 12 incubation vials. Peptide release stabilized after approximately 60 min. *$p < 0.01$, **$p < 0.001$ vs. the preceding (240 min) basal collection.

CRH-41, SRIF, GHRH, AVP, and oxytocin stabilizes approximately 60 min after commencement of incubation, as shown in Figs. 1 and 2 for SRIF and AVP, respectively. Therefore, an 80-min preincubation period is allowed, during which time the medium is aspirated every 20 min and replaced with fresh medium. After preincubation, the tissue is usually incubated in fresh medium for a 20-min control period, followed by another 20-min period in either medium alone (control group) or in medium containing test substances (test group). Viability of the tissue is always tested by incubation in the presence of 56 mM KCl at the end of each experiment. In studies investigating the inhibitory effects of drugs, submaximal stimulation of peptide release can be achieved by adding 28 or 40 mM KCl (Figs. 1 and 2).

Media collected throughout the studies are immediately placed on dry ice, and at the completion of each experiment stored at −20°C until assay.

The assays coupled to the system (RIAs) are usually performed on the same tubes used for collecting the medium to minimize peptide loss.

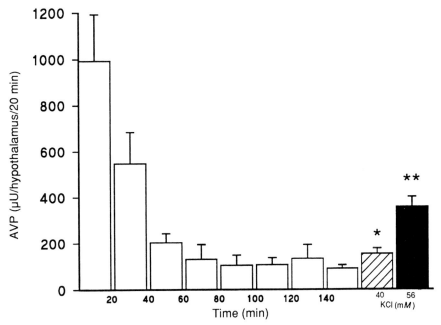

FIG. 2   Spontaneous secretion of arginine vasopressin (AVP) from hypothalami incubated over 160 min, and the effect of 40 and 56 mM KCl. Each bar represents the mean ± SEM of concentrations from 7 to 13 vials. AVP release stabilized after 80 min. *$p < 0.05$, **$p < 0.01$, vs. the preceding (160 min) basal collection.

Processing of Results

Usually, the effects of any substance added to the test incubation vials are compared in a preliminary analysis (e.g., by one-way analysis of variance) to the parallel control vials from which the substance had been excluded (a "per test" comparison). Once established whether an effect does occur, individual comparisons are made by post hoc *t* tests. Alternatively, individual test results may be compared to the control by means of Dunnett's test, or multiple comparisons made with correction factors, such as Bonferroni's, Tukey's, or Duncan's. The magnitude of release is conventionally expressed as either peptide concentration/hypothalamus/20 min or percentage over control release, the latter being more suitable when variations between experiments are found. Another way to express the hypothalamic release is the ratio of secretion (B_2/B_1 or S_2/S_1), calculated by dividing the absolute value during a collection (B_2) by the value of the preceding basal collection (B_1), or the value from the stimulated collection (S_2) by the value of the previous-stimulated collection (S_1).

A minimum of four experimental vials is considered necessary, although on most occasions considerably larger numbers are obtained over a series of studies.

Limits and Advantages of Technique

A system that provides information regarding neuroendocrine regulation in the rat hypothalamus should simulate the physiological situation with the maximum approximation possible. Even so, much care must be taken in extrapolating the findings to the *in vivo* context, and particularly to results from humans. Indeed, the major objection to the technique that can be put forward is that investigations are performed on the isolated hypothalamus, which is a structure removed from its natural environment; thus, its function *in vitro* does not necessarily mirror what actually occurs *in vivo*. Although the incubation devices (temperature, oxygen, and nutrient supplies) tend to recreate the physiological conditions as far as possible in a CSF-like milieu, inputs from the supra- and extrahypothalamic brain areas are inevitably removed. Moreover, by their very nature, the preparations are no longer subject to the diverse and complex neuronal feedback controls that are known to operate *in vivo*. Although such characteristics may be advantageous when assessing putative modulatory substances, the true physiological relevance of the *in vitro* set-up should be borne in mind in the investigation of the control of neuropeptide release. In other words, results obtained from this technique can define intrinsic biological mechanisms in a reliable manner, but to a limited extent, and regardless of their systemic consequences. As suggested by Robbins and Reichlin (18), combination of these data with those from complementary *in vivo* studies is indispensable, and may allow one to relate *in vivo* expression to *in vitro* changes.

Another major point regarding such tissue incubation is the actual time of survival of the tissue in the medium. Studies on oxygen consumption and maintainance of cellular integrity on histology have shown that incubation (or perifusion) in CSF-like media allows the whole hypothalamus to survive for at least 3 hr (19). The major limiting factor for adequate maintainance of the hypothalamus is the size, and possibly the shape, of the tissue examined. There appears to be a gradient of diffusion of nutrients into, and of toxic metabolites out from, the central part as opposed to the periphery of the explant. Although some investigators may continue to use the isolated hypothalamus as a whole, many others have tried to circumvent this major problem by employing fragmented materials, such as quartered hypothalami (20), or slices of various width (21, 22). These preparations are advantageous in terms of nutrient diffusion, but the procedures inevitably lead to loss of interneuronal connections. In this respect, we have found the use of halved hypothalami more satisfactory, the volume of the tissue actually decreasing but the neuronal projections remaining largely unaffected (15). It should be added, however, that there is still controversy regarding data obtained from whole tissue as opposed to those from hypothalamic halves, as will be reported below for cytokines. The bisection of the tissue, in our experience, allows for a larger surface to be exposed to the medium, thus prolonging cell survival and facilitating the access of test substances to the neuronal nuclei close to the midline. This is supported by the observation that the average survival of hypothalamic explants in our system exceeds 4 hr, as indicated by good responses to incubation with 56 mM KCl seen at least up to this time (see Fig. 1 for SRIF). Although addition of KCl does not represent a specific stimulus for the release of a particular hormone, it is universally considered as a reliable tool to check the residual viability of the system. Indeed, the dose-dependent effects of KCl on the release of various hormones have been established; Fig. 3 shows KCl-induced CRH-41 secretion. Therefore, only those hypothalami that respond to depolarization at the end of each experiment are selected for analysis. We conventionally (and to some extent arbitrarily) regard a hypothalamus as viable when at least a twofold increase in peptide secretion occurs in the presence of 56 mM KCl. However, far higher responses (up to 10-fold increases) are most frequently observed by using either 56 mM KCl or other depolarizing agents, such as veratridine. The phenomenon has been shown to depend strictly on the presence of Ca^{2+} in either the medium or the hypothalamic tissue (23).

One open question is to what extent the hormone release measured in this system reflects that destined to reach the median eminence, and thus the pituitary. Hypothalamic neurons known to synthesize and release hypophysiotrophic factors also project to intrahypothalamic regions distinct from the median eminence, and to extrahypothalamic sites. For instance, the axons of the vast majority of CRH-41-producing neurons of the parvocellular part of the PVN terminate in the proximity of the median eminence. However, CRH-41 immunoreactivity has also been found in subpopulations of PVN cells that project to autonomic-related cell groups and to the posterior pituitary. On the other hand, it must be added that *en passant* axons arising in the magnocellular division of the PVN are capable of releasing hormones (AVP and oxytocin) in the median eminence. This means that although the median eminence acts as the final common path for secretions from different hypothalamic areas, a fraction of the hormones assayed in the incubation medium may not be destined to reach the median eminence. In the case of CRH-41, this amount has been quantified as about 50% of the total secretion

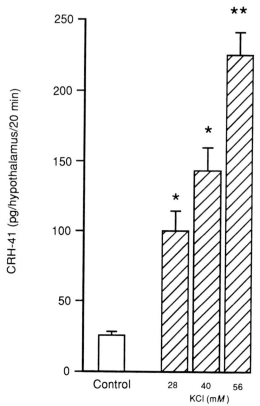

FIG. 3   Dose–response effect of KCl on CRH-41 release. Bars represent the mean ± SEM of values from eight incubation vials. $*p < 0.01$, $**p < 0.001$, compared to control.

(P. Sawchenko, personal communication). This phenomenon must therefore be borne in mind when discussing the relevance of hormonal secretion measured in our system to the functional regulation of pituitary activity.

Another acknowledged limit of this system depends on the possible differential diffusion of test drugs through the tissue, which may well account for discrepancies between studies in the literature. In addition, when static incubations such as the present one are used, accumulation of secretory products in the medium may also affect neurosecretion and provide confounding results. The use of perifusion or superfusion of tissue would partially overcome this problem, ensuring a rapid removal of interfering substances. Indeed, discrepant results from incubated or perifused pituitaries have been shown to depend on this phenomenon (24).

In our system, the times of incubation were dictated by experiments carried out to determine the optimal incubation duration. As secretion of peptides is rapid during the first few minutes (10 min in the case of CRH-41), with a further slower increase after 20 min of total incubation, we chose 20 min as the ideal time for each incubation step. This time was particularly adequate for accumulation of peptide sufficient to be measurable in our assay system, without the need for prior extraction. Studies performed on CRH-41 showed that negligible degradation of the peptide occurred with 20-min incubations, provided the medium was supplemented with aprotinin at a concentration of 100 kIU/ml.

The shaking pace of the water bath also appears to be of some importance, as it enables the medium to wet the surface and continuously remove the products of secretion. It has been suggested that differences in the speed of shaking may affect hormone release and explain differences between studies (25).

Among the advantages of this system, it must be mentioned that minimal trauma to the tissue is ensured by extreme care in the brain removal and dissection procedures, as well as by the CSF-like fluid surrounding the preparations in the vials. Then, during the experiments, any damage to the hypothalami is carefully avoided by the experimenter while collecting and renewing the incubation medium. Moreover, the system guarantees the retention of a high degree of cellular integrity and the preservation of the constituents of the tissue, such as the intrinsic neuronal networks, the supporting glia, and other neuronal cells. Therefore compared to other systems, such as synaptosomes or incubated slices, this method seems to mirror more closely the prior physiological state. Another advantage is that the technique allows precise control of the composition of the medium, and thus allows the study of the effects of various neuroactive substances. Finally, the running of the system is relatively inexpensive. Table II summarizes the main advantages and disadvantages of the technique.

As mentioned above, the use of this incubation system has provided data on the mechanisms of the hypothalamic release of different peptides. In

TABLE II   Major Advantages and Disadvantages
of *in Vitro* Incubation System

Advantages	Disadvantages
Minimal trauma	Absence of inputs
Defined structural system	Presence of interneurons
Functional integrity	Diffusion insufficiency

TABLE III   Role of Different Substances (except Cytokines) in Regulation of CRH-41 Secretion from Rat Hypothalamus in *in Vitro* System[a]

Excitatory	Inhibitory	No effect
Noradrenaline (β)	GABA	MCH
Serotonin	Opioids (μ, κ)	EGF
Acetylcholine (M)	ANP	NGF
NPY	Substance P	Melatonin
	Nitric oxide	EAA

[a] The receptors involved and/or the mediating factors are reported in parentheses. GABA, γ-Aminobutyric acid; MCH, melanin concentrating hormone; ANP, atrial natriuretic peptide; NPY, neuropeptide Y; EGF, epidermal growth factor; NGF, nerve growth factor; EAA, excitatory amino acids; M, muscarinic receptor.

Table III the main results that we have obtained regarding the mechanisms of CRH-41 secretion over the past few years are briefly reported.

As the purpose of this article is to deal with the hypothalamic hormones with particular respect to the effects of cytokines, results concerning these are reported in the next section.

Effects of Cytokines on Endocrine Hypothalamus

Cytokines and Hypothalamo–Pituitary–Adrenal Axis

There is an increasing body of evidence for reciprocal interactions between immune and endocrine responses. The two major biological systems involved appear to be linked via bidirectional and well-integrated circuits (26), the hypothalamus most likely representing the interface for the majority of immunoneuroendocrine connections. Cytokines hve been shown to play a key role in mediating communication between the two systems. Interleukin 1 (IL-1) is a cytokine produced by many cells, but especially monocytes, which activates both B and T lymphocytes and appears to mediate many of the changes seen during the acute-phase response (27). On the basis of extensive studies, IL-1 has been shown to exert a stimulatory effect on the hypothalamo–pituitary–adrenal (HPA) axis (28, 29), and has been proposed to be a major messenger from the immune system to the brain, possibly through the activation of other factors such as classic neurotransmitters (30). Besedovsky *et al.* (31) reported that IL-1, administered intravenously, acutely stimulated adrenocorticotropic hormone (ACTH) and glucocorticoid secretion in the rat. It has long been known that increased secretion of glucocorticoids during severe infective stress such as endotoxemia is essential to the survival of the organism, and this may result in part by increased secretion of IL-1. However, the precise site of action of IL-1 in mediating this response has been controversial. Several early studies provided evidence in favor of IL-1 stimulating ACTH release directly from the pituitary (32, 33), but these studies involved incubation of cultured pituitary cells for several hours with IL-1, conditions unlikely to relate to the rapid pituitary–adrenal responses seen *in vivo*. Most acute studies, including those involving perifusion of freshly dispersed rat anterior pituitary cells, showed no direct action of cytokines on ACTH release. It therefore appears that the receptors present on the corticotrophs (if any) are either relatively insensitive to cytokines, or are not immediately responsive to IL-1. A central site of action of IL-1 in stimulating the HPA axis has therefore been proposed by several studies. It has been demonstrated that rats treated with anti-CRH-14 antiserum before IL-1 injection did not show the expected increase in ACTH (34). Furthermore, CRH-41 concentrations in the nerve terminals of the median eminence have been found to decrease in response to IL-1, provided replenishment of CRH-41 was prevented by blocking axonal transport with colchicine (34). Sapolsky *et al.* (29) observed that, in blood samples obtained from the hypothalamo–hypophyseal portal system after IL-1 injection, CRH-41 levels were increased. The IL-1-induced ACTH release is relatively specific in that plasma levels of prolactin, growth hormone, and oxytocin are not affected (28), although others have shown that lower doses than those that stimulate ACTH secretion may affect growth hormone and thyrotrophin-stimulating hormone (35). These studies pointed to an activation of CRH-41 secretion as a final common path in response to IL-1; however, they did not directly prove that IL-1 acts at the level of hypothalamus.

We applied the previously described incubation system to the investigation of any direct effects of IL-1 and other cytokines on the release of hypothalamic CRH-41. Interleukin 1 is a polypeptide that exists in at least two different forms, IL-1α and IL-1β; the forms share approximately 25% homology, but are thought to act through the same receptor, at least in the periphery. In our studies, both forms of human recombinant IL-1 were tested *in vitro*. IL-1α was found to produce a dose-dependent increase in the release of CRH-41 in the dose range 1–100 U/ml. The maximum and minimum stimulations occurred at 10 and 5 U/ml, respectively (36). The use of IL-1β provided substantially similar results, with a significant stimulation in the same dose–response fashion (Fig. 4). As the recombinant products of both interleukins were expressed in *Escherichia coli*, which may synthesize endotoxin, IL-1β was also tested after denaturation by heating at 95°C for 60 min,

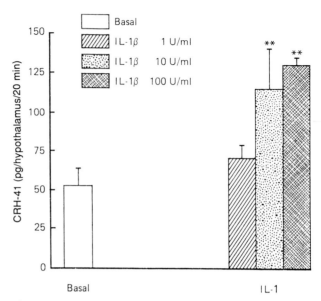

FIG. 4   Dose-dependent stimulation of CRH-41 release by IL-1β. Each bar represents the mean ± SEM of CRH-41 release in four to six experimental vials per group. **$p < 0.01$ vs. control at 10 and 100 U/ml.

treatment known not to affect endotoxin but that destroys interleukin activity. This procedure abolished the CRH-41 response, suggesting that endotoxin itself was not responsible for the increase in hormone secretion. Attempts to block interleukin action with specific antisera failed because of interference with the CRH-41 assay, emphasizing the need to assess assay cross-reactivity in all such studies (36).

Thus the hypothalamus appears to be extremely sensitive to low concentrations of IL-1, and this would agree with studies showing that IL-1 stimulates ACTH release at subpyrogenic doses (29, 34). Interleukin 1 has been shown to exert different actions on the brain, and although our findings are in favor of a direct effect on the hypothalamus, they do not necessarily indicate a primary action on the CRH-41 neurons. This is, however, supported by the finding of the presence of IL-1β-immunoreactive neuronal fibers in the human brain, including the hypothalamus. These fibers run to the median eminence and are also in close proximity to CRH-41 cell bodies in the PVN (37).

The effect of IL-1 on CRH-41 release may be mediated by noradrenaline (30), this neurotransmitter showing a direct stimulatory effect on CRH-41 neurons (23). It is not known whether circulating IL-1 has privileged access to the CNS, but parts of the medial basal hypothalamus appear to be outside the blood–brain barrier. It is therefore possible that pituitary–adrenal activity may be under the direct control of circulating IL-1 acting directly/indirectly at a hypothalamic level. Interleukin 1 concentrations that stimulate CRH-41 release are similar to those found circulating during the acute-phase response (38). The candidate sites for this effect are either the median eminence (although we were unable to show direct effects at this site) or the organum vasculosum of the lamina terminalis (OVLT) (28, 39).

Alternatively, an indirect effect through stimulation of hypothalamic prostaglandin (particularly PGE_2) secretion was suggested by one group (40). Interleukin 1 stimulates PGE_2 synthesis in several brain areas *in vitro,* including the hypothalamus, and can stimulate the astroglial release of PGE_2 (41). Prostaglandins, in turn, are known to stimulate ACTH release when injected in the median eminence (28). Using our incubation system, a series of studies were undertaken to investigate the role of prostaglandins in CRH-41 secretion, along with the central neuroendocrine effects of other cytokines. As shown in Fig. 5, the effects of IL-1β were found to be antagonized by blockade of the eicosanoid cyclooxygenase pathway by indomethacin and naproxen, but not by blockade of the lipoxygenase system by the selective inhibitor BW A4C (42). Interleukin 6 stimulated CRH-41 release (Fig. 6) in the dose range of 10–100 U/ml, in agreement with other findings (43), suggesting an ACTH-increasing effect in the rat. As found for IL-1, mediation by prostaglandins was observed, whereas IL-6 showed no effect on the isolated median eminences incubated under the same conditions (42), suggesting a different site of action.

Our findings on bisected hypothalami are in agreement with other studies on the intact hypothalamus reporting a stimulatory effect of IL-1 on PGE_2 release, and of IL-6 on CRH-41 release (44). The latter group was unable to show any effect of IL-1 on the intact hypothalamus (45), the different preparations possibly accounting for the discrepancies. On the other hand, most other studies have also shown a direct effect of IL-1 on CRH-41 release (46, 47).

Interleukin 2 has been shown to increase ACTH secretion in patients with neoplasia (48), but not in most animal studies (31, 49), although a stimulatory effect on CRH-41 in *in vitro* long-term incubated explants has been reported (46). Unlike IL-1, we found that incubation of hypothalami with IL-2 in the dose range of 1–10.00 U/ml had no effect in activating CRH-41 release (42), this discrepancy possibly being due to the different duration of incubation system, which may affect the receptor populations. Similarly, no effect was found for IL-8 (0.1–10 nM), tumor necrosis factor (TNF) (10–1000 U/ml), interferon α_2 (10–1000 U/ml), or interferon γ (10–1000 U/ml), at variance with both *in vivo* and *in vitro* studies showing a stimulatory effect on the HPA axis for TNF (50, 51) and the interferons (52, 53). However, different

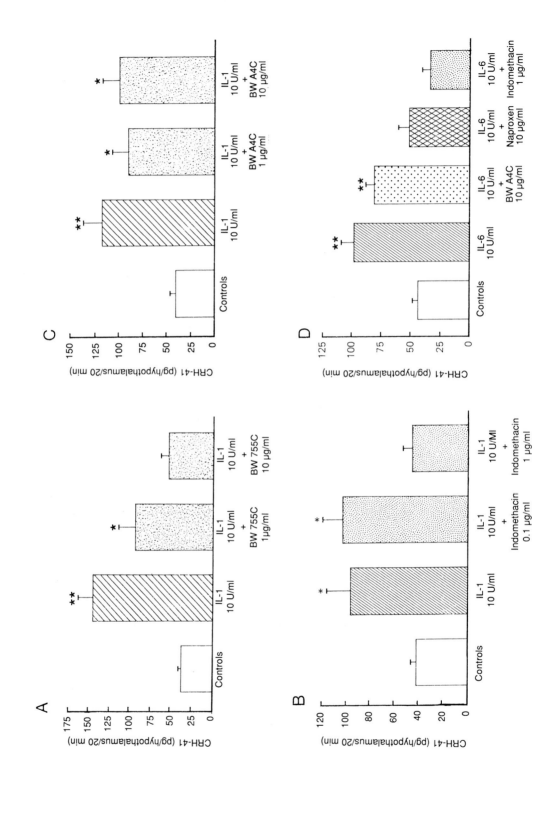

stabilization periods were used in the reported *in vitro* studies, and this may possibly explain the discrepancies. Other authors (31) were unable to demonstrate any acute effect of γ-interferon on cortisol levels *in vivo* in the rat.

Thus, both IL-1 and IL-6 are able to activate CRH-41 release by specific mechanisms involving cyclooxygenase products, in agreement with other *in vitro* studies (54); such a stimulatory effect appears to take place at sites within the hypothalamus but outside the median eminence, and is not shared with IL-2, IL-8, TNF, or with interferons-α_2 or -γ. These findings further support the existence of sites of communication between endocrine and immune systems. Moreover, it would appear that CRH-41 plays a role of physiological significance in the mechanisms of fever, as it has also been shown that administration of the CRH-41 antagonists in the CSF of rat treated with intracerebroventricular (icv) IL-1 blocks the stimulatory effects of the latter on body temperature, metabolic rate and brown adipose tissue (55).

More recently, we have investigated the direct effect of cytokines on the secretion of AVP, the other main ACTH-stimulating peptide. Indeed, AVP may well be involved in the mechanisms of fever, and there is evidence that it may be an endogenous antipyretic (56). By contrast, a pyretic action mediated peripherally by prostaglandins has also been claimed for AVP (57).

In our system, IL-1β, at doses of 10–100 U/ml, stimulated AVP release, with a maximum effect at 100 U/ml (Fig. 7), suggesting that cytokines may activate the HPA axis via the release of AVP, in addition to that of CRH-41. The IL-1β effect was then tested in the presence of L-arginine, a precursor of nitric oxide (NO) synthesis. Nitric oxide is a ubiquitous molecule that may act as an inhibitory neurotransmitter in the brain, and that has been shown to be primarily involved in the control of blood pressure, but also in the regulation of endocrine and immune processes (58). Interestingly, L-arginine at concentrations of 10–100 μM significantly reduced interleukin-induced AVP release. Furthermore, the addition of the specific L-arginine antagonist N^G-monomethyl-L-arginine (L-NMMA) restored the AVP response to IL-1β, suggesting that the mechanisms of NO formation may modulate the action of at least IL-1β in the supraoptic nucleus of hypothalamus (59).

We have also extended the use of this incubation system to investigate the effects of cytokines on prostaglandin and prostacyclin release. Both IL-1

FIG. 5   Effects of BW 755C (A), indomethacin (B), and BW A4C (C) on the release of CRH-41 induced by IL-1β. (D) Effects of indomethacin, naproxen, and BW A4C on the release of CRH-41 induced by IL-6. Each bar represents the mean $\pm$ SEM of 6 to 12 experimental vials per group. $*p < 0.05$, $**p < 0.01$ vs. control.

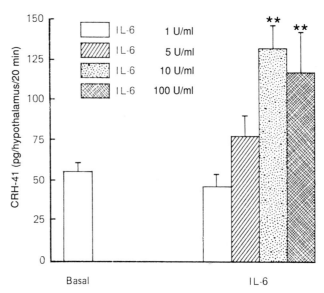

FIG. 6   Dose–response effect of IL-6 on CRH-41 release from incubated hypothalami. Each bar represents the mean ± SEM of secretion in four to six experimental vials per group. **$p < 0.01$ vs. control.

and IL-6 specifically stimulated the hypothalamic release of PGE_2, while leaving PGF_{2a}, 6K PGF_{1a} (the principal metabolite of prostacyclin), and thromboxane B_2 unchanged (60). However, as PGE_2 does not per se stimulate CRH-41 release, the significance of this finding to neuroendocrine regulation remains unclear.

Effect of Cytokines on Growth Axis

Somatostatin and GHRH represent the two major regulators of growth so far known, via their control of GH release from the pituitary.

Previous studies had suggested that cytokines might mediate the release of SRIF *in vitro* (61, 62); there was, however, no report on the direct effect of cytokines on the release of GHRH. The effect of IL-1β, IL-6, and TNF on both peptides was investigated in our system (63). Interleukin 1β (1–100 U/ml) caused a pronounced dose-dependent stimulation of SRIF (Fig. 8), with a modest but significant increase in GHRH in the dose range of 10–100 U/ml, whereas no effect on either peptide was shown in the isolated median eminence or in the mediobasal hypothalamus. Furthermore, the effects of IL-1 were antagonized by the cyclooxygenase inhibitor, indomethacin (10

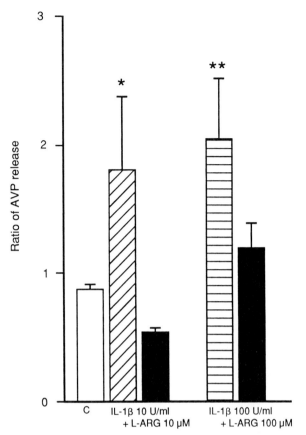

FIG. 7   Effect of IL-1β, either alone or with L-arginine, on AVP release. Bars represent the mean ± SEM of the ratio of secretion, calculated by dividing the absolute values from the stimulated collection by the value from the preceding basal collection. Data refer to 4 to 15 experimental vials. $*p < 0.05$, $**p < 0.01$ vs. control.

μg/ml), but not by α-helical CRH(9–41). By contrast, neither IL-6 (10–100 U/ml) nor TNF-α (10–10.000 U/ml) showed any effect on SRIF and GHRH secretion (63).

Thus, only IL-1β seems to stimulate the release of hypothalamic GH-regulating hormones, via the formation of cyclooxygenase products but regardless of any concomitant effect on CRH-41 secretion. As no effect on median eminence is detectable, IL-1 is likely to act at a higher level in the hypothalamus, this being consistent with our previous findings on CRH-41 (36), and with the fact that few IL-1 receptors are expressed in the median

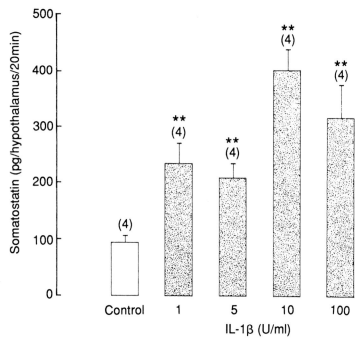

FIG. 8   Dose-dependent effect of IL-1β on SRIF release. Values are expressed as means ± SEM. Numbers in parentheses are the numbers of experimental vials. **$p < 0.01$.

eminence (64). As in the case of CRH-41, the precise site of action of IL-1 is still uncertain. The reciprocal interactions between SRIF- and GHRH-containing neurons in the hypothalamus, with SRIF apparently suppressing the release of GHRH (65), may complicate the interpretation of these findings. However, it is possible that the marked stimulation of SRIF may override the minor increase in GHRH.

The absence of any effect of IL-6 on both SRIF and GHRH is in agreement with a previous study (62), and suggests that the observed increase in GH secretion from anterior pituitary cells following IL-6 (66) may occur by a direct effect at the pituitary level. Tumor necrosis factor was found to be ineffective on both SRIF and GHRH secretion, similar to our findings for CRH-41, although a previous study with a different system had shown a stimulatory effect of chronic exposure to TNF on SRIF release (67).

In the first instance, these *in vitro* findings provide further evidence for communication between the immune and neuroendocrine systems, possibly at a hypothalamic level, and also outside the HPA axis. Moreover, it is well established that chronic inflammatory conditions of childhood (juvenile rheumatoid arthritis, inflammatory bowel disease) often produce a failure to thrive and an inhibition of growth velocity (68, 69). From this viewpoint, our data would suggest that cytokines (at least IL-1) not only regulate stress-dependent activation of the HPA axis and the mechanisms of thermogenesis, but are also involved in growth processes.

Conclusions

Numerous effects of cytokines on the hypothalamus *in vitro* have been observed in our system, most of which are consistent with the findings of current research in the field. This system, previously validated for the investigation of the effect of more "traditional" neuroendocrine regulators (classic neurotransmitters and hormonal peptides), has indeed also proved to be a reliable model for the study of the effects of cytokines on the hypothalamus, the principal CNS station for immunoendocrine interactions.

Over the past few years, the products of activated immune cells have been found to possess potent neuroendocrine effects, in addition to many others in the brain. Cytokines, and especially interleukins, appear to act as messengers that provide the CNS with instantaneous information regarding events that are taking place in the periphery. Thus their action enables the brain to react appropriately to the situation by activating the relevant neuroendocrine mechanisms.

As far as the precise site of action of cytokines within the hypothalamus is concerned, this still remains unclear, although there is some evidence supporting the existence of specific receptors in the hypothalamus. It is equally not fully understood whether cytokines (mainly IL-1 and IL-6) affect the release of hypothalamic hormones principally either as regulatory factors produced locally or as circulating agents. Studies have shown a limited number of receptors for IL-1 in the median eminence (64) and, consistently, no secretion of CRH-41 or SRIF from the eminence incubated with interleukin was seen in our system. The effect of interleukins may therefore occur within the hypothalamus itself. The OVLT, where the blood–brain barrier is absent, would be a reliable candidate as a site for the cytokines to penetrate the CNS. Additionally, the local release of prostanoids, particularly PGE_2, which may in turn activate endogenous hypothalamic IL-1, may act to "relay" the cytokine message to hypothalamic CRH-41.

The role that circulating cytokines play in activating the neuroendocrine system may, however, be of limited importance; in this respect, their presence within the CNS should not be underestimated. Interleukin 1 is known to be synthesized in the brain by astroglial cells (70) and IL-6 expression may also be induced in such cells (71). Thus it remains uncertain whether the actions performed by interleukins are to be viewed mainly as endocrine or paracrine.

Studies are currently in progress to characterize further the actions of cytokines on the hypothalamus *in vitro*. There is indeed little doubt that such techniques, when integrated with *in vivo* data, have greatly expanded our understanding of neuroimmune interactions.

References

1. C. Kordon, M. T. Bluet-Pajot, H. Clauser, S. Drouva, A. Enjalbert, and J. Epelbaum, *Prog. Brain Res.* **72,** 27 (1987).
2. T. Hokfelt, D. Johansson, and M. Goldstein, *Science* **225,** 1326 (1984).
3. E. De Robertis, A. DeLores, L. Salganicoff, A. De Irladi, and L. M. Zieher, *J. Neurochem.* **10,** 225 (1963).
4. J. Epelbaum, P. Brazeau, D. Tsang, J. Brawer, and J. Martin, *Brain Res.* **126,** 309 (1977).
5. R. B. Kelly, J. W. Deutch, S. S. Carlson, and J. A. Wagner, *Annu. Rev. Neurosci.* **2,** 399 (1979).
6. C. D. Sladek and C. R. Joynt, *Endocrinology (Baltimore)* **104,** 148 (1979).
7. S. B. Richardson, C. S. Hollander, R. D'Eletto, P. W. Greenleaf, and C. Thaw, *Endocrinology (Baltimore)* **107,** 122 (1980).
8. A. Gyevai, P. J. Chapple, and W. H. J. Douglas, *J. Cell Sci.* **34,** 159 (1978).
9. A. Tixier-Vidal, R. Picart, C. Loudes, and A. Faivre-Bauman, *Neuroscience* **17,** 115 (1986).
10. M. F. Scanlon, R. J. Robbins, J. L. Bolaffi, I. M. D. Jackson, and S. Reichlin, *Neuroendocrinology* **37,** 269 (1983).
11. M. A. Smith, G. Bissette, T. A. Slotkin, D. L. Knight, and C. B. Nemeroff, *Endocrinology (Baltimore)* **118,** 1997 (1986).
12. M. C. Holmes, F. A. Antoni, K. J. Catt, and G. Aguilera, *Neuroendocrinology* **43,** 245 (1986).
13. T. Suda, F. Yajima, N. Tomori, H. Demura, and K. Shizume, *Life Sci.* **37,** 1499 (1985).
14. A. E. Calogero, W. T. Gallucci, R. Bernardini, C. Saoutis, P. W. Gold, and G. P. Chrousos, *Neuroendocrinology* **47,** 303 (1988).
15. A. M. Lengyel, A. Grossman, A. C. Nieuwenhuizen-Kruseman, J. Acland, L. Rees, and G. M. Besser, *Neuroendocrinology* **39,** 31 (1984).
16. M. T. Jones, E. W. Hillhouse, and J. L. Burden, *J. Endocrinol.* **69,** 1 (1976).
17. G. Fink, *in* "Neuroendocrine Perspectives" (E. E. Muller and R. M. MacLeod, eds.), Vol. 5, p. 23. Elsevier, Amsterdam, 1986.
18. R. Robbins and S. Reichlin, *in* "Neuroendocrine Perspectives" (E. E. Muller and R. M. MacLeod, eds.), p. 111. Elsevier, Amsterdam, 1982.
19. M. W. B. Bradbury, J. Burden, E. W. Hillhouse, and M. T. Jones, *J. Physiol. (London)* **239,** 269 (1974).
20. K. Maeda and L. A. Frohman, *Endocrinology (Baltimore)* **106,** 1837 (1980).

21. C. Yamamoto and H. McIlwain, *J. Neurochem.* **13,** 1333 (1966).

22. M. J. Kelly, T. P. Condon, J. E. Levine, and O. K. Ponnekleiv, *Brain Res.* **345,** 264 (1985).

23. S. Tsagarakis, J. M. P. Holly, L. H. Rees, G. M. Besser, and A. Grossman, *Endocrinology (Baltimore)* **123,** 1962 (1988).

24. J. Price, A. Grossman, G. M. Besser, and L. H. Rees, *Neuroendocrinology* **36,** 125 (1983).

25. S. Wibullaksanakul and D. Handelsman, *J. Neuroendocrinol.* **3,** 185 (1991).

26. J. E. Blalock and E. M. Smith, *Fed. Am. Soc. Exp. Biol. Fed. Proc.* **44,** 108 (1985).

27. C. A. Dinarello, *N. Engl. J. Med.* **311,** 1413 (1984).

28. A. Bateman, A. Singh, T. Kral, and S. Solomon, *Endocr. Rev.* **10,** 92 (1989).

29. R. Sapolsky, C. Rivier, G. Yamamoto, P. Plotsky, and V. Vale, *Science* **238,** 522 (1987).

30. A. J. Dunn, *Life Sci.* **42,** 429 (1988).

31. A. Besedovsky, A. Del Rey, E. Sorkin, and C. A. Dinarello, *Science* **233,** 652 (1986).

32. B. M. R. N. J. Wolowsky, E. M. Smith, W. J. Meyer, G. M. Fuller, and J. E. Blalock, *Science* **230,** 1035 (1985).

33. E. W. Bernton, J. E. Beach, and J. W. Holaday, *Science* **238,** 519 (1987).

34. F. Berkenbosch, J. Van Oers, A. Del Rey, F. Tilders, and H. Besedowsky, *Science* **238,** 524 (1987).

35. V. Rettori, J. Jurcovicova, and S. M. McCann, *J. Neurosci. Res.* **18,** 179 (1987).

36. S. Tsagarakis, G. Gillies, L. H. Rees, M. Besser, and A. Grossman, *Neuroendocrinology* **49,** 98 (1989).

37. C. D. Breder, C. A. Dinarello, and C. B. Saper, *Science* **240,** 321 (1988).

38. A. Luger, H. Graf, H. P. Schwarz, H. K. Stummroll, and T. A. Luger, *CRC Crit. Care Med.* **14,** 458 (1986).

39. G. Katsuura, A. Arimura, K. Koves, and P. E. Gottschall, *Am. J. Physiol.* **258,** 163 (1990).

40. G. Katsuura, P. E. Gottschall, R. R. Dall, and A. Arimura, *Endocrinology (Baltimore)* **122,** 1773 (1988).

41. G. Katsuura, P. E. Gottschall, R. R. Dall, and A. Arimura, *Endocrinology (Baltimore)* **124,** 3125 (1989).

42. P. Navarra, S. Tsagarakis, M. S. Faria, L. H. Rees, G. M. Besser, and A. B. Grossman, *Endocrinology (Baltimore)* **128,** 37 (1990).

43. Y. Naitoh, J. Fukata, T. Tominaga, Y. Nakay, S. Tamai, K. Mori, and H. Imura, *Biochem. Biophys. Res. Commun.* **155,** 1459 (1988).

44. N. G. N. Milton, C. H. Self, and E. W. Hillhouse, *J. Endocrinol.* **132,** Suppl. 214 (1992).

45. N. G. N. Milton, C. H. Self, and E. W. Hillhouse, *J. Endocrinol.* **129,** Suppl., 238 (1991).

46. R. Bernardini, A. E. Calogero, G. Mauceri, and G. P. Chrousos, *Life Sci.* **47,** 1601 (1990).

47. J. C. Cambronero, J. Borrel, and C. Guaza, *J. Neurosci. Res.* **24,** 470 (1989).

48. C. Bindon, M. Czerniecki, P. Ruell, A. Edwards, W. H. McCarthy, R. Harris, and P. Hersey, *Br. J. Cancer* **46,** 123 (1983).

49. A. Del Rey, H. Besedovsky, E. Sorkin, and C. A. Dinarello, *Ann. N.Y. Acad. Sci.* **496,** 85 (1987).

50. B. M. Sharp, S. G. Matta, P. K. Peterson, R. Newton, C. Chao, and K. McAllen, *Endocrinology (Baltimore)* **124,** 3131 (1989).

51. R. Bernardini, T. C. Kamilaris, A. E. Calogero, E. O. Johnson, M. T. Gomez, P. W. Gold, and G. P. Chrousos, *Endocrinology (Baltimore)* **126,** 2876 (1990).

52. F. Holsboer, G. K. Stalla, U. von Bardeleben, K. Hamman, H. Miler, and O. A. Miller, *Life Sci.* **42,** 1 (1988).

53. J. Roosth, L. B. Pollard, S. Lori Brown, and W. J. Meyer, *J. Neuroimmunol.* **12,** 311 (1986).

54. R. Bernardini, A. Chiarenza, A. E. Calogero, P. W. Gold, and G. P. Chrousos, *Neuroendocrinology* **50,** 708 (1989).

55. N. J. L. Rothwell, *Neurosci. Behav. Rev.* **14,** 263 (1988).

56. N. W. Kasting, *Brain Res.* **14,** 143 (1990).

57. A. S. Milton, E. W. Hillhouse, and N. G. N. Milton, *J. Endocrinol.* **132,** Suppl., 211 (1992).

58. S. Moncada, R. M. J. Palmer, and E. Higgs, *Pharmacol. Rev.* **43,** 109 (1991).

59. S. Yasin, A. Costa, A. Grossman, and M. Forsling, unpublished observations (1992).

60. P. Navarra, G. Pozzoli, L. Brunetti, E. Ragazzoni, M. Besser, and A. Grossman, *Neuroendocrinology* **56,** 61 (1992).

61. D. E. Scarborough, S. L. Lee, C. A. Dinarello, and S. Reichlin, *Endocrinology (Baltimore)* **124,** 549 (1989).

62. B. L. Spangelo, A. M. Judd, R. M. MacLeod, D. W. Goodman, and P. C. Isakson, *Endocrinology (Baltimore)* **127,** 1779 (1990).

63. J. Honegger, A. Spagnoli, R. D'Urso, P. Navarra, S. Tsagarakis, G. M. Besser, and A. Grossman, *Endocrinology (Baltimore)* **129,** 1275 (1991).

64. W. L. Farrar, P. L. Kilian, M. R. Ruff, J. M. Hill, and C. B. Pert, *J. Immunol.* **139,** 459 (1987).

65. N. Kitajima, K. Chihara, H. Abe, Y. Okimura, Y. Fujii, M. Sato, S. Shakutsui, M. Watanabe, and T. Fujita, *Endocrinology (Baltimore)* **124,** 69 (1989).

66. B. L. Spangelo, A. M. Judd, P. C. Isakson, and R. M. MacLeod, *Endocrinology (Baltimore)* **125,** 575 (1989).

67. D. E. Scarborough and C. A. Dinarello, *Proc. 71st Annu. Meet. Endocr. Soc.,* Abstr., p. 103 (1989).

68. T. McCaffery, N. Khosrow, A. Lawrence, and J. Kirsner, *Pediatrics* **45,** 386 (1970).

69. M. J. G. Farthing, C. A. Campell, J. Walker-Smith, C. R. W. Edwards, L. H. Rees, and A. M. Dawson, *Gut* **22,** 933 (1981).

70. D. Giulian, D. G. Young, J. Woodwars, D. C. Brown, and L. B. Lachman, *J. Neurosci.* **8,** 709 (1988).

71. T. Kishimoto, *Blood* **74,** 1 (1989).

[18] Effects of Interleukin 1 on β-Endorphin Secretion in AtT-20 Pituitary Cells: Methods and Overview

Mirela O. Făgărăşan

Introduction

In AtT-20 cells, a mouse anterior pituitary cell line, corticotropin-releasing factor (CRF), vasoactive intestinal peptide (VIP), β-adrenergic agonists, forskolin, and phorbol 12-*O*-tetradecanoate 13-acetate (TPA) rapidly stimulate adrenocorticotropic hormone (ACTH) and β-endorphin secretion (1). In contrast, we determined that the treatment of AtT-20 cells with the cytokine interleukin 1 (IL-1) increases β-endorphin release after many hours (2).

Our previous work has also shown that prolonged pretreatment with IL-1 also potentiates the secretion induced by secretagogues such as CRF, VIP, forskolin (2), norepinephrine, and isoproterenol (3). It has been demonstrated that IL-1 can increase the formation of mRNA for proopiomelanocortin (POMC) only after treatment with the cytokine for a long period of time (4). The late-induced secretion of β-endorphin by IL-1 did not require the continuous presence of the cytokine (5). This suggests that the interaction of IL-1 with its receptors generates a cascade of early and intermediate signals that results in the late secretion of β-endorphin.

Information concerning the early signals that IL-1 generates and biochemical events following IL-1 receptor interaction is scanty. Some of the data described appear to be contradictory and no clear picture has yet emerged (6). The phosphorylation of a cytosolic 65-kDa protein induced by IL-1 in glucocorticoid-pretreated normal human peripheral blood mononuclear leukocytes has been reported (7). Interleukin 1 was found to stimulate the production of diacylglycerol and phosphatidic acid in cultured rat mesangial cells (8) and prostaglandin synthesis in fibroblasts (9). The cytokines were found to stimulate immediate-early protooncogenes, such as c-*fos*, c-*myb*, and c-*myc* (10). Several transcription factors have been implicated in the action of IL-1 on gene expression (11).

We demonstrated that the treatment of AtT-20 cells with IL-1 causes phosphorylation of 19-, 20-, and 60-kDa proteins within minutes (5) and induces early and transient expression of mRNAs for c-*fos* and c-*jun* (12).

Also, we examined whether c-*jun* or c-*fos* is involved in IL-1 induction of late β-endorphin release from AtT-20 cells. We provided evidence that c-*jun* and c-*fos* are essential to IL-1 stimulation of β-endorphin release (12).

Methods

Cell Culture

AtT-20/D16-16, a line of mouse anterior pituitary tumor cells (obtained from S. Sabol, National Institutes of Health, Bethesda, MD), was grown in Dulbecco's modified Eagle's medium (DMEM) containing glucose (4.5 g/liter), 10% fetal bovine serum (FBS), penicillin (100 units/ml), and streptomycin (100 μg/ml). The cells were maintained in a humidified atmosphere of 10% CO_2 at 37°C and subcultured as described previously (2, 5, 12). The cells were used 5–7 days later (80–90% confluency).

For studies in normal corticotrophs, anterior pituitary cells from adult female Sprague–Dawley rats were enzymatically dispersed and cultured in 24-well plates at a density of 500,000 cells/well at 37°C, in an atmosphere of 5% CO_2/95% air in bicarbonate-buffered medium 199 containing 10% horse serum, streptomycin (1 μg/ml), and penicillin (100 U/ml). The normal pituitary cells were used after 3 to 5 days of culture.

β-Endorphin Release Experiments

At the onset of each experiment, freshly prepared 10% FBS–DMEM with or without IL-1 was added to the cells and the incubation was continued for the times indicated. Then AtT-20 cells were washed twice with 1 ml of 0.2% bovine serum albumin (BSA)–DMEM and incubated in identical serum-free medium in the presence or absence of IL-1 with or without other secretagogues for 60 min. Normal pituitary cells, after pretreatment with IL-1β for 48 hr, were washed with serum-free medium and further incubated with serum-free medium containing streptomycin (1 μg/ml), penicillin (100 U/ml), aprotonin (100 kallikrein units/ml), ascorbic acid (30 μg/ml), and 0.1% BSA for 1 hr, with agonists and drugs. The test medium was collected separately from each well, centrifuged, and the supernatant fluids were stored at -20°C until analysis by radioimmunoassay (13). Results were expressed as nanograms per well per hour. Data representing β-endorphin secretion induced by secretagogues were calculated by subtracting the amount of β-endorphin release by untreated cells.

Phosphorylation Experiments

AtT-20 cells were preincubated for 15 min in phosphate-free medium and then labeled for 45 min with 100 μCi of ^{32}P$_i$/ml in phosphate-free DMEM or phosphate-free Krebs–Ringer buffer. Secretagogue solutions were added and, after incubation periods ranging from 5 to 120 min, the cells were dissolved in a buffer containing 50 mM Tris-phosphate, 100 mM NaF, 10 mM ethylenediaminetetraacetic acid (EDTA), 5 mM ethylene glycol-bis (β-amminoethyl ether)-N,N,N',N'-tetraacetic acid (EGTA), leupeptin (4 mg/liter), and 1% (v/v) Triton X-100, pH 7.4. Cytosolic fractions were obtained by centrifugation of cell homogenates (15,000 rpm, 5 min) followed by collection of the supernatants. After precipitation of proteins with ice-cold 6% trichloroacetic acid and a second centrifugation step (15,000 rpm, 5 min), the resulting pellets were homogenized twice in 50% ethanol–50% diethyl ether with a sonicator, followed each time by centrifugation (15,000 rpm, 5 min). Pellets were then resuspended in phosphate-buffered saline, aliquots were removed for determination of protein concentration, and the remaining samples were lyophilized and stored overnight at $-30°$C. Two-dimensional gel electrophoresis was performed as described previously (5).

RNA Isolation and Northern Analysis

At selected time points after treatment, cytoplasmic RNA was isolated from cells washed with ice-cold phosphate-buffered saline (PBS) and lysed with guanidinium isothiocynate buffer. Total cellular RNA was extracted by cesium chloride centrifugation and fractionated on 1% agarose gel containing formaldehyde. Blots were hybridized with ^{32}P-labeled mouse c-*fos* and human c-*jun* probes. Hybridization with human actin cDNA probes verified uniformity of loaded RNA (12).

Oligonucleotides

Antisense c-*fos* (5'-TGC-GTT-GAA-GCC-CGA-GAA 3') and c-*jun* (5'-CGT-TTC-CAT-CTT-TGC-AGT 3') unsubstituted oligodeoxynucleotides (PO-ODNs) were synthesized on a multiple-column DNA synthesizer (model 8750; Biosearch, San Rafael, CA), purified on denatured acrylamide gels, electroeluted, and further purified by several cycles of ethanol precipitation. The nucleotide sequences were complementary to the first 18 bases following the AUG sequence of c-*fos* (14) and c-*jun* (15) mRNAs. These small synthetic oligonucleotides actively penetrate into the cells without any treatment (16) complex with their corresponding mRNAs, and probably accelerate degradation of the specific mRNA, resulting in a reduction in the amount of specific protein produced. The corresponding sense oligonucleotides were used as a control.

Results

Induction of β-Endorphin Secretion from AtT-20 Cells in a Time- and Dose-Related Manner

Human recombinant IL-1α and IL-1β stimulated β-endorphin release only after a prolonged period of incubation. There was no measurable β-endorphin secretion after 12 hr of pretreatment. However, after 18 hr of pretreatment, a small but significant increase in β-endorphin release was observed, reaching a maximum at 24 hr. Both IL-1α and IL-1β induced β-endorphin secretion with similar potency and in a dose-dependent manner (2). A significant stimulation of β-endorphin release was observed at 10^{-12} M IL-1, whereas maximum stimulation occurred at 10^{-9} M (Fig. 1).

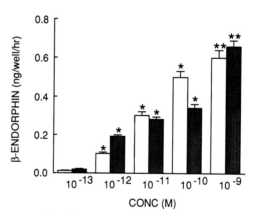

FIG. 1   Dose–response data for IL-1-induced β-endorphin secretion. AtT-20 cells were pretreated with IL-1α (open bars) or IL-1β (hatched bars) for 23 hr and then washed and serum-free medium with IL-1 was added. After a 1-hr incubation, medium from each well was collected and β-endorphin release was assayed. The secretion for different concentrations of IL-1α and IL-1β is shown after subtracting the amount of β-endorphin released by untreated cells. The results are the mean ± SEM from one of four similar experiments. $^{*}p < 0.05$; $^{**}p < 0.01$ (vs control).

Enhancement of Corticotropin-Releasing Factor, Vasoactive Intestinal Peptide, Norepinephrine, Isoproterenol, Forskolin, 12-O-Tetradecanoate 13-Acetate-Induced β-Endorphin Secretion in AtT-20 Cells

After treating AtT-20 cells with CRF alone for 1 hr, there was the expected increase in the release of β-endorphin. In cells pretreated with IL-1 for 23

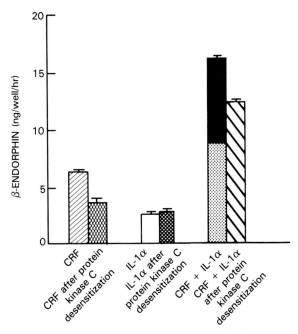

FIG. 2 Interleukin 1 potentiation of CRF-induced β-endorphin secretion in AtT-20 cells is only partly dependent on protein kinase C (PKC). AtT-20 cells were incubated in the absence or presence of 10^{-9} M IL-1α for 24 hr and then washed twice. The medium was removed by aspiration and fresh medium was added either without any drug or with TPA alone (10^{-7} M), IL-1 alone (10^{-9} M), or IL-1 plus TPA. The incubation continued for an additional 8 hr. The cells were washed and the untreated cells were incubated in serum-free medium with 10^{-7} M CRF. Interleukin 1-pretreated cells were incubated either with IL-1 or with IL-1 together with CRF. TPA-pretreated cells were incubated with TPA plus CRF. Interleukin plus TPA-pretreated cells were incubated either with IL-1 plus TPA or with IL-1 plus TPA plus CRF. Incubations were continued for an additional hour and β-endorphin concentrations were measured in aliquots from media. Solid bar represents the enhancement produced by IL-1 on β-endorphin release induced by CRF. Data represent the mean ± SEM from four experiments.

hr, CRF induced more than an additive secretion as compared to that produced by neuropeptide or lymphokine when incubated separately. Desensitization of protein kinase C (PKC) by prolonged treatment with TPA only partly abolished the effect of CRF alone as well as the potentiating effects induced by IL-1 (Fig. 2). Interleukin 1 pretreatment for 23 hr also resulted in enhanced β-endorphin release by VIP, forskolin, TPA (2), norepinephrine, and isoproterenol (3).

Induction of Vasopressin-Induced β-Endorphin Release in AtT-20 Cells

In contrast to its action in normal pituitary cells, arginine vasopressin (AVP) does not stimulate the secretion of ACTH and β-endorphin in AtT-20 cells. Thus no detectable increase in β-endorphin secretion was observed after incubation of AtT-20 cells with AVP for 1 hr. However, after pretreatment

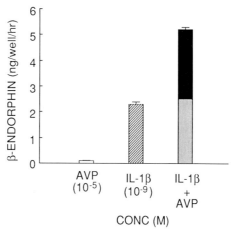

FIG. 3 Interleukin 1 activates arginine vasopressin (AVP)-mediated release of β-endorphin in AtT-20 cells. AtT-20 cells were incubated in the presence or absence of IL-1β for 48 hr. For PKC desensitization another group of cells was pretreated with 10^{-7} M TPA overnight before IL-1 treatment, then washed twice with serum-free medium. The untreated cells were incubated in 0.2% BSA/DMEM for another hour either with vehicle alone or with 10^{-5} M AVP. The cells pretreated with IL-1β were also divided into two groups after washing. One group was incubated with IL-1β alone and another group with IL-1β plus AVP. After 1 hr, medium was collected from each well and β-endorphin release into the medium was determined. Solid bar represents the enhancement produced by IL-1β alone. Data are the mean ± SEM of six observations from one of four similar experiments.

with 10^{-9} M IL-1β for 48 hr, exposure of AtT-20 cells to IL-1β (10^{-9} M) plus AVP (10^{-5} M) markedly stimulated β-endorphin release (17) (Fig. 3). After desensitization of PKC by prolonged pretreatment with 100 nM TPA, this effect of IL-1β was abolished.

Potentiation of Corticotropin-Releasing Factor-Induced β-Endorphin Release by IL-1 in Normal Pituitary Cells

The effects of IL-1 pretreatment on basal and agonist-stimulated secretion of β-endorphin were studied in primary cultures of normal anterior pituitary cells. Pretreatment with IL-1β for 48 hr caused a minor but significant increase in β-endorphin release, and potentiated the β-endorphin responses to CRF (Fig. 4b). The enhancement of the secretagogue-induced responses by IL-1 was even greater than observed in AtT-20 cells (17). In some cell cultures in which β-endorphin responses to CRF were relatively small, treatment with IL-1β for 48 hr still caused prominent enhancement of the secretory response to CRF (Fig. 4a).

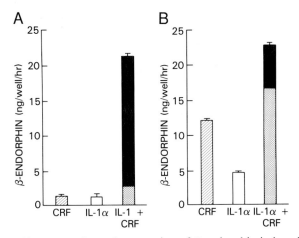

FIG. 4 Interleukin 1 potentiates the secretion of β-endorphin induced by CRF and activates CRF-mediated secretion in rat anterior pituitary cells. After 48 hr of incubation with or without IL-1, the cells were washed twice and then incubated with serum-free medium with 10^{-7} M CRF, 10^{-9} M IL-1α alone, or with IL-1 plus CRF. After 1 hr medium was collected and β-endorphin release was determined. Solid bars represent the enhancement by IL-1 of CRF-induced β-endorphin secretion over the additive effects of the individual secretagogues. Stimulated β-endorphin release minus basal values is shown. Results are the mean ± SEM of data from three experiments.

Induction of Early Protein Phosphorylation in AtT-20 Cells

We studied the effects of IL-1 alone on the activation of protein kinases by determining its action on protein phosphorylation in AtT-20 cells, using two-dimensional gel electrophoresis. Treatment of the cells with IL-1α for 15 min resulted in increased ^{32}P incorporation in several acidic cytosolic proteins with the relative molecular masses of 60, 43, 39, 20, and 19 kDa. A subset of these proteins, the 60-, 20-, and 19-kDa species, exhibited marked (fivefold) increases in phosphorylation levels (Fig. 5). The 87-kDa protein showed a smaller increase in phosphorylation levels, after a 1-hr treatment of the cells with IL-1.

The effect of desensitization of PKC on phosphorylation of the 20-, 60-, and 87-kDa proteins induced by a 15-min treatment with IL-1 was then studied. AtT-20 cells were pretreated for 24 hr with TPA, washed, and then exposed to IL-1α for 15 min. Densensitization of PKC by TPA pretreatment

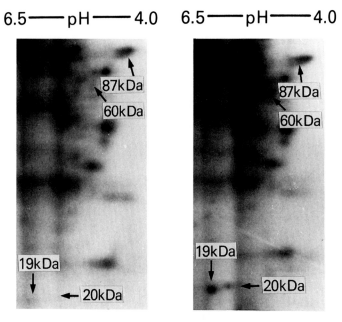

FIG. 5   Early protein phosphorylation induced by IL-1 in AtT-20 cells. The cells were preincubated with ^{32}P$_i$ and then stimulated with 10^{-9} M IL-1α for 15 min. *Left:* A representative control autoradiogram. *Right:* An autoradiogram from IL-1-treated cells. Arrows indicate phosphoproteins that were investigated in this study.

had no effect on the ability of IL-1 to induce the phosphorylation of the 20- and 60-kDa proteins (Fig. 6).

Continuous Presence of IL-1: Not Necessary for Late Induced β-Endorphin Secretion

The early signal, protein phosphorylation by IL-1, appears to generate a cascade of events that does not require the continuous presence of IL-1. We examined whether the continuous presence of IL-1 was necessary for the late induced secretion of β-endorphin. After 6 hr of treatment of AtT-20 cells with IL-1α, there was no increase in β-endorphin secretion induced by IL-1. At that time the cells were thoroughly washed to remove IL-1, and IL-1-free medium was added. Eighteen hours after the cells were washed, those cells that were initially treated with IL-1 secreted a significantly greater

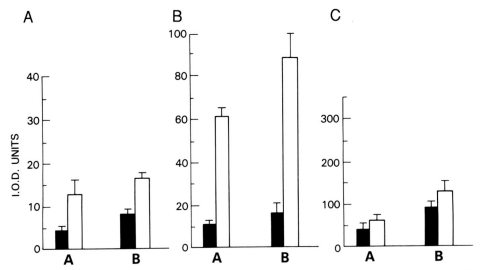

FIG. 6   Interleukin 1-induced protein phosphorylation persists after PKC densensitization. AtT-20 cells were preincubated with $^{32}P_i$ and then stimulated with 10^{-9} M IL-1α alone for 15 min (A). Another group of cells was pretreated with TPA for 24 hr to desensitize PKC, washed, preincubated with $^{32}P_i$, and treated with 10^{-9} M IL-1α for 15 min (B). After 15 min the cells were homogenized, centrifuged, and processed for two-dimensional gel autoradiography. The results are expressed as the mean ± SEM and each treatment condition was repeated at least three times. Black bars, control cells incubated only in medium; open bars, IL-1-treated cells.

amount of β-endorphin than the basal levels and at the same magnitude as was found when IL-1 was continuously present (Table I).

Induction of an Early and Transient Expression of c-fos and c-jun mRNAs in AtT-20 Cells

AtT-20 cells were treated with IL-1α and c-*jun* and c-*fos* mRNA levels were examined. Induction of c-*jun* mRNA by IL-1 appeared within 15 min, was highest after 30–60 min, and reached basal levels at 2 hr. Interleukin 1 also induced c-*fos* mRNA, which was maximum at 30 min and returned to the basal levels at 2 hr (Fig. 7).

Inhibition of IL-1-Induced β-Endorphin Secretion by Antisense Oligonucleotides to c-jun and c-fos

We examined whether either one of the protooncogenes, or both, are necessary for IL-1-induced β-endorphin secretion, using antisense c-*jun* and c-*fos* oligonucleotides. As shown in Fig. 8, the addition of either antisense c-*jun* or c-*fos* to AtT-20 cells did not inhibit IL-1-induced β-endorphin secretion. However, when AtT-20 cells were treated with antisense to both c-*jun* and c-*fos*, IL-1-induced β-endorphin secretion was blocked. This blockade was specific for the antisense sequences, because the corresponding sense oligonucleotides had no effect.

TABLE I   IL-1 Induces Secretion of β-Endorphin 18 hr after Its Removal[a]

Treatment	β-Endorphin (ng/well/hr)	
	6 hr[b]	24 hr
Control	3.43 ± 0.2	4.08 ± 0.2
IL-1α (6-hr treatment)	3.13 ± 0.3	7.32 ± 0.58*
IL-1α (maintained for 24 hr)		7.11 ± 0.4*

[a] AtT-20 cells were incubated in the presence or absence (control) of IL-1α (10^{-9} M) for the times indicated and β-endorphin release was determined, as described in Methods. A group of cells was treated for 6 hr with IL-1, washed four times to remove IL-1 totally, and β-endorphin release was measured after a further 18-hr incubation. Data are the mean ± SEM from five experiments. *$p < 0.05$ (vs control).

[b] Hours after addition of β-endorphin to the cells.

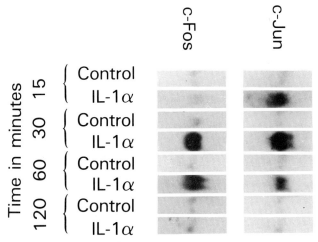

FIG. 7   The time course of c-*fos* and c-*jun* mRNA induction by IL-1. AtT-20 cells were treated with 10^{-9} M IL-1α for the indicated periods of time, lysed, and 10 μg of extracted RNA analyzed by Northern hybridization with c-*fos* and c-*jun* cDNA probes. There was a uniform loading of the samples as demonstrated by actin blotting (not shown). The gel is representative of three different experiments.

IL-1-Induced c-fos and c-jun mRNA Expression and β-Endorphin Secretion: Independent of Protein Kinase C

To assess the role of PKC in activation of early gene expression by IL-1, AtT-20 cells were pretreated with TPA for 24 hr. After 24 hr of TPA pretreatment, the cells were washed and exposed to IL-1α for 30 min, then analyzed for c-*fos* and c-*jun* mRNA levels. Desensitization of PKC by prolonged treatment with phorbol ester had no effect on IL-1-induced expression of c-*fos* and c-*jun* mRNA (Fig. 9).

Discussion

The cytokine IL-1 has been shown to stimulate β-endorphin release directly and to potentiate the effects of several secretagogues in the mouse anterior pituitary cell line, AtT-20. This action of IL-1 on β-endorphin release from AtT-20 cells develops over a period of 18–24 hr, and is accompanied by enhancement of the secretory responses to CRF, VIP, forskolin, phorbol ester (2), catecholamines (3), and vasopressin (17). The enhancement of the CRF-induced β-endorphin response was greater in normal pituitary cells (17)

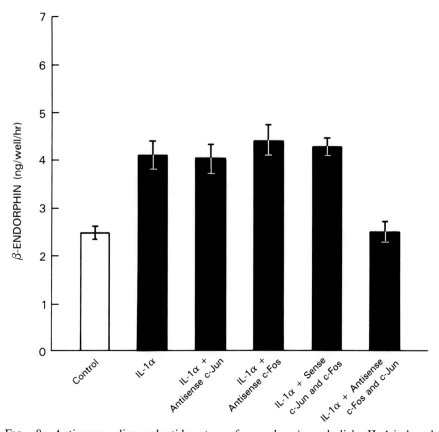

FIG. 8 Antisense oligonucleotides to c-*fos* and c-*jun* abolish IL-1-induced β-endorphin secretion. AtT-20 cells were incubated in the presence or absence of 10 μM antisense oligodeoxynucleotide to c-*fos* and/or c-*jun* for 5 hr. Then 10^{-9} M IL-1α was added. After 23 hr the cells were washed, and serum-free medium with IL-1 was added. After a 1-hr incubation, medium from each well was collected and release of β-endorphin measured. The data are the mean ± SEM of six observations from one of four similar experiments.

than in AtT-20 cells. AtT-20 pituitary tumor cells, like normal corticotrophs, have receptors for both CRF and vasopressin. However, the vasopressin receptors of AtT-20 cells are not coupled to biological responses, including expression of POMC mRNA, secretion of peptides (ACTH), and enhancement of CRF-induced cAMP formation and ACTH release (18). Likewise, vasopressin did not stimulate β-endorphin release from AtT-20 cells in the present study. However, after treatment of AtT-20 cells with IL-1β for 48

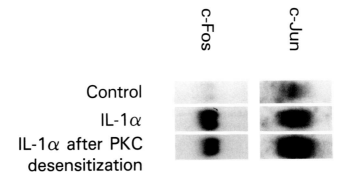

FIG. 9   Interleukin-1 induced c-*fos* or c-*jun* mRNA expression persists after PKC densensitization. AtT-20 cells were pretreated with 100 n*M* TPA for 24 hr and then stimulated with IL-1α for 30 min. RNA was analyzed by Northern analysis as described in Methods. The results are representative examples of three experiments.

hr, vasopressin markedly stimulated β-endorphin secretion (17). The induction of vasopressin responses by IL-1 was not accompanied by an increase in the number of vasopressin receptors. The abolition of this effect of IL-1 after overnight treatment with TPA is consistent with the known role of protein kinase C in the action of vasopressin on ACTH secretion from pituitary corticotrophs (19). Interleukin 1α has also been reported to induce a secretory response to CRF in AtT-20 cells that were insensitive to the neuropeptide, and to cause an increase in POMC mRNA and ACTH synthesis (4). Interleukin 1 receptors were identified in brain with characteristics similar to IL-1 receptors in immune and neuroendocrine tissues (20). It is noteworthy that treatment with IL-1 influences the expression of adrenergic receptors on A549 human lung adenocarcinoma cells (21) and augments GABA$_A$ receptor function in brain (22). These findings demonstrate that IL-1 amplifies receptor-mediated biological responses in normal as well as tumoral pituitary cells.

It was previously shown that secretagogues, such as CRF, norepinephrine and forskolin, can induce early secretion of neuropeptides via protein kinase A and/or protein kinase C. Because IL-1 also stimulates the secretion of β-endorphin in AtT-20 cells, we studied if these kinases might be involved in early signals generated by IL-1. Phorbol ester (TPA), an activator of PKC, causes the secretion of β-endorphin presumably via PKC activation and its effect is abolished after prolonged incubation with phorbol ester. Desensitization of PKC abolished the potentiating effect of IL-1 on TPA-induced β-endorphin secretion and partly reduced the potentiating effect of IL-1 on CRF-induced β-endorphin secretion. This suggests that PKC, as well as other kinases, could be involved in early IL-1 signaling mechanisms. However, treatment with phorbol ester had no effect on IL-1-induced β-endorphin secretion (Fig. 2). Treatment of cells with staurosporine, an inhibitor of protein kinases with selectivity for protein kinase C at low doses, further decreased the enhancement of CRF-induced β-endorphin release by IL-1. These observations suggest that induction of β-endorphin secretion by IL-1 involves a different mechanism than that by which it potentiates the effects of secretagogues.

Interleukin 1 did not generate cAMP, suggesting that cAMP activation of protein kinase A (PKA) is not involved in IL-1 signal transduction. We have also shown that IL-1 did not affect forskolin-induced cAMP generation but enhanced the effect of forskolin on β-endorphin secretion. This suggests that IL-1 does not induce adenylate cyclase and that forskolin causes the secretion of β-endorphin by a mechanism independent of cAMP.

An examination of protein phosphorylation induced by IL-1 in AtT-20 cells indicated that this effect does not directly involve PKC or cAMP-dependent protein kinases. We have observed that IL-1 can activate other protein kinases in AtT-20 cells, which then markedly phosphorylate 19-, 20-, and 60-kDa proteins within minutes, in a time-dependent manner (Fig. 5). Prolonged treatment with TPA, which was found to abolish 87-kDa protein phosphorylation, had no effect on IL-1-induced phosphorylation of the 20-, 60-, and 87-kDa proteins, indicating that the phosphorylation of these proteins is independent of PKC activation (Fig. 6). The removal of IL-1 from the cells after a 6-hr treatment period, followed by a further 18-hr incubation in IL-1-free medium, led to an increase in β-endorphin levels as compared with those cells that were not treated with IL-1.

From these observations it appears that IL-1 generates an early signal that activates protein kinases other than PKC or cAMP-dependent protein kinase to phosphorylate 20- and 60-kDa proteins. These phosphoproteins may then contribute to complex biochemical events, involving intermediate-early gene products, that lead to late induced secretion by activating POMC gene expression and secretion. Although the mechanism of the potentiating effects of IL-1 is not well defined, it also appears to involve internalization of IL-1 (23). Treatment of AtT-20 with IL-1 induced a transient and early stimulation of mRNA from both immediate-early protooncogenes c-*fos* and c-*jun*. It does not appear that either PKA or PKC is involved in early and transient induction of c-*jun* and c-*fos* mRNA in AtT-20 cells.

Induction of both c-*jun* and c-*fos* mRNA expression by IL-1 appears to be a critical step in the late secretion of β-endorphin in AtT-20 cells. This was demonstrated by addition to the cells of antisense oligonucleotides to c-*fos* and c-*jun* mRNA. Antisense oligonucleotides were made complementary to a region near the initiation sequence of c-*fos* and c-*jun* mRNA. They are presumed to prevent the translation of messages by forming duplexes with mRNAs of interest (24). Another mechanism of these oligonucleotides appears to involve RNase H, which specifically degrades the RNA partner in DNA–RNA duplexes, freeing the oligonucleotide to hybridize another mRNA (25). When both antisense oligonucleotides were introduced into the cells, the secretion of β-endorphin induced by IL-1 was abolished (Fig. 8).

Fos and Jun proteins have been shown to form a heterodimer, via leucine zippers, which can serve as the AP-1 transcription factor. When both of the early-immediate genes are blocked, IL-1-induced β-endorphin secretion is abolished. The AP-1 factor, resulting from the combination of Fos and Jun, would increase the transcription of one or more genes that are involved in subsequent release of β-endorphin. β-Endorphin is one of the products of the POMC gene. Whether this AP-1 transcription factor acts on the POMC gene directly or on other gene products that participate in translation, processing, or secretion of POMC gene products remains to be established.

References

1. J. Axelrod and T. D. Reisine, *Science* **224,** 452 (1984).
2. M. O. Făgărăşan, R. Eskay, and J. Axelrod, *Proc. Natl. Acad. Sci. U.S.A.* **86,** 2070 (1989).
3. M. O. Făgărăşan and J. Axelrod, *Int. J. Neurosci.* **51,** 311 (1990).
4. J. Fukata, T. Usui, Y. Naitoh, Y. Nakai, and H. Imura, *J. Endocrinol.* **122,** 33 (1989).
5. M. O. Făgărăşan, J. F. Bishop, M. S. Rinaudo, and J. Axelrod, *Proc. Natl. Acad. Sci. U.S.A.* **87,** 2555 (1990).
6. C. A. Dinarello and N. Savage, *CRC Crit. Rev. Immunol.* **9,** 1 (1989).
7. K. Matsushima, Y. Kobayashi, T. D. Copeland, T. Akahoshi, and J. J. Oppenhein, *J. Immunol.* **139,** 3367 (1987).
8. M. Kester, M. S. Simonsen, P. Mene, and J. R. Sedor, *J. Clin. Invest.* **83,** 718 (1989).
9. A. Raz, A. Wyche, and P. Needleman, *Proc. Natl. Acad. Sci. U.S.A.* **86,** 1657 (1989).
10. W. L. Farrar, D. K. Ferris, and A. Harel-Bellan, *CRC Crit. Rev. Ther. Drug Carrier Syst.* **5,** 229 (1989).
11. K. Muegge and S. K. Durum, *New Biol.* **1**(3), 239 (1989).
12. M. O. Făgărăşan, F. Aiello, K. Muegge, S. Durum, and J. Axelrod, *Proc. Natl. Acad. Sci. U.S.A.* **87,** 7871 (1990).
13. G. P. Meuller, D. J. Pettibone, J. M. Farah, and D. Sapun-Malcolm, *Proc. Soc. Exp. Biol. Med.* **179,** 338 (1985).
14. C. Beveren, F. Straateen, T. Curran, R. Muller, and I. M. Verma, *Cell (Cambridge, Mass.)* **32,** 1241 (1983).
15. K. Ryder and D. Nathans, *Proc. Natl. Acad. Sci. U.S.A.* **85,** 8464 (1988).
16. S. L. Loke, C. A. Stein, X. H. Zhang, K. Mori, M. Nakanishi, C. Subasinghe, J. S. Cohen, and M. L. Neckers, *Proc. Natl. Acad. Sci. U.S.A.* **86,** 3474 (1989).

17. M. O. Făgărăşan, J. Axelrod, and K. J. Catt, *Biochem. Biophys. Res. Commun.* **173**(3), 988 (1990).

18. B. Lutz-Bucher, L. Jeandel, S. Heisler, J. L. Roberts, and B. Koch, *Mol. Cell. Endocrinol.* **53,** 161 (1987).

19. A. B. Abou-Samra, J. P. Harwood, K. J. Catt, and G. Aguilera, *Endocrinology (Baltimore)* **118,** 212 (1986).

20. T. Takao, D. E. Tracey, M. Mitchell, and E. B. De Souza, *Endocrinology (Baltimore)* **127**(6), 3070 (1990).

21. L. Stern and G. Kunos, *J. Biol. Chem.* **263,** 15876 (1988).

22. L. G. Miller, W. R. Galpern, K. Dunlap, C. A. Dinarello, and T. J. Turner, *Mol. Pharmacol.* **39**(2), 105 (1992).

23. M. O. Făgărăşan, P. K. Arora, and J. Axelrod, *Prog. Neuro-Psychopharmacol. Biol. Psychiatry* **15,** 551 (1991).

24. E. S. Kawaski, *Nucleic Acids Res.* **13,** 4991 (1985).

25. P. Dash, I. Lotan, E. R. Kandel, and P. Goelet, *Proc. Natl. Acad. Sci. U.S.A.* **84,** 7896 (1987).

Index

Acetylcholine, IL-2 modulatory role, 180–182
Adrenocorticotropic hormone
  direct effects of cytokines, 271–274
  hypothalamic control, 196
  IL-1 effects, 197–198, 315
  IL-1β-induced secretion, 271–274
  IL-2 effects, 317–318
  IL-6 effects, 201–202
  INF-γ effects, 200–201
  summary of cytokine actions, 206
  thymosin-α effects, 203
  TNF effects, 199
  in vitro effects of cytokines
    assay systems, 235–237
    plasma levels, 238–242
Affinity cross-linking
  cytokine receptors, 20–23
  IL-1, 131–132
  IL-1α, 137–139
Antibodies, *see also* Antiserum
  anti-IL-1ra, ELISA detection, 37
  anti-ligand, for hematopoietin receptor complexes, 58–59
  monoclonal, *see* Monoclonal antibodies
  phosphostyrosine, for immunoblotting, 56–57
  receptor-specific, for hematopoietin receptor complexes, 57–58
Antigen localization, with diaminobenzidine reaction, 103, 105
Antiserum, *see also* Antibodies
  for immunocytochemistry, 107–108
  for passive immunization studies, 222–225
Arginine vasopressin
  IL-1β effects, 319
  in vitro effects of cytokines
    assay systems, 235–237
    plasma levels, 238–242
Association reactions, equation for, 16
AtT-20 pituitary tumor cells
  early protein phosphorylation induction, 334–335

β-endorphin secretion
  cell culture, 328
  CRF-induced, 331–332
  forskolin-induced, 331–332
  isoproterenol-induced, 331–332
  norepinephrine-induced, 331–332
  oligonucleotide synthesis, 329–330
  phosphorylation experiments, 329
  release experiments, 328
  RNA isolation, Northern analysis, 329
  time and dose relationship, 330
  TPA-induced, 331–332
  vasopressin-induced, 332–333
  VIP-induced, 331–332
  c-*fos* and c-*jun* mRNA expression, 336
  in vitro assessment of cytokine actions, 244
  in vitro modulation of IL-1 receptors, 149–150
Autoradiography
  cytokine receptors, 20
  IL-1, 132–133
  IL-1 and IL-1 receptor antagonist, 97
  IL-1 type I mRNA, 121–125
  IL-2 immunoreactive neurons, regional localization, 174–175
Avidin–biotin–immunoperoxidase method, c-*fos* transcription factor localization, 159–162
8-Azido-ATP binding, identification of protein kinases, 63–64

Biotinylated ligands, for hematopoietin receptor complexes, 59
Blood–brain barrier
  cytokine disruption of, 75–76
  cytokine passage across, 204–205
    amounts entering brain, 73–74
    brain distribution after peripheral administration, 74
    brain perfusion through carotid artery, 70
    integrity of injected material, 74–75

multiple time regression analysis, 70–73
  saturable transport, 73
diffusion across, 56
leakiness of, 68
saturable transport across, 68–69
Blood collection
  hypophysial portal blood, 190–191
  for IL-1 effects, 259–260
Brain
  cerebroventriclar microinjections, 276–279
  intracerebroventricular microinjections, 258
  microinjections, 188–189
  push–pull cannulas, 189–190
  third ventricular injections, 255–256

Cachectin, *see also* Tumor necrosis factor
  effect on hypothalamic–pituitary function, 199–
    200
Cameras, CCD, 108–109
Cannulation
  intraatrial, 258–259
  lateral ventricle, 256–258
    push–pull, *see* Push–pull cannulation
  third ventricle, 255–256
CCD cameras, 108–109
Cell cultures, pituitary
  aggregate, 194
  hemipituitary system, 193–194
  monolayers, 193
  short-term, 193
Cerebroventricle, microinjections, 276–279
Charge-coupled device cameras, 108–109
Chemical affinity cross-linking, IL-1 to receptors,
    131–132
Chemiluminescent development, immunoblots, 56–
    57
Chloramine-T method, for cytokine radiolabeling, 8
Ciliary neurotropic factor receptors, classification,
    3
Circumventricular organs, cytokine passage into
    brain via, 74, 204–205
CL2MDP liposomes
  administration, 220
  preparation, 219–220
Cloning, cytokine receptors
  expression cloning, 24–28
  purification strategy, 23–24
  vectors for, 26–27
Colorimetric development, immunoblots, 56

Complementary DNA, probes for *in situ* hybridiza-
    tion histochemistry, 82–83
Complementary RNA
  for *in situ* hybridization histochemistry, 82–83,
    116–118
  ^{35}S-labeled probes, for IL-1 *in situ* hybridization
    histochemistry, 89
Computer programs, for binding analysis, 17–18
Corticotropin-releasing hormone
  β-endorphin induction
    enhancement, 331–332
    by IL-1, 333
  IL-1 actions and, 197–198
  IL-2 effects, 203
  IL-6 effects, 202
  mediation of IL-1 effects on LH release, 254–
    255
  thymosin-α effects, 203
  in vitro stimulation by cytokines, 244–245
Corticotropin-releasing hormone 41
  cytokine effects, 321–323
  IL-1 effects, 315, 316, 319
  IL-6 effects, 319
COS cells, cytokine receptor cloning in, 25–28
Cytokine receptors
  binding assays
    autoradiography, 20
    computer programs, 17–18
    data analysis, 15–20
    equations for, 15–20
    flow cytometry, 20
    phthalate oil method, 10–13
    Scatchard equation, 17
    strategy for binding analysis, 13–15
  characterization by affinity cross-linking, 20–23
  combinatorial structures, 5
  cooperativity between, 19–20
  families, 3–4
  molecular cloning, 23–28
  monoclonal antibodies, production, 28–29
  soluble, 5–6
Cytokines
  blood-borne, site of action determination
    direct effects on anterior pituitary hormone
      secretion, 271–274
    pituitary cell cultures, 270–271
  disruption of blood–brain barrier, 75–76
  hypothalamic–pituitary
    immunocytochemistry, 194–195

overview of actions, 195–196
receptor autoradiography, 194–195
in situ hybridization, 194–195
in vitro studies, 191–192
in vivo studies, 187–191
passage across blood–brain barrier, 204–205
amounts entering brain, 73–74
brain distribution after peripheral administration, 74
brain perfusion through carotid artery, 70
integrity of injected material, 74–75
multiple time regression analysis, 70–73
saturable transport, 73
production, pituitary, 205
recombinant, production and radiolabeling, 6–7
Bolton–Hunter reagent, 7–8
Enzymobead method, 8–10
in vitro effects
assay systems, 233–237
on pituitary hormone secretion, 243–246
in vitro system for effects on hypothalamus
acute explants, 305
advantages and limitations, 310–314
animals, 305
decapitation and brain removal, 305–306
growth axis, 320–323
hypothalamic dissection, 306
hypothalamo–pituitary–adrenal axis, 314–320
results processing, 309–310
static tissue incubation, 306–307
in vivo effects on
ACTH plasma levels, 238–242
AVP plasma levels, 238–242
OT plasma levels, 238–242
in vivo methods for neuroendocrine effects, 274–275
brain sites for ACTH release, 279–282
glial cultures, 288–290
hypothalamic hypophysiotropic hormones in portal blood, 286–288
microinjections into cerebroventricle, 276–279
microperfusion for immune signal transmission sites, 282–286

DESIGN program, 18
Diaminobenzidine reaction
for double-label immunocytochemistry, 105
for single-label immunocytochemistry, 103

Dicholoromethylene diphosphonate, liposome-mediated delivery to phagocytic cells, 218–220
Diffusion, across blood–brain barrier, 68
Dissociation reactions, equation for, 16
DNA, complementary, *see* Complementary DNA
Double-immunohistochemical analysis, Fos and dopamine-β-hydroxylase, 165

Electrophoresis, thin-layer, *see* Thin-layer electrophoresis
Emulsion detection, IL-1 type I mRNA, 121–125
Endogenous opioid peptides, role in IL-1-induced suppression of LH surge, 254
β-Endorphin, secretion in AtT-20 cells
cell culture, 328
CRF-induced, 331–332
forskolin-induced, 331–332
isoproterenol-induced, 331–332
late secretion, IL-1 role, 335–336
norepinephrine-induced, 331–332
oligonucleotide synthesis, 329–330
phosphorylation experiments, 329
release experiments, 328
RNA isolation, Northern analysis, 329
time and dose relationship, 330
TPA-induced, 331–332
vasopressin-induced, 332–333
VIP-induced, 331–332
Endotoxin-induced responses, liposome-mediated macrophage suicide technique, 217–220
Enzyme-linked immunosorbent assay, identification of anti-IL-1ra antibodies, 37
Enzymobead method, for cytokine radiolabeling, 8–10
Estradiol, circulating, RIA quantitation, 265–266
Expression cloning, cytokine receptors
advantages and drawbacks, 24–25
eukaryotic
direct ligand-binding method, 25–28
panning method, 25, 27

Fibroblast growth factor receptors, classification, 4
Film detection, IL-1 type I mRNA, 121
Flow cytometry, cytokine receptors, 20
Fluorescence, measurements for IL-1 determination, 228–229

Follicle-stimulating hormone
  IL-1 effects, 198–199
  IL-2 effects, 203
  summary of cytokine actions, 206
Folliculostellate cells, IL-6 production, 205
Formalin, for tissue preparation, 113
Forskolin, β-endorphin induction enhancement,
    331–332
Fos transcription factor
  c-*fos* antisense oligonucleotides, inhibition of IL-
      1-induced β-endorphin secretion, 336–337
  c-*fos* mRNA expression
    in AtT-20 cells, 336
    protein kinase C role, 337
  functional mapping with IL-1β
    dose–response relationships, 162–163
    IL-1 immunoreactive neurons, 163–165
    systemic administration, 156–158
    time course, 158–162
FSH, *see* Follicle-stimulating hormone

Gel filtration, TNF-α *in vitro* effects, 297–298
Genes, *jun*
  antisense oligonucleotides, inhibition of IL-1-
      induced β-endorphin secretion in AtT-20
      cells, 336
  mRNA expression
    in AtT-20 cells, 336
    protein kinase C role, 337
GH, *see* Growth hormone
Glucose oxidase–lactoperoxidase method, for
    cytokine radiolabeling, 8–10
Gonadal steroids, RIA quantitation, 265–266
Gonadotropin, IL-1 effects, 198–199
Granulocyte colony-stimulating factor receptors,
    classification, 3
Granulocyte–macrophage colony-stimulating factor
  effect on IL-1ra production, 43–46
  receptor classification, 3
Growth hormone, *see also specific growth hor-
    mones*
  hypothalamic control, 196
  IL-1 effects, 198
  IL-1β-induced secretion, 271–274
  IL-2 effects, 203
  IL-6 effects, 201–202
  INF-γ effects, 201
  summary of cytokine actions, 206

  thymosin-α effects, 203
  TNF effects, 199, 298–300
Growth hormone-releasing hormone, cytokine
    effects, 320–323

Hematopoietin receptor complexes, purification
    strategies, 57–59
Hemipituitary system, 193–194
High-performance liquid chromatography, TNF-α
    in vitro effects, 297
Hippocampus
  ^{125}I-Ilα and ^{125}I-IL-1ra binding, autoradiographic
      localization, 142–145
  quinolinic acid lesions, 133, 145–146
Human mononuclear cells
  cultures, 39–41
  IL-1ra production, 42–46
Hybridization histochemistry, *in situ*
  c-*fos* mRNA, 159–162
  cytokines in hypothalmic–pituitary system, 194–
      195
  general precautions, 82–83
  hypothalamic–pituitary system, 194–195
  IL-1 mRNA
    autoradiography, 91, 96
    brain removal, 83–89
    hybridization procedure, 89–90
    IL-1 receptor antagonist mRNA, tissue stain-
        ing, 91, 97
    probe synthesis, 89
    RNase treatment, 90–91
    sectioning, 83–89
    tissue preparation, 83–89
  IL-1 receptor antagonist mRNA
    autoradiography, 96
    brain removal, 91–94
    hybridization procedure, 95–96
    synthetic oligodeoxynucleotide probe, 94–95
    tissue preparation, 91–94
    tissue staining, 97
    washing and dehydration, 91, 96
  IL-1 type I mRNA
    autoradiography, 121–125
    controls, 125–126
    data analysis, 125–126
    hybridization procedure, 118–119
    posthybridization, 119–120
  probe types for, 82–83

Hybridomas, for IL-1ra detection, 36–37
Hypophysectomy, effects on *in vivo* modulation of
  IL-1 receptors, 146–148
Hypothalamic–pituitary system
  actions of mono- and cytokines, overview, 195–
    196
  immunocytochemistry, 194–195
  intravenous injections, 187
  receptor autoradiography, 194–195
  response to infection, 197
  in situ hybridization, 194–195
  third ventricular injections, 187
  in vitro studies, 191–194
  in vivo studies, 187
Hypothalamo–pituitary–adrenal axis, cytokine
  effects, 314–320
Hypothalamus
  acute explants, *in vitro* system
    advantages and limitations, 310–314
    animals, 305
    dissection, 306
    results processing, 309–310
    sampling procedure, 307–308
    static tissue incubation, 306
  control of pituitary secretion, 197
  cytokine actions, *in vitro* assessment, 244–245
  LHRH RIA, 264–265
  paraventricular nucleus, c-*fos* induction by IL-
    1β, 159–161
  in vitro hormone release, 191–192, 303–304

IL-1ra, *see* Interleukin-1 receptor antagonist
Image analysis, computerized, for immunocytochemistry, 108–109
Immunization, passive, for IL-1, requirements and
  methods, 222–225
Immunoblotting, with antiphosphtyrosine antibodies, 56–57
Immunocytochemistry
  antisera, 107–108
  computerized image analysis, 108–109
  controls, 107–108
  cytokines in hypothalmic–pituitary system, 194–
    195
  data analysis, 108–109
  double-label, 105–106
  electron microscopy, 106–107
  fixation protocols, 102

hypothalamic–pituitary system, 194–195
  quantitative, for IL-1, 228–229
  single-label, 103–105
Immunoglobulin G, effect on IL-1ra production, 44
Immunohistochemistry
  IL-2-like immunoreactivity in brain, 173–174
  peroxidase–anti-peroxidase, IL-2-like immuno-
    reactivity, 175–179
  Tac antigen-like immunoreactivity, 178–179
Immunoperoxidase method, 106–107
Immunoprecipitation
  IL-1ra protein detection, 38–39
  protein phosphorylation analysis, 50–54
  protein tyrosine phosphorylation analysis, 56–57
Incubation systems
  hypothalamus, 191–192
  hypothalamus, static tissue, 306–307
  pituitary, 192–194
  in vitro static, 261–263
Indomethacin, effects on cachectin, 199
INF, *see* Interferons
Infection, response of hypothalamic–pituitary
  system, 197
Injections, *see also* Microinjections
  into brain, 188–189
  intracerebroventricular, 258
  intravenous, 187–188
  into pituitary, 188–189
Interferon γ, effect on hypothalamic–pituitary
  function, 200–201
Interferons, classification, 4
Interleukin-1
  autoradiography, 132–133
    quantification and data analysis, 132–133
  chemical affinity cross-linking to receptors, 131–
    132
  circulation concentrations, determination, 211–
    212
  direct effects on pituitary cells, 271–274
  effects on
    ACTH, 315, 316
    CRH-41, 319
    hypothalamic–pituitary function, 197–199
    LHRH, 260–261
  human type II, monoclonal antibodies to, 28–29
  intraatrial cannulation, 258–259
  localization, 204
  mechanism of action, 225–226
    peptide turnover determination, 226–227

quantitative immunocytochemistry, 228–229
in vivo methods, 274–275
mRNA, *in situ* hybridization histochemistry
autoradiography, 91, 96
brain removal, 83–89
hybridization procedure, 89–90
probe synthesis, 89
RNase treatment, 90–91
sectioning, 83–89
tissue preparation, 83–89
tissue staining, 91, 97
passive immunization studies, 222–225
potentiation of CRF-induced β-endorphin release, 333
radioimmunoassay
displacement curves, 215–216
extraction of plasma samples, 214–215
plasma samples, 216–217
radioiodination of recombinant IL-1β, 213–214
recombinant protein storage, 212–213
receptor-binding assay, 131
role as tissue corticotropin-releasing factor, 271–
274
role in late induced β-endorphin secretion, 335–
336
stereotaxic procedures
intracerebroventricular injection, 258
lateral ventricle cannulation, 256–258
third ventricle cannulation, 255–256
Interleukin-1β
direct effects on hypothalamic neurostimulatory
neurons, 244–246
effects on AVP, 319
Fos mapping after iv injection
dose–response, 162
experimental manipulations, 165–167
phenotyping of immunoreactive neurons, 163–
165
systemic administration, 156–158
time course, 158–162
neuroendocrine effects, 271–274
Interleukin-1α, recombinant
affinity cross-linking, 139–142
binding at equilibrium, 137
brain regions assayed, 135–136
choice of species for binding assays, 131–135
pharmacological specificity, 137–139
radioligands, 134
Interleukin-1 receptor antagonist
affinity cross-linking, 139–142

autoradiographic localization, 142–145
binding
autoradiographic localization, 142–145
at equilibrium, 137
brain regions for binding assays, 135–136
cell culture production
mRNA determination, 35–36
U937 cells, 34–35
induction in human monocytes
mononuclear cell cultures, 39–41
procedure, 42–46
mRNA, *in situ* hybridization histochemistry
autoradiography, 96
brain removal, 91–94
hybridization procedure, 95–96
synthetic oligodeoxynucleotide probe, 94–95
tissue preparation, 91–94
tissue staining, 97
washing and dehydration, 91, 96
pharmacological specificity, 137–139
protein detection
ELISA, 37
hybridoma generation, 36–37
immunoprecipitation, 38–39
Western blots, 37–39
radioligand for, 134
species for binding assays, 134–135
tissue protein concentration effects, 135–137
uses of, 220–221
Interleukin-1 receptors
heterogeneity, 128–129
localization, 204
in vitro modulation, in AtT-20 pituitary tumor
cells, 149–150
in vivo modulation
hypophysectomy effects, 146–148
lipopolysaccharde treatment effects, 148–149
Interleukin-1α receptors
autoradiographic localization, 142–145
tissue protein concentration effects, 136–137
Interleukin-2
disruption of blood–brain barrier, 75–76
effects on ACTH secretion, 317–318
immunoautoradiography, 174–175
immunohistochemical detection, 173–174
role in acetylcholine release, 180–182
Interleukin-2 receptors
quantitative autoradiography, 179–180
Tac antigen-like immunoreactivity, 178–179
Interleukin-3, effect on IL-1ra production, 44–46

Interleukin-6
  effects on
    CRH-41, 319
    hypothalamic–pituitary function, 201–202
  production
    by folliculostellate cells, 205
    IL-1-induced *in vitro*, 205
Interleukin-8, classification, 4–5
Interleukin receptors
  classification, 4
  type I mRNA, *in situ* hybridization histochemistry
    autoradiography, 121–125
    controls, 125–126
    cRNA probe synthesis, 116–118
    data analysis, 125–126
    hybridization procedure, 118–119
    posthybridization, 119–120
    prehybridization, 115–116
    tissue preparation, 113–114
Intracerebroventricular injections, 258
Intravenous injections, 187–188
Iodogen method
  for cytokine radiolabeling, 8
  for IL-1β labeling, 213–214
Isoproterenol, β-endorphin induction enhancement, 331–332

Kidney, ^{125}I-Ilα and ^{125}I-IL-1ra binding, autoradiographic localization, 142–145
Kinase renaturation assay, identification of proteins kinases, 64–65

Lateral ventricle cannulation, 256–258
Leakiness, blood–brain barrier, 68
LH, *see* Luteinizing hormone
LHRH, *see* Luteinizing hormone-releasing hormone
LIGAND program, 18, 132–133
Lipopolysaccharde treatment effects
  in vitro, on IL-6, 204
  in vivo, modulation of IL-1 receptors, 148–149
Liposome-mediated macrophage suicide technique
  CL2MDP liposomes
    administration, 220
    preparation, 219–220
  cytochemical identification of macrophages, 220
Liposomes, CL2MDP
  administration, 220
  preparation, 219–220

Luteinizing hormone
  IL-1 effects, 198–199
    central actions, 250–255
    mode of action, 252–253
    peripheral actions, 249–250
    on proestrous rats, 250–252
    steroid-induced surges, 252
    in vitro actions, 249–250
  IL-1β-induced secretion, 271–274
  IL-2 effects, 203
  plasma levels, RIA, 264
  summary of cytokine actions, 206
  surge, IL-1 suppression
    CRF mediation, 254–255
    role of endogenous opioid peptides, 254
Luteinizing hormone-releasing hormone
  hypothalamic, RIA, 264–265
  IL-1 effects, 260–261
  IL-2 effects, 203
Luteinizing hormone-releasing hormone–LH, inhibition, IL-1 effects, 253–255

Macrophages, liposome-mediated macrophage suicide technique, 217–220
α-Melanocyte-stimulating hormone, effects on IL-6-induced CRH , 202
Messenger RNA
  c-*fos* transcription factor, *in situ* hybridization histochemistry, 159–162
  IL-1, *in situ* hybridization histochemistry
    autoradiography, 91, 96
    brain removal, 83–89
    hybridization procedure, 89–90
    probe synthesis, 89
    RNase treatment, 90–91
    sectioning, 83–89
    tissue preparation, 83–89
    tissue staining, 91, 97
    washing and dehydration, 91
  IL-1 receptor antagonist, *in situ* hybridization histochemistry
    autoradiography, 96
    brain removal, 91–94
    hybridization procedure, 95–96
    synthetic oligodeoxynucleotide probe, 94–95
    tissue preparation, 91–94
    tissue staining, 97
    washing and dehydration, 96
  IL-1 type I, *in situ* hybridization histochemistry
    autoradiography, 121–125

controls, 125–126
data analysis, 125–126
hybridization procedure, 118–119
posthybridization, 119–120
Microfluorometry, IL-1 fluorescence determination, 228–229
Microinjections, *see also* Injections
into brain or pituitary, 188–189
Monoclonal antibodies
cytokine receptor, production, 28–29
to human type II IL-1, 28–29
Monokines, hypothalamic–pituitary, overview of actions, 195–196
Mononuclear cells, human, *see* Human mononuclear cells
Multiple time regression analysis, detection of cytokine passage from blood to CNS, 70–73

Nerve growth factor receptors, classification, 4
Nickel-enhanced diaminobenzidine reaction, 103
Norepinephrine, β-endorphin induction enhancement, 331–332
Nucleus of the solitary tract, c-*fos* induction by IL-1β, 161

Oligonucleotide probes
c-*jun* and c-*fos*, inhibition of IL-1-induced β-endorphin secretion, 336–337
for *in situ* hybridization, 82–83
synthetic, for IL-1 receptor antagonist *in situ* hybridization histochemistry, 94–95
Opioid peptides, endogenous, *see* Endogenous opioid peptides
Organum vasculosum lamina terminalis, cytokine passage into brain via, 204–205
Oxytocin, *in vitro* effects of cytokines
assay systems, 235–237
plasma levels, 238–242

Panning method, for cytokine receptor expression cloning, 25, 27
Paraformaldehyde, for tissue preparation, 113
Paraventricular nucleus, hypothalamic, c-*fos* induction by IL-1β, 159–160
Passive immunization, for IL-1, requirements and methods, 222–225
Peptides, prolactin receptor-associated p120, *in vitro* phosphorylation, 62
Peptide turnover, for IL-1 mechanism of action, 226–227

Perfusion systems, for *in vitro* assessment of neuropeptide release, 263–264
Peroxidase–antiperoxidase method, for cellular localization of IL-2-like immunoreactivity, 175–179
Phenotyping, Fos immunoreactive neurons, 163–165
Phosphoamino acids
determination by protein hydrolysis and thin-layer electrophoresis, 54–55
from renatured protein kinases, 65
Phosphotyrosyl proteins, receptor-associated, analysis, 57–59
Phthalate oil method, cytokine receptor binding, 10–13
Pituitary
AtT-20 cells, *see* AtT-20 pituitary tumor cells
cytokine production, 205
direct effect of cytokines of hormone secretion, 271–274
hypothalamic control, 197
^{125}I-Ilα and ^{125}I-IL-1ra binding, autoradiographic localization, 142–145
incubation systems, 192–194
LH release, IL-1 effects
central, 250–255
peripheral, 249–250
microinjections, 188–189
normal cells, CRF-induced β-endorphin release by IL-1, 333
push–pull cannulas, 189–190
TNF-α *in vitro* effects
cell culture, 295–296
cell dispersion, 295
cell perfusion method, 296
choice of pituitaries, 294–295
fragments, 296
gel filtration, 297–298
HPLC analysis, 297
RIAs, 298
sample preparation, 296–297
Platelet-derived growth factor receptors, classification, 4
Portal blood, hypophysial, collection, 190–191
Probes, *see also* Complementary DNA; Oligonucleotide probes; Riboprobes
for *in situ* hybridization, 82–83
Progesterone, circulating, RIA quantitation, 265–266
Prolactin
hypothalamic control, 196, 197

IL-1 effects, 198
IL-2 effects, 203
IL-6 effects, 201–202
INF-γ effects, 201
prolactin-inhibiting factors, 196
summary of cytokine actions, 206
TNF effects, 200
Prostacyclin, cytokine effects, 319–320
Prostaglandin, cytokine effects, 319–320
Prostaglandin E_2, IL-1 effects, 317
Protein hydrolysis, phosphoamino acid determination, 54–55
Protein kinase C, role in c-*jun* and c-*fos* mRNA expression, 337
Protein kinases
    signal transduction, identification
        phosphoamino acid determination, 54–55
        receptor-associated phosphotyrosyl proteins, 57–59
        in vitro kinase assay, 59–62
    substrates in signal transduction
        phosphoamino acid determination, 54–55
        protein phosphorylation analysis, 50–54
        receptor-associated phosphotyrosyl proteins, 57–59
Protein phosphorylation
    analysis by $^{32}P_i$ labeling and immunoprecipitation, 50–54
    early, induction in AtT-20 cells, 334–335
    tyrosine-specific, immunoprecipitation and immunoblotting, 56–57
Push-pull cannulation
    brain, 189–190
    pituitary, 189–190

Quantitative autoradiography, IL-2 receptors, 179–180
Quantitative immunocytochemistry, for IL-1 mechanism of action, 228–229
Quinolinic acid lesions, hippocampus, 133, 145–146

Radioimmunoassays
    gonadal steroids, 265–266
    IL-1
        displacement curves, 215–216
        extraction of plasma samples, 214–215
        plasma samples, 216–217
        radioiodination of recombinant IL-1β, 213–214
        recombinant protein storage, 212–213
    LH plasma levels, 264

LHRH, 264–265
    progesterone, 265–266
    TNF-α *in vitro* effects, 298
Radioiodination, recombinant IL-1β, 213–214
Radiolabeling
    cytokines
        Bolton–Hunter reagent, 7–8
        Enzymobead method, 8–10
        with $^{32}P_i$, for protein phosphorylation, 50–54
    recombinant IL-1α, 134
Receptor autoradiography, cytokines in hypothalamic–pituitary system, 194–195
Recombinant cytokines
    IL-1 storage, 212–213
    production and radiolabeling, 6–7
        Bolton–Hunter reagent, 7–8
        Enzymobead method, 8–10
Regression analysis, multiple time, *see* Multiple time regression analysis
Riboprobes
    for *in situ* hybridization histochemistry, 82–83, 116–118
    ^{35}S-labeled, for IL-1 *in situ* hybridization histochemistry, 89
RNA
    complementary, *see* Complementary RNA
    messenger, *see* Messenger RNA

Saturable transport
    across blood–brain barrier, 68–69
    cytokines across blood–brain barrier, 73
Scatchard equation, for cytokine binding, 17
Signal transduction
    protein kinases in
        8-azido-ATP binding, 63–64
        kinase renaturation assay, 64–65
        in vitro kinase assay, 59–62
    protein kinase substrates
        phosphoamino acid determination, 54–55
        protein phosphorylation analysis, 50–54
        receptor-associated phosphotyrosyl proteins, 57–59
Soluble cytokine receptors, 5–6
Somatostatin, cytokine effects, 320–323
Spleen, ^{125}I-IIα and ^{125}I-IL-1ra binding, autoradiographic localization, 142–145
Steroid hormones, RIA quantitation, 265–266
Streptavidin–agarose affinity purification, hematopoietin receptor complexes, 59

Tac antigen-like immunoreactivity, in CNS, 178–179

Testis, ^{125}I-IIα and ^{125}I-IL-1ra binding, autoradiographic localization, 142–145

Testosterone, circulating, RIA quantitation, 265–266

12-*O*-Tetradecanoate 13-acetate, β-endorphin induction enhancement, 331–332

Thin-layer electrophoresis, determination of phosphoamino acids, 54–55

Thymosin α, effect on hypothalamic–pituitary function, 203–204

Thyroid-stimulating hormone
  hypothalamic control, 197
  IL-1 effects, 198
  IL-2 effects, 203
  IL-6 effects, 201–202
  INF-γ effects, 201
  summary of cytokine actions, 206
  thymosin-α effects, 203
  TNF effects, 199

TPA, *see* 12-*O*-Tetradecanoate 13-acetate

Transmembrane diffusion, across blood–brain barrier, 68–69

Tumor necrosis factor
  effect on hypothalamic–pituitary function, 199–200
  receptor classification, 4

Tumor necrosis factor-α
  effects on GH, *in vitro* analysis, 298–300
  pituitary effects

in vitro methods
  cell perfusion method, 296
  collection of pituitaries, 294–295
  gel filtration, 297–298
  HPLC analysis, 297
  pituitary cell cultures, 295–296
  pituitary cell dispersion, 295
  pituitary fragments, 296
  protocol, 296
  RIAs, 297–298
  sample preparation, 296–297
in vivo methods, 298–300

Tyrosine phosphorylation, immunoprecipitation and immunoblotting, 56–57

UJ937 cells
  culture method, 34–35
  IL-1ra mRNA determination, 35–36

Vasoactive intestinal peptide, β-endorphin induction enhancement, 331–332

Vasopressin
  arginine, *see* Arginine vasopressin
  induction of β-endorphin release in AtT-20 cells, 332–333

Ventricle, third
  cannulation, 255–256
  injections, 187–188, 255–256

Western blotting, IL-1ra protein detection, 37–38